Tissue and Organ Regeneration in Adults

Springer

New York
Berlin
Heidelberg
Barcelona
Hong Kong
London
Milan
Paris
Singapore
Tokyo

Ioannis V. Yannas

Tissue and Organ Regeneration in Adults

With 50 Illustrations

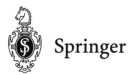 Springer

Ioannis V. Yannas
Massachusetts Institute of Technology
Cambridge, MA 02139-4307
USA

Cover illustration: The cover illustration was provided by Wayne Hsiao.

Library of Congress Cataloging-in-Publication Data
Yannas, Ioannis V.
    Tissue and organ regeneration in adults / Ioannis V. Yannas.
        p.   cm.
    Includes bibliographical references and index.
    ISBN 0-387-95214-4 (alk. paper)
        1. Regeneration (Biology)   2. Skin—Regeneration.   3. Nerves—Regeneration.
    I. Title.
QP90.2.Y36   2001
571.8′891—dc21   00-053199

Printed on acid-free paper.

Production coordinated by Chernow Editorial Services, Inc., and managed by Francine McNeill; manufacturing supervised by Jeffrey Taub.
Typeset by Best-set Typesetter Ltd., Hong Kong.
Printed and bound by Maple-Vail Book Manufacturing Group, York, PA.
Printed in the United States of America.

9 8 7 6 5 4 3 2 1

ISBN 0-387-95214-4   SPIN 10791572

Springer-Verlag   New York Berlin Heidelberg
A member of BertelsmannSpringer Science+Business Media GmbH

*To Tania and Alexi
and
to Nichola's kitchen*

Preface

Why This Volume?

The title of this volume reads like an oxymoron. After all, it is well known that, whether animal or human, adults do not spontaneously regenerate any of their organs that have been lost to accidental trauma or to surgery. If mammals could somehow regenerate organs such as the skin of a hand lost to a burn or a breast lost to mastectomy, scars should not fill the anatomical site of the lost organ; instead, a regrown organ should emerge. If regeneration were possible, treatments might also be developed for potentially lethal degenerative conditions such as a scarred heart muscle or a cirrhotic liver.

The concept of induced organ regeneration in adults is relatively new. The deliberate modification of healing to achieve regrowth of lost tissue structures does not follow directly from current mainstream paradigms of biological research. The first tentative recognition that the healing process could be modified to induce regeneration of the dermis, a tissue that does not spontaneously regenerate in adults, appeared in reports published in the early 1980s. Eventually, other organs, including peripheral nerves and the eye conjunctiva, were induced to regenerate in anatomical wounds known to be incapable of supporting spontaneous regeneration.

The data on induced regeneration are scattered in a variety of journals, book chapters, abstracts, and theses. It is time to marshal the extensive evidence. This is the main reason for writing this volume.

Generic Methodology

The emphasis throughout this volume is on systematic development of the viewpoint that regeneration is an instance of synthesis of tissues and organs. Although somewhat self-evident, this proposition has been hardly employed. It has three simple consequences. The first is the requirement for a special kind of experimental reactor, free of tissues that do not spontaneously regenerate. The second calls for meticulous physicochemical and biological characterization of the end products of such a reaction. The third requires the use of appropriate nondiffusible regulators in the experimental reactor. These insoluble matrices induce adult cells to abandon their normal proclivity in closing up adult wounds in exchange for synthesizing physiological tissues.

This approach appears to be independent of the organ under study. It is developed in substantial depth during the first several chapters by limiting the discussion to just two organs that are quite different from each other, namely, skin and peripheral nerves. The conclusions from this analysis apply to either organ with roughly equal strength. This intriguing result clearly suggests a generic methodology for synthesis of other organs.

In Vitro or In Vivo?

Many researchers in tissue engineering have preferred to carry an organ synthesis in vitro as extensively as possible before implanting the resulting construct in an experimental animal model. The methodology developed in this volume applies whether the bulk of the synthetic process is being carried in vitro or in vivo. Irrespective of whether the organ being synthesized in vitro is in advanced state of completion or is simply a matrix seeded with cells, it is still necessary to eventually implant it by inflicting a traumatic (surgical) injury at the correct anatomical site. Once more, the implantation site can be construed as an experimental reactor and the process of remodeling or regeneration that follows can be looked at as a synthetic process. In short, the methodology of organ synthesis developed in this volume should apply in a large variety of protocols used in tissue and organ synthesis.

Who Should Benefit by Reading This Volume?

A second reason for writing this volume is the need for a single-author textbook on organ synthesis. Lack of a unifying text has frustrated both university students and practitioners in industry. For years my graduate students have had to confront a motley array of lecture notes. This volume is partly based on the author's notes for undergraduate and graduate classes in biomaterials–tissue interactions, tissue engineering, and design of medical devices at Massachusetts Institute of Technology.

This work should be of interest to three groups of investigators: biologists, experimental surgeons, and biomedical engineers. Biologists should be interested in the molecular biological basis of induced regeneration, a process that appears to reverse the developmental process that normally converts the wound-healing response of the fetus to that of the adult. Experimental surgeons interested in organ regeneration should benefit from a fresh approach toward making their experimental protocols more quantitative and standardized. Biomedical engineers will gain a new look at the treatment of old ailments. In particular, it is hoped that the generic organ-blind methodology described in this volume should be useful to most students and practitioners of tissue engineering.

Outline

This volume is divided into four major sections. Loss of organ function, the basic medical problem treated in this volume, is defined in Chapter 1. The basic methodology of organ synthesis in vivo is described in Chapters 2 through 4. Application to adult skin and peripheral nerves is treated in detail in Chapters 5 through 7. Finally, detailed mechanistic hypotheses of induced tissue and organ regeneration are presented in Chapters 8 through 10, leading to generic methodology for organ regeneration.

IOANNIS V. YANNAS
Newton, Massachusetts

Acknowledgments

I have benefited greatly from the seminal writings of Paul Flory and Arthur Tobolsky in polymer chemistry; the pioneers of connective tissue research, Jerome Gross, Alexander Rich, Frank Schmitt, and David Swann; the fascinating treatises on amphibian and mammalian regeneration by Richard Goss, Elizabeth Hay, David Stocum, Panagiotis Tsonis, and H. Wallace; the early studies of Abercrombie, Billingham, Medawar, and their coworkers in the area of skin wound-healing research; the penetrating discoveries in the area of wound contraction, as well as those relating to the role of myofibroblasts and smooth muscle cells, by Alexis Desmoulière, Giulio Gabbiani, Guido Majno, and Russell Ross; the powerful insights on cell-matrix interactions afforded by the studies of Fred Grinnell, Elizabeth Hay, and Richard Hynes; the original studies of Eugene Bell, Howard Green, John Hansbrough, and Dennis Orgill, who charted new directions in the treatment of skin loss; the seminal contributions of Patrick Aebischer, Simon Archibald, Göran Lundborg, Roger Madison, and Xavier Navarro in the area of peripheral nerve regeneration; my beginner's tutorship in nerve electrophysiology with Christian Krarup, in neurosurgery with Thor Norregaard and Nicholas Zervas, and in neuropathology with William Schoene; the immensely useful compilations of the literature of wound healing by Richard Clark, as well as by I. Kelman Cohen, Robert Diegelmann, and William Lindblad; my early, unforgettable collaboration with John Burke, who first taught me about the treatment of burn patients with clarity and authority; the thorough morphological studies of partly regenerated skin by Carolyn Compton and George Murphy; and the inspired mentoring I received from MIT bioengineers Robert Mann, Edward Merrill, and Ascher Shapiro.

I thank my former students or research associates Lila Chamberlain, Albert Chang, Elizabeth Chen, Jude Colt, Ariel Ferdman, Martin Forbes, Philip Gordon, Chor Huang, Susan Izatt, James Kirk, Elaine Lee, Dennis Orgill, Fred Silver, Eugene Skrabut, Mark Spilker, Nak-Ho Sung, and Karen Troxel, who prepared the ECM analogs over the years, took care of the animals, and made the measurements on regenerated tissues. Most of the illustrations were prepared by Wayne Hsiao. I thank Alexi Yannas, who closed the door to procrastination.

IOANNIS V. YANNAS
Newton, Massachusetts

Contents

6 Regeneration of a Peripheral Nerve

1
The Irreversibility of Injury

1.1 Repair versus Regeneration

Organ regeneration is distinct from organ repair as an endpoint of a healing process following injury. Repair is an adaptation to loss of normal organ mass and leads to restoration of the interrupted continuity by synthesis of scar tissue without restoration of the normal tissues. In contrast, regeneration restores the interrupted continuity by synthesis of the missing organ mass at the original anatomical site, yielding a regenerate. Regeneration restores the normal structure and function of the organ; repair does not.

An adult typically responds to chronic as well as acute injury (trauma) by repairing the injured anatomical site. Trauma is injury caused by an external energy source, usually acting destructively for seconds or minutes. Chronic injury is the end result of a prolonged sequence of biochemical insults, typically extending over years, such as those leading to liver cirrhosis. Acute and chronic injury often have a common outcome: loss of organ function. Response to chronic injury, caused by viral or toxic agents, is much harder to study experimentally than the response to acute injury; for this reason, the emphasis in this volume will be on response to trauma.

Regeneration may take place unaided by the experimenter (spontaneous regeneration) or it may be deliberately provoked using exogenous agents (induced regeneration). Although spontaneous regeneration is a basic topic that is treated in this volume, the major focus is the phenomenon of induced regeneration following acute injury.

1.2 Tissues and Organs

The anatomical terms used in this volume usually follow the nomenclature used either in *Wheater's Functional Histology* (Burkitt et al., 1993) or in the volume *Pathology*, edited by Rubin and Farber (Rubin and Farber, 1988).

Tissues are collections of individual cells that become specialized (differentiated) to perform specific functions in multicellular organisms. A tissue comprises either cells alone or cells and extracellular matrix (ECM); provided that the tissue is not undergoing active development or healing, all cells in the tissue are of similar morphology, and the tissue itself is often relatively homogeneous in structure throughout its mass (e.g., bone, cartilage, epidermis, muscle, epineurium). Anatomically distinct assemblies of tissues comprise organs that perform specialized functions of far greater complexity than those of individual tissues comprising them (e.g., lung, kidney, peripheral nerve, skin, liver, eye, testis). Organs and tissues arrange themselves in organ systems, major anatomical networks that integrate the functions of several organs (e.g., respiratory system, central nervous system, immune system, circulatory system, gastrointestinal tract).

Classification according to cell type is often used to divide tissues into epithelial, supporting/connective/stroma, nervous, and muscle cell types; several authors have distinguished blood as a fifth tissue type rather than including it with connective tissues. The term "connective tissue" has been traditionally applied to tissues of mesodermal origin that provide structural and metabolic support for other tissues and organs throughout the body. These tissues are carriers of blood vessels (vasculature) and, as a result, mediate the transport of metabolites, nutrients, and waste products between the circulatory system and tissues or organs as well as providing mechanical support. Such a wide range of functions transcends the simple connection of organs and has prompted several authors to employ the term "supporting tissue" or "stroma" instead (Martinez-Hernandez, 1988; Burkitt et al., 1993). Stroma will be used to indicate the normally functioning tissue; connective tissue will typically refer to a product of repair. In many organs, three tissue layers (epithelia, basement membrane and stroma) are grouped together, comprising a reference structure that is used extensively in this volume to compare the response of organs to injury.

1.3 Spontaneous and Induced Regeneration

Certain individual tissues, such as epithelial tissues, are capable of spontaneous regeneration following injury, even in the adult mammal; other tissues are not. A detailed account of this important phenomenon will be presented later in this chapter and in the next one. Organs are assemblies both of tissues that spontaneously regenerate (regenerative) and those that do not (nonregenerative).

Induced regeneration is the recovery of physiological structure and function of nonregenerative tissues in an organ. Organ regeneration may be induced in an adult by use of external means, typically by application of the appropriate cells, matrices, cytokines, or a combination, to the site of injury. In the literature, the progress of induced regeneration of tissues has been often observed only by morphological methods whereas organ regeneration has frequently been monitored by functional methods as well. The practice and theory of induced tissue and organ regeneration, and the general principles that emerge from such practice, are the topics treated in this volume.

1.4 Diversity of Spontaneously Regenerative Phenomena

A survey of the literature shows use of the term "regeneration" in a variety of contexts, which have been reviewed (Goss, 1992; Stocum, 1995; Tsonis, 1996). "Physiological regeneration" (Hay, 1966) has been used to describe the processes by which living organisms engage in continuous self-renewal or turnover. For instance, progenitor cells are continuously produced in the bone marrow and replace older blood cells; basal cells are continuously produced in the innermost layer of the epidermis and replace older cells in the outermost layer of skin. These ubiquitous "cell turnover" phenomena (Brockes, 1997) do not result directly from acute or chronic injury. Loss of blood from a hemorrhage or loss of the epidermis due to a sunburn are reversible losses of tissue following injury and the response to these losses has been referred to as "reparative regeneration" (Hay, 1966).

"Compensatory growth" is the adjustment of the mass and corresponding function of an organ to the changed mass of an organ or to the changed needs of the organism as a whole (Goss, 1992). It does not always follow injury: Overuse of an organ leads to hypertrophy while disuse leads to atrophy. Examples are the reversible hypertrophy of heart muscle or the increase in bone mass resulting from increased physical activity. Organ hypertrophy is a systemic response that can result not only from functional overload but also as a response to injury, such as surgical removal of part of the organ. A well-known example involves the liver, which responds to surgical deletion of a fraction of its mass by growth of the remainder so as to compensate roughly for lost organ mass and function. The kidney offers another example of compensatory growth; following incapacitation or removal of one of the kidneys, the remaining one grows to almost double its original mass, largely compensating thereby for the mass lost by the other (Goss, 1992). Neither the excised liver nor the kidney recover the lost mass at the original anatomical site where the injury occurred. Compensatory growth is referred to only incidentally here since the focus in this volume is on responses to injury that are local rather than extending outside the injured site (systemic).

Certain amphibians are capable of truly spectacular feats of regeneration (see Figure 1.1). Almost perfect regeneration occurs after amputation of a limb in many larval and adult newts and salamanders, as well as in the larvae (tadpoles) of frogs (Wallace, 1981; Stocum, 1995; Tsonis, 1996). This phe-

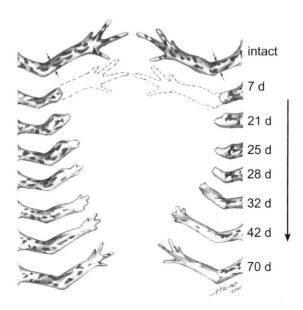

FIGURE 1.1. Montage of individual newt limbs amputated across the lower or upper arms, photographed at indicated times and regenerating spontaneously. (From Goss, 1992.)

nomenon has been termed "epimorphic regeneration," the replacement of an amputated appendage by a direct outgrowth from the severed cross section (Goss, 1992; Stocum, 1995). Limb regeneration is widespread in metazoan phylogeny, but the adult urodeles appear to comprise the exceptional vertebrate species that is capable of this feat (Brockes, 1997). Rare instances of epimorphic regeneration in mammals have been described (Goss, 1992). An often-cited case is the regeneration of crushed or lost distal tips of fingers in young children (Illingworth, 1974). Other examples that have been particularly well documented include the capacity of rabbits to fill in holes that were punched through their external ears and the annual regrowth of deer antlers from the wound that forms when the old antlers are shed in the spring (Goss, 1980; Stocum, 1995). In this volume, epimorphic regeneration will be regarded as the response to a special case of traumatic organ loss (loss of limb) rather than as a qualitatively distinct regenerative response.

Provided they are at an early enough point along the fetal stage of development, mammals appear capable of regeneration. Surveys of organ healing in the mammalian fetus have emphasized the absence of scarring in several animal models of injury during the early stages of gestation (Mast et al., 1992b).

1.5 Anatomical and Phylogenetic Focus of Regeneration

Much of the literature of regeneration and repair appears to have crystallized around a few, well-known, experimental paradigms: limb regeneration in amphibians, mainly urodeles and reptiles; skin wound healing in the adult mammal and its comparison to healing in the mammalian fetus; and peripheral nerve healing in the rodent.

The paradigm of limb amputation in the urodeles, young frogs (tadpoles), and lizards has been treated in a large number of studies as an instance of spontaneous regeneration (Hay, 1966; Goss, 1969; Wallace, 1981; Stocum, 1995; Tsonis, 1996). In this paradigm of epimorphic regeneration, the progress of regeneration of an entire limb can be studied unambiguously; however, the wound itself is quite complex, reflecting loss of an entire hierarchy of tissues and organs. Due to the large scale of injury, study of limb amputation and its aftermath has been restricted to small amphibians and is rarely conducted experimentally with larger mammals.

Skin wound healing in the adult mammal has been the classical paradigm of organ repair throughout history (Majno, 1982). Skin is the first line of defense of the organism to exogenous insults; consequently, skin is the organ that is most often injured, either accidentally, as in a cut or a burn, or intentionally, as part of surgical operations on the internal organs. Being exposed to direct view, the healing of skin is also easier to study than is the healing of internal organs. Consequently, references to "wound healing" in the literature usually imply studies of skin wounds, and "scar" typically refers to scar in skin. Studies of skin wound healing in the mammalian fetus have likewise fashioned a paradigm for spontaneous organ regeneration (Mast et al., 1992a; Stocum, 1995). Because of the wealth of reports in the literature concerned with skin wound healing (Peacock and Van Winkle, 1976; Clark and Henson, 1988; Mast, 1992; Clark, 1996b), this paradigm forms an invaluable source of information on the macroscopic as well as molecular biological phenomena that comprise repair.

Another well-known paradigm of wound healing, studied about as frequently as skin, is peripheral nerve healing in adult mammals following complete transection (Lundborg, 1987; Madison et al., 1992; Valentini, 1995; Fu and Gordon, 1997). The data is somewhat more quantitative in this field than in skin, and typically comprises measurements of the properties of nerve regenerates that result when the healing process is deliberately modified.

Skin and peripheral nerves are distinctly different from each other; and so are also the experimental conditions employed to study regeneration of each organ. One of my tasks in writing this volume is to show the intrinsic relation between wound healing phenomena and induced regeneration in skin and in peripheral nerves, in order to elicit "trans-organ" rules that can be used to study these processes in other organs as well.

1.6 Wounds, Lesions, and Defects

The term "wound" suggests to most people the result of an injury in skin; use of the term in relation to organs other than skin (e.g., peripheral nerves) usually requires some explanation. It is uncommon to find this term used to describe what is frequently referred to as a "lesion" in an internal organ, such as the heart, lung, or liver. In the next two chapters we seek to identify a type of wound that is suited to the study of induced regeneration, not only in skin but in other organs as well.

There is a further reason to seek a special term describing wounds in which investigators have carried on studies of induced regeneration. The outcome of an injury in any organ depends profoundly on the precise type of wound that has been generated. Investigators have studied a large variety of wound types, most of them not suited to the study we wish to undertake in this volume. In order to elicit useful generalizations from data based on independent studies, it is necessary to select experiments that have been conducted with the appropriate type of wound. For this reason, the vast majority of experimental data on spontaneous or induced regeneration described in this volume have been drawn from these investigations in which a specific type of anatomically well-defined wound, uniquely suited to the study of induced regeneration, was studied.

In order to emphasize the restrictions applied in selecting a particular kind of wound, as well as to discuss wounds in organs other than skin, I will consistently use the term "defect" as shorthand to represent the anatomically well-defined wound that is appropriate for study of induced regeneration. Definition of the anatomically well-defined defect, or simply defect, in skin and peripheral nerves will be made in the next two chapters. Use of this term will hopefully provide instant and relatively precise information to the reader about the anatomical site in which the process of interest is taking place. The term "wound" will be retained to denote the result of injury without specification of the type or extent of injury.

1.7 All Organs Can Be Irreversibly Injured

Although the focus in this volume is on skin and peripheral nerves, the experimental evidence shows that all organs in the adult can be irreversibly injured. In this section and the next, we review the outcome of healing in a variety of tissues and organs following injury. Only studies of spontaneous healing events in adult mammals, unaided by devices, are reviewed below.

We begin this survey with an internal organ, the *liver*. After surgical removal of 70% of its mass, the liver regrows, attaining its original size by seven to ten days. Such regrowth is recognized as an example of compensatory hyperplasia, which restores the optimal mass in relation to body size (Higgins and Anderson, 1931; Michalopoulos, 1990; Steer, 1995). In this

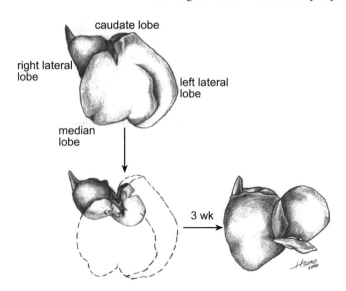

caudate lobe

right lateral
lobe

left lateral
lobe

median
lobe

3 wk

FIGURE 1.2. Liver does not regenerate at the anatomical site of injury. When the median and left lateral lobes of a rat liver are removed (broken line shows shape of intact organ), only the caudate and right lateral lobes remain, representing about one-third of the intact organ. After three weeks, these lobes enlarge to a mass equivalent to the initial size of the liver. The shape of the intact liver is not restored. (From Goss, 1992.)

well-studied experimental paradigm, amputation of three of five lobes of rat liver leads to hypertrophy of the two intact lobes until the original liver cell mass has been restored (Bucher, 1963). The three resected lobes never grow back (Michalopoulos and DeFrances, 1997). Since the residual lobes enlarge, the restored organ has a distinctly different shape from that of the intact organ (Goss, 1992). The nature of the tissues that result from healing of each lobe at the site of amputation does not appear to have been studied extensively. However, following chronic injury of liver with viral or toxic agents (cirrhosis), fibrous tissue is deposited in areas where liver cells have died (Vracko, 1974; Seyer and Raghow, 1992). Although liver is often cited routinely in the literature as the exceptional organ in the adult mammal that regenerates completely, the observations cited here define a healing process that is clearly different from spontaneous regeneration as defined above by the paradigm of limb regeneration in certain amphibians (see Figure 1.2).

Shifting our attention from the liver to the cardiovascular system, we find that the *blood vessel wall* can be injured not only by direct trauma but by chronic hypertension as well. The formation of atherosclerotic plaque appears to be a pathologic response to intimal injury (Stemerman, 1973). One of the results of such chronic abuse is accumulation of elastin, as well as the formation of fibrotic tissue based on collagen

(Davidson et al., 1992). The combined effects of the repair process are increased stiffness of the blood vessel wall and stenosis, or even occlusion, of the lumen (Stemerman and Ross, 1972; Davidson et al., 1992).

In another example from the diverse cardiovascular system, we find that cardiac *muscle* has been reported to be strongly resistant to regeneration (Polezhaev, 1972; Stocum, 1995). The cytology of death of heart muscle due to lack of oxygen (ischemia) has been studied extensively and the results of the healing process appear to be nearly identical to findings obtained following surgical incisions of this tissue. In none of these cases was new muscle formation observed; fibrous tissue repair was instead observed universally (McMinn, 1969).

Tissues of the *central nervous system* (spinal cord, brain) are notoriously resistant to regeneration (Cajal, 1928; Hay, 1966; Stocum, 1995). Unlike the response to injury in the peripheral nervous system, a crush injury in the spinal cord apparently is not followed by any measure of spontaneous regeneration (Eng et al., 1987; Liuzzi and Lasek, 1987); instead, scar formation has been reported (Cajal, 1928) and has been considered a major cause of lack of regeneration in the injured spinal cord (Kiernan, 1979). It has been suggested that there is an intrinsic difference between the healing patterns of lesions in the peripheral (PNS) and central nervous systems (CNS): The endoneurial tubes that are ubiquitously present in peripheral nerves, and that are often credited with the small but finite amount of regeneration in the PNS, are absent in the CNS. Accordingly, it has been hypothesized that spinal axon elongation fails to occur because nonneuronal (glial) cells in the CNS lack appropriate guiding tracks (Rutka et al., 1988).

Additional examples of the irreversibility of injury can be found in the musculoskeletal system. *Articular cartilage*, the thin but tough tissue layer that lines the surfaces of bones in a joint, lacks blood flow. Accordingly, when cartilage is injured, there is little evidence of the classical inflammatory response that normally supplies the defect site within minutes with blood elements as well as with a variety of growth factors and tissue cell types. The cartilage cell (chondrocyte) is the lone defender of tissue integrity in cartilage and a very limited amount of synthesis of new tissue occurs (Campbell, 1969). Much more exuberant is the response to a deeper injury, extending underneath cartilage and into the subchondral bone region (Stocum, 1995). An inflammatory response does in fact result from this deeper injury. Eventually, the cartilage defect is filled in with tissue that appears to be partly hyaline cartilage, suggesting partial regeneration, and partly fibrocartilage, indicating repair (Wornom and Buchman, 1992).

Transection of *skeletal muscle* has been studied extensively in connection with the healing of surgical incisions. After a clean cut, sarcoplasm retracts over a short distance inside the sarcolemma, leaving an empty tube that is soon filled by invading leukocytes and macrophages. Provided that the cut ends are held closely together, budding and union of cut fibers occurs, suggesting that effective regeneration has taken place across the very short gap length (McMinn, 1969). On the other hand, evidence of scar formation has been reported when the distance between the cut ends has been greater than a few millimeters (Volkman, 1893; Allbrook, 1962). It has been hypothesized that scar formation in the gap effectively prevents connection of muscle fibers (McMinn, 1969). In contrast, injury of skeletal muscle by methods (freezing, ischemia) that killed the cells without disorganizing the matrix, was followed by repopulation of the defect with new cells and recovery of physiological structure after three weeks (Vracko and Benditt, 1972).

The examples in this section illustrate the prevalence of irreversible injury in several, distinctly different, anatomical sites in the adult mammal. No organ, not even liver, is spared the irreversible loss of its structure and function at the site of injury (see Figure 1.3).

1.8 Critical Size of Defect versus Nature of Injured Tissue

It often appears that the size of the wound, or the severity of injury, dictates the outcome of the healing process. Wounds that are deep or extensive in volume are frequently considered to be irreversible. In this section, we will review tissues in different organs in order to answer the question: What makes an injury irreversible? Is it the size of the resulting wound or the identity of injured tissues?

Epithelial and endothelial tissues in all parts of the anatomy are widely reported to be capable of spontaneous regeneration without apparent loss of structural or functional characteristics (Hay, 1966). For example, the epidermis of skin, a cellular tissue layer about 100 µm thick, comprises several cell layers at states of increased differentiation. A reproducible and reversible injury that is confined to the epidermis can be produced by tape stripping (Pinkus, 1952; Stoschek et al., 1992). In one study, when the tape was applied ten times to the mouse tail, almost all of the stratum corneum and a few layers of the stratum granulosum were removed; however, the basal and spinous layers remained intact. Three days later, the epidermis had become three times thicker (hyperplasia) and the stratum corneum began to reappear; by day 7, the epidermis returned to its preinjury thickness and the epidermis was apparently also restored (Stoschek et al., 1992). However, an increase in the depth of injury to include the underlying dermis led to irreversible injury (Billingham and Medawar, 1955; Ross and Benditt, 1961; Luccioli et al., 1964; Dunphy and Van Winkle, 1968; Madden, 1972; Peacock and Van Winkle, 1976; Goss, 1992). Corneal epithelium provides another example where the precise depth of injury determines the outcome. After a superficial injury, resulting in complete removal of the epithelial layer, the surface becomes covered by conjunctival cells and the

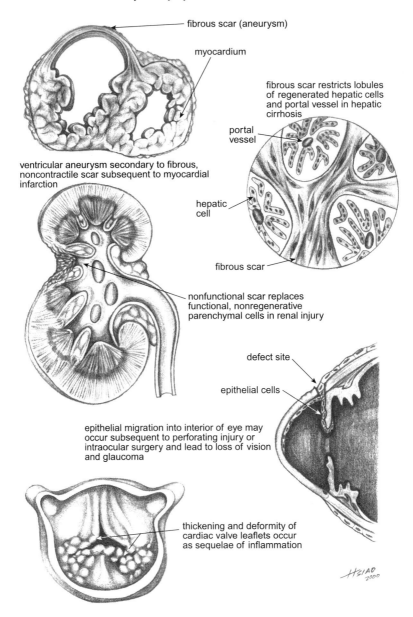

fibrous scar (aneurysm)

myocardium

fibrous scar restricts lobules of regenerated hepatic cells and portal vessel in hepatic cirrhosis

portal vessel

ventricular aneurysm secondary to fibrous, noncontractile scar subsequent to myocardial infarction

hepatic cell

fibrous scar

nonfunctional scar replaces functional, nonregenerative parenchymal cells in renal injury

defect site

epithelial cells

epithelial migration into interior of eye may occur subsequent to perforating injury or intraocular surgery and lead to loss of vision and glaucoma

thickening and deformity of cardiac valve leaflets occur as sequelae of inflammation

FIGURE 1.3. Most organs heal irreversibly (i.e., by repair rather than by regeneration) after extensive acute trauma or following chronic insults. The examples shown here illustrate repair processes in (clockwise from top left) the heart muscle, liver, eye, heart valve, and kidney. (Copyright, 1977. ICON learning Systems. Adapted with permission from ICON learning Systems, a subsidiary of Havas MediMedia USA Inc., illustrated by Frank H. Netter, MD. All rights reserved.)

latter become transformed eventually into typical corneal epithelium. However, a somewhat deeper injury, extending into the underlying supporting tissue (stroma), causes formation of scar and opacity of the eye (McMinn, 1969).

A further example of a cell lining is afforded by the intima, the endothelial lining of blood vessels with large diameter. Superficial scraping of the endothelium by balloon angioplasty is followed by proliferation of cells in the intact lining adjacent to the denuded area and by resurfacing of the lumenal surface. However, an injury extending deeply into the tissue layer underneath (media) leads to accumulation of scar-like connective tissue (Stemerman and Ross, 1972). Still another example of cell lining is found in the gut. Gastric epithelium responds to superficial injury (erosion) by rapid reepithelialization. A much deeper wound that has penetrated through the thin basement membrane into the underlying layers (submucosa and muscularis propria) leads to scar formation (ulcers) (Graham et al., 1992). Similarly, while the surface epithelia or endothelia of the gall bladder and the urinary bladder readily regenerate, the stroma underneath does not (Goss, 1964).

The response to injury of other organs also suggests that the nature of the injured tissue is a critical factor in the response. The outcome of injury to *lung* ranges from a mild and reversible response to light injury, caused by exposure to 100% oxygen for a few hours, to a lethal process in which the tiny hollow sacs responsible for gas exchange processes (alveoli) undergo irreversible changes leading to massive fibrosis. As with other organs, the early stage of acute lung injury is characterized by an inflammatory process. The initial inflammatory stage leads either to limited formation of fibrotic tissue with subsequent resumption of lung function, or to massive fibrosis that causes the lung to become nonfunctional (Hertz et al., 1992). However, the extent of injury as well as its tissue specificity are undoubtedly factors here as well. In studies of dog lung, one-half of the volume of the lung was injected intravenously with oleic acid, leading to death of epithelial and endothelial cells but not to destruction of the basement membrane in the affected volume. In these studies, repopulation of "dead" tissue started within about three days; most of the structure and all functional measurements returned to normal in three weeks (Vracko, 1972). On the other hand, formation of a lung abscess, a process in which it has been inferred that the pulmonary basement membrane was destroyed, has been generally observed to heal by scar formation (Vracko, 1974).

The response of *pancreas* to injury has been studied using a variety of protocols. In one study, following excision of as much as about 55% of rat pancreas, no reconstitution of the excised part was observed as late as 12 months after the trauma; however, the residual organ increased in weight, suggesting that compensatory hyperplasia had occurred (Lehv and Fitzgerald, 1968). In contrast, following ligation of the main pancreatic duct, a much less traumatic injury, pancreatic cells became atrophic; although the ducts dilated during the period two to seven weeks after the trauma, they remained largely intact; organ function returned to normal after four to ten weeks (Tiscornia et al., 1965). In another study, rats were fed a protein-free diet while being given intraperitoneal injections of ethionine for 10 days. While this regimen caused many pancreatic cells to die, the basement membrane that lines the cells and the pancreatic ducts remained intact. Two to three weeks after injury, pancreatic cells had been replenished and the normal structure of pancreas had been restored (Fitzgerald et al., 1968).

The *kidney* is, like the liver, capable of compensatory growth. Following excision of one kidney, the remaining organ increases its functional mass, although doubling of mass is not observed (Goss, 1992). These observations do not provide information about the local response of the organ to injury; however, it is universally assumed that no significant regrowth is observed at the site of the excised kidney. One study of the local response to injury was based on a protocol of destruction of cells in the outer portion of rat kidney (cortex) by freezing and thawing. Although the injury resulted in destruction of most cells, the scaffolding of the basement membrane in the compact arrays of interconnected capillary loops (glomeruli) was preserved. Repopulation by cells, probably originating from uninjured cells in the glomeruli, began within three days; eventually, the capillary side of the basement membrane became repopulated with endothelial cells while cells repopulating the epithelial side of the basement membrane became differentiated to podocytes (Cuppage et al., 1967; Madrazo et al., 1970). In a study of the response of renal tubules to acute tubular cell necrosis, it was observed that uninjured cells reepithelialized the surfaces of the basement membrane, leading to completely functional tubules, provided that the injury had not caused rupture of the basement membrane. Tears in the basement membrane prevented reconstitution of tubules into functioning units, apparently due to inability of tubular epithelial cells to bridge large enough gaps in the membrane (Oliver, 1953; Vracko, 1974). The data from these studies of cell necrosis have been interpreted to suggest that failure to preserve the basement membrane surfaces of tubules or glomeruli prevents repopulation by cells and eventual recovery of kidney function (Vracko, 1974).

The preceding examples emphasized the importance of tissue identity to its response to injury. However, the response of *bone* to fracture is an instance where the scale of injury rather than the nature of tissue injured appears to control the outcome of the healing process. The site of a fracture or osteotomy that had been anatomically reduced and mechanically stabilized has been described as a very fine line corresponding to a defect of order 0.1 mm (Shapiro, 1988). Under such highly controlled experimental conditions, lamellar bone formed across the interfragmentary space in a direction parallel to the long axis of the bone (contact healing). Larger defects, up to 0.5 mm, may also heal by formation of lamellar bone; however, the new bone tissue that is formed is deposited perpendicularly to the long axis of the bone and originates from marrow and periosteal cells (gap healing) (Shapiro, 1988). Defects that significantly exceed the 0.5-mm size heal by formation of nonmineralized connective tissue (soft callus), which later becomes mineralized, forming hard callus (union) (Ham, 1965; Hay, 1966). Larger gaps or smaller gaps that have not been mechanically stabilized may not heal by formation of osseous tissue (nonunion). In the adult rat, a clear gap larger than about 2 mm is not bridged with new mineralized tissue (nonunion) (McMinn, 1969).

Data supporting the existence of a critical-sized defect (i.e., a defect of a size that does not heal by reconnection during the lifetime of the organism) have been collected; for example, following an increase in bone defect size in the skull of the rat from 4 to 8 mm there was significantly less bridging by bone formation than with smaller defects (Schmitz and Hollinger, 1986; Schmitz et al., 1990). The minimum gap that can be bridged is not a constant for a given species but appears to vary with age and with the precise anatomical nature of the lesion. Generally, when bone loss is extensive, the fibrous tissue that forms does not suffice to fill the defect (Wornom and Buchman, 1992).

Peripheral nerves are another organ that heals in a manner suggesting the existence of a critically sized defect. Following complete transection of the nerve trunk, the stumps are typically inserted inside a tube (tubulation) in order to induce reconnection. It has been observed that reconnection of stumps does not take place when a critical gap length between the stumps has been exceeded (Lundborg et al., 1982a; Butí et al., 1996). Since, however, tubulation induces regeneration, this experimental configuration is disqualified from consideration as an example of spontaneous healing.

The survey presented above is far from an exhaustive review of all organs. Nevertheless, the combined evidence clearly shows that, depending on the organ, the identity of injured tissue is at least as useful a predictor of irreversibility as is size of injury. Evidence from several organs has shown that an injury of the epithelial and endothelial cell layers that cover the surfaces of an organ appears to be always reversible; injuries that reach much deeper appear to be irreversible. A more precise identification of the limiting tissue depth that is consistent with reversible injury in skin and peripheral nerves will be discussed in the next chapter.

1.9 A Universal End Product of Repair Processes in All Organs?

The spontaneous outcome of most injuries in adult mammalian tissues and organs is repair rather than regeneration. It is now appropriate to briefly examine the nature of tissues that are produced in repair processes. Is repair an organ-specific process, leading to synthesis of tissues with a structure characteristic of the organ undergoing repair or, rather, a nonspecific trans-organ process resulting in synthesis of just one type of tissue independently of anatomical location?

Investigators have usually identified simply as "scar" the fibrous tissues that result from injury or disease in a very large number of anatomical sites (Nimni, 1983; Diegelmann et al., 1988; Rudolph et al., 1992). The term "scar" has been used to describe the response to extensive injury in tissues as different as skin (Mast, 1992), tympanic membrane (McMinn, 1969), tendon (Amadio, 1992), peripheral nerves (Nimni, 1983), spinal cord (Kiernan, 1979), urethra (Rudolph et al., 1992), palmar fascia of fingers (Rudolph, 1980), skeletal muscle (McMinn, 1969), and others. However, a review of the literature reveals that the long-term outcome to various traumatic injuries and to a number of degenerative conditions in adult mammals is described not only as scar but also by the following terms: fibrosis, elastosis, retrocorneal fibrous membrane, fibrous tissue, adhesions, matrix calcification, pulmonary fibrosis, hepatic fibrosis, scar contracture, ulceration, neuroma, and fibrous capsule. Does the end product of irreversible injury vary from one organ to another or is there just one "universal" tissue product of repair processes in all organs?

The morphology and function of the tissue resulting from repair have not been popular topics of study by researchers. There is general lack of controlled studies in which tissues resulting from repair processes in different organs of a given species have been compared. Three examples of products of repair processes in skin, tendon, and peripheral nerve will be described briefly here to show that, in these three organs at least, the architecture of tissues resulting from the respective repair processes is not identical. Following healing of a full-thickness guinea pig skin wound, the fibrous tissue that eventually filled the site of the lesion comprised collagen fibers with an average diameter of $11 \pm 8 \mu m$ that were arranged in a pattern characterized by strong orientation of fiber axes in the plane of the epidermis, unlike fibers oriented in a basketweave pattern in the normal dermis (Ferdman and Yannas, 1993). By comparison, the collagen fibers in the connective tissue present in a healed rabbit tendon wound following complete transection were highly aligned along the tendon axis, as was also the case with normal tissue, but had an average diameter of just 0.2 to $0.4 \mu m$, almost two orders of magnitude lower than fibers in the healed skin wound (Ippolito et al., 1980). In a third example of repair, following complete transection of the rat sciatic nerve, the proximal stump was transformed into a bulbous mass with diameter typically 1.5 times that of the parent nerve (neuroma); unlike scar in the other two organs, the bulbous mass comprised primarily bundles of fine unmyelinated fibers (axons) meandering through disorganized fibrous tissue (Wall and Gutnick, 1974).

We conclude from these studies that, although the tissue products of repair in skin, tendon, and peripheral nerve comprised mostly connective tissue, they appeared to be distinguished by significant morphological differences. The few available data do not support the hypothesis that there is a tissue with unique morphology that could conceivably be considered as the universal product of repair processes in all organs.

1.10 Theoretical Views of Adult Failure to Regenerate

The ability of a few species (e.g., certain urodeles) to regenerate while most species do not is a central question in studies of limb regeneration in vertebrates (Tsonis, 1996). At the other end of phylogenetic development, where limb amputation is not used experimentally, investigators have attempted to explain why adults heal their wounds irreversibly. Hypothetical explanations have often been inspired by instances where the opposite outcome was observed (i.e., examples of spontaneous regeneration in mammalian fetal defects or sporadic cases of organ regeneration in the adult mammal).

Vertebrate limb regeneration has been often interpreted by use of the lucidly presented paradigm of the highly dedifferentiated cluster of cells (blastema) (Hay, 1966) that leads spectacularly to limb regeneration once given the chance to form at the apex of an amputated limb. The blastema paradigm has been used to explain adult response to healing, mostly by invoking the absence of blastema formation in cases of failed regeneration. These views were summarized in the form of recommendations for an improved effort to accomplish the goal of limb regeneration in the adult: The overall strategy was described as production of a blastema, while the detailed steps consisted of upregulating cell dedifferentiation, stimulating cell division, and delaying redifferentiation (Wallace, 1981). A similar hypothesis was presented in an effort to explain the lack of regeneration in amputated nonregenerating limbs of vertebrates. It was postulated that scar formation at the limb tips of such vertebrates is the result of a "nonfunctional" defect epidermis that does not maintain dedifferentiated and undifferentiated cells in the cell cycle over a sufficiently long period; instead, differentiation occurs early, producing scar and preventing blastema formation (Tassava and Olsen, 1982).

Lack of blastema formation due to interference from synthesis of scar was invoked to explain the difference between regenerative and nonregenerative ears in various species (Goss and Grimes, 1975). The basic paradigm was the full-thickness hole in the rabbit ear, a hole known to regenerate fully, including formation of hair follicles and sebaceous glands. In this model of dermis-free defect, contraction is not observed and the hole fills up entirely by the synthesis of new physiological tissues (Joseph and Dyson, 1966). While holes in the ears of lagomorphs, including rabbits, hares and pikas, regenerate fully with blastema formation, similar holes in sheep and dogs form scar tissue (Goss and Grimes, 1972, 1975). Comparison of morphological features of regenerating and nonregenerating ear holes highlighted transient epidermal downgrowths located between the original intact dermis of the skin and the tissues that gave rise to the blastema (Goss and Grimes, 1975; Goss, 1980, 1992). In the rabbit, but not in the sheep or dog, these transient epidermal tissues were presumptively involved in interaction with the underlying cartilage (epidermal-chondrogenic interaction), which hypothetically inhibited scar formation. These epidermal tissues were thought to play the same critical role in blastema formation as did the "functional epidermis" proposed independently, which prevents differentiation of cells indefinitely in the cell cycle (Tassava and Olsen, 1982). Not only rabbit ears but deer antlers, which are shed and regrown annually, are regenerated spontaneously (Goss, 1980, 1987). These examples suggested that being a mammal is not necessarily incompatible with spontaneous regeneration (Goss, 1980, 1992). The failure of most mammalian skin structures to regenerate was accordingly attributed to interference of scar with the interaction between epithelial tissues and underlying mesodermal tissues in the defect, thereby preventing the step that was considered critical to blastema formation (Goss, 1980).

Fetal skin wound healing has commonly provided the most common model of scarless healing (Lorenz et al., 1992; Mast et al., 1992a; Stocum, 1995). Many investigators who have looked for clues that might account for such often flawless healing have emphasized the relative lack of inflammatory response in models of fetal healing (McCallion and Ferguson, 1996; Martin, 1997). The ontogenetic transition in defect healing from fetal to adult is apparently characterized by at least three major changes: increased expression of the fibroblast phenotype associated with contraction of granulation tissue (Lanning et al., 1999, 2000; Chin et al., 2000), decreasing levels of hyaluronic acid synthesis (Clark, 1996b; McCallion and Ferguson, 1996; Sawai et al., 1997; Chin et al., 2000), as well as increasing importance of closure by contraction rather than by regeneration with increasing development (Yannas et al., 1996). In another approach, tissue regeneration during scarless skin healing in the fetus was considered to be similar to urodele regeneration, requiring neural stimulation in its early stages (Stelnicki et al., 2000). The genetic basis of the fetal-to-adult transition has been studied with emphasis on modulation of homeobox genes (Stelnicki et al., 1998), an approach that has been extensively pursued in studies of the developing limb (Tsonis, 1996). The results of a study of RNA differential display suggested the hypothesis that downregulation of chaperonins in fetal wounds may inhibit the formation of myofibroblasts, a differentiated fibroblast that has been implicated in wound contraction (Darden et al., 2000).

Interference with formation of scar in adult skin wounds has often been considered as a means of controlling the outcome of the healing process. It has been hypothesized that such control could be applied either to the self-assembly of collagen fibers (Ehrlich, 2000) or to formation of covalent crosslinks in these fibers (Tanzer, 1973). Following collagen synthesis, fibroblasts pack collagen molecules into cellular clefts that have been formed by a process of compartmentalization of the extracellular space. Self-assembly of collagen molecules takes place in these compartments, followed by polymerization into fibrils and organization into packets of fiber bundles (Birk and Trelstad, 1985). It has been hypothesized that embryonic fibroblasts, as well as fibroblasts inside an adult defect, release these bundles of collagen fibers quite differently; the former assemble fiber bundles that are oriented randomly, as in the intact adult dermis, whereas the bundles formed by the latter are oriented, as in scar (Ehrlich, 2000). Following formation, collagen bundles undergo crosslinking (Kivirikko and Myllylä, 1984; Yamauchi and Mechanic, 1988). Since the strength of scar depends on formation of covalent crosslinks in newly deposited collagen fibrils, it has been hypothesized that synthesis of crosslinked scar might be prevented by use of chemical inhibitors that block crosslinking (Tanzer, 1973). Other investigators have hypothesized that scar synthesis might be suppressed by interfering with each of several cellular activities that precede its deposition, such as integrin expression, protease activity, collagen matrix deposition, and cell apoptosis (Xu and Clark, 2000). In another approach, neutralization of transforming growth factor β (TGF-β) by an appropriate antibody has been proposed as a method for controlling scarring (Shah et al., 1992, 1994, 1995).

The specific organ under consideration has historically dictated the nature of theoretical interpretations of regeneration or repair. In an intriguing example of such an organ-specific viewpoint, theories of peripheral nerve regeneration have differed from those of skin in at least one important respect: While the failure of skin to regenerate spontaneously has been often explained in terms of the inhibiting presence of scar, failure to regenerate in the peripheral nervous system (PNS) has been rarely considered to be associated with the presence of neuroma. As it happens, PNS regeneration has been historically studied in a model of induced regeneration, the tubulated transected nerve, where neuroma formation is usually absent. In contrast, the untubulated model of healing of the transected nerve, the true model of spontaneous wound healing, has not been studied as much as the dermis-free defect, the model of spontaneous healing in skin wounds. The overwhelming choice of the tubulated model as an experimental paradigm in PNS studies may have disposed most theories of nerve regeneration subtly away from consideration of the presumptive role of nerve scar (neuroma); instead, the search was directed toward new conditions of tubulation that could extend and magnify a rudimentary regenerate that formed rather readily inside the tube. This historical difference in viewpoint may be used to explain why regeneration processes are so commonly referred to and accepted in the PNS literature while being so cautiously and infrequently alluded to in the literature of skin wound healing.

Theories that have been proposed to account for insufficient regeneration of transected peripheral nerves across a tubulated gap have historically followed two major lines of thought. In the first, elongation of axons and nonneuronal supporting cells from the proximal stump was thought to require diffusion of growth-promoting (trophic) soluble factors from the distal stump across the gap; in a slightly different version, cells in the distal stump were thought to exert an attractive (tropic) effect on regenerating axons (Cajal, 1928; Lundborg et al., 1982b,d; Politis et al., 1982; Longo et al., 1983a,b; Fu and Gordon, 1997). The second major direction of research in peripheral nerve regeneration evolved from the hypothesis that regeneration requires guidance by contact with an appropriate substrate (contact guidance) (Weiss, 1944; Weiss and Taylor, 1944b; Williams, 1987; Williams et al., 1987; Yannas et al., 1987a; Chang and Yannas, 1992; Whitworth et al., 1995; Lundborg et al., 1997; Chamberlain et al., 1998b).

A related hypothesis has focused on the detailed binding interactions between the growth cones of neurons and domains on the surface of adjacent ECM (Carbonetto et al., 1983). In an apparent combination of the two basic approaches, substrates have been thought to promote regeneration by binding on their surfaces these growth factors that are believed to facilitate the process (Madison et al., 1988). The presence of antibodies directed against structures that normally facilitate regeneration, such as an active site on laminin and an integrin receptor for laminin and collagen, has also been cited as a factor that may suppress regeneration (Carbonetto, 1991). Other theories have attributed the regenerative effect of tubulation either to prevention of fibroblast migration into the gap from tissues lying outside it or to prevention of axonal escape outside the gap or else in enhancement of concentration of growth factors inside the gap space (Madison et al., 1992). All of these hypotheses appear to share the common view that axon elongation along a tubulated gap should be interpreted as an instance of incompletely facilitated regeneration rather than as instances where neuroma had been suppressed.

Clearly, theories of regeneration of skin and of peripheral newes have followed different paradigms. One of the topics that will be discussed in this volume is the construction of a theory of regeneration that is not organ specific.

1.11 The Missing Organ and How to Replace It

The irreversibility of injury manifests itself strikingly as loss of normal function. Whether the injury is acute or chronic, its consequences vary from life-threatening symptoms (e.g., ischemic heart muscle, cirrhotic liver) to loss of mobility (e.g., neuroma, tendon adhesions) or to severe lack of social acceptance (e.g., disfiguring facial scars from extensive burns) (Boykin and Molnar, 1992; Rudolph et al., 1992). While a defect at the molecular scale can frequently be dealt with by use of one or more drugs, a defect at the scale of an entire organ requires radically different strategies. These considerations usher in the problem of the essentially nonfunctional organ, referred to as the "missing organ" (Yannas, 1988).

Six approaches appear to have been used in order to cope with the problem of the missing organ: transplantation, autografting, implantation of a permanent prosthesis, use of stem cells, in vitro synthesis of organs, and induced regeneration have all been developed to an extent. The last two methodologies have been compiled collectively in the literature under the title "tissue engineering" (Lanza et al., 1997b).

1.11.1 Transplantation

The transfer of an organ, or fraction thereof, from a donor to a host was introduced in the early twentieth century by Alexis Carrel (Brown, 1992). The successful transplantation of skin homografts between identical twins was demonstrated while the storage and rejection of skin homografts was studied in depth (Medawar, 1944, 1954). Successful transplantation of a kidney to an identical twin was reported (Murray et al., 1955). It is a currently widespread therapeutic strategy. Spectacular successes in patient survival have been reported following a host of transplantation events, involving a large variety of organs (e.g., kidney, liver, lungs) (Cooper et al., 1997; Lanza and Chick, 1997).

Overcoming the formidable immunological barrier has obviously been the main target of research in the field of xenotransplantation (Medawar, 1944; Bach et al., 1995). Exceptionally, the eye and testis contain "immune-privileged" sites and transplants at these sites are safe from rejection. Strategies that center around immunosuppression of the host by use of drugs have been pursued and successes have been reported; however, the immunosuppressed host becomes vulnerable to infections and cancer (Wickelgren, 1996). Advances in genetic engineering have led to cloning of muscle cells which express a protein (the Fas ligand) that induces immune cells to commit apoptosis (Lau et al., 1996; Wickelgren, 1996), suggesting the future possibility of using these cells in the vicinity of transplants for the purpose of restricting immunosuppression to the environment of the graft. In an effort to mask the antigens, heterologous cells have been encapsulated in appropriate materials, such as spheres manufactured from natural or synthetic polymers (Lim and Sun, 1980; Avgoustiniatos and Colton, 1997; Lanza and Chick, 1997).

An extensive effort has been mounted to develop transgenic pigs that could be used as immunocompatible donors for humans (xenotransplantation). Evidence that certain pig viruses are capable of infecting human cells (Patience et al., 1997) has introduced the risk of producing novel viral infections in the recipient (Kaiser, 1996; Sikorski and Peters, 1997). Currently, transplantation using human donors is a process burdened with substantial social cost, often requiring acts of altruism by relatives or other immuno-compatible individuals; and demand for organs has been greatly outpacing the supply (Lanza et al., 1997a).

1.11.2 Autografting

The problem of organ rejection is prevented by use of autografting. In this procedure, in which the donor and the host are the same individual, a fraction of a tissue or organ is surgically removed from an uninjured site and is grafted at the site of a nonfunctioning organ of the same individual (Medawar, 1944). Even though the graft is usually harvested by subjecting the individual to severe trauma, the transfer is justified when the primary loss of organ function threatens with excessive morbidity or death. Well-known examples of this approach are skin grafting in massively burned individuals (Burke et al., 1974), the coronary artery bypass operation, in which an autologous vein graft is excised and used to shunt blood circulation around blocked coronary arteries (Grondin et al., 1989), and the use of sural and other nerves to bridge a severe injury in a nerve of the hand as an alternative to direct suturing of transected nerves (Millesi, 1967; Millesi et al., 1972, 1976; Sunderland, 1978; Terzis, 1987). Although used extensively, this procedure is ultimately limited by the occasional unavailability of an autograft of suitable size or type.

1.11.3 Permanent Prosthesis

Implantation of a permanent prosthesis does not provoke an immunological rejection or problems of availability. Such prostheses are manufactured from ceramics, metallics, or synthetic polymers. In this approach, the physical function of the missing organ is replaced by implanting a biologically inactive device. Examples are artificial hip prostheses (Kohn and Ducheyne, 1992), cardiac pacemakers (Neuman, 1998), and contact lenses (Peppas and Langer, 1994). By and large, these devices are fabricated from materials that are clearly not part of the biosphere and are designed to remain biologically inert. In practice, the biological milieu surrounding the implant adapts in a manner that creates long-term complications. Examples of such responses are the stress shielding of bone supporting a hip prosthesis, that eventually leads to bone tissue resorption (Spector et al., 1993) and the formation of a fibrous capsule of scar tissue around a silicone breast implant (Ginsbach et al., 1979; Rudolph et al., 1992). These diverse phenomena are manifestations of the fundamental incompatibility generated by the presence of a biologically irrelevant device inside host tissue. They also alert the investigator to the importance of the active remodeling processes with which the host greets any implant.

1.11.4 Stem Cells

The use of stem cells has introduced a relatively new concept in the field: the synthesis of tissues starting from the least differentiated cells in the body. Various strategies for the potential use of stem cells to replace a missing organ have been suggested (Prockop, 1997; Solter and Gearhart, 1999). In one of these, cells are harvested from the patient, expanded in culture, and implanted directly into the anatomical site of the missing tissue or organ. In another, genes for selected proteins are introduced into stem cells followed by systemic infusion of the cells in an attempt to return them back to the bone marrow where they will presumably synthesize the proteins that have been selected. In a third strategy, stem cells are infused under conditions in which they will repopulate the marrow and provide stimulus for repopulation of the tissue targeted for treatment. The methodology for stem cell culture is developing rapidly. There appears to be a lack of protocols that have been used in more than one laboratory; accordingly, it is not clear whether investigators have even isolated the same cells (Prockop, 1997). Some of the greatest challenges in this field are due to the powerful drive of these cells to differentiate into something else (Vogel, 1999). In another report, cells that have the characteristics of human mesenchymal stem cells have been isolated from marrow aspirates of volunteer donors and have displayed a stable phenotype, remaining as a monolayer in vitro (Pittenger et al., 1999). Progress has been reported in studies of epithelial stem cells (Slack, 2000) and neural stem cells (Gage, 2000).

1.11.5 In Vitro Synthesis

Early successful efforts towards in vitro synthesis focused on culturing epithelial cells to produce a physiological epidermis (Compton, 1994). These studies initially focused on the growth of keratinocyte (KC) sheets from skin explants, followed by transplantation to skin wounds with subsequent observation of formation of a fully stratified epidermis (Karasek, 1966, 1968). In a later study, KC sheet grafts were produced from disaggregated epidermal cells that had been grown to confluence in vitro and were transplanted as cell sheets on skin wounds to eventually yield a fully differentiated, normally stratified epidermis (Worst et al., 1974). A significant advance in KC cultivation methods was marked by development of in vitro procedures for rapid growth and serial subcultivation from disaggregated suspensions of epidermal cells (Rheinwald and Green, 1975a,b; Green and Rheinwald, 1977; Green et al., 1979). This procedure has been used extensively to prepare sheets of autologous KC that have been used to cover skin wounds in severely burned patients (Green et al., 1979; Gallico et al., 1984; Eldad et al., 1987; Compton et al., 1989; Munster, 1992, 1996).

In vitro synthesis of a more complicated system, consisting of an epithelial-mesenchymal bilayer, was the focus of another early series of studies for the eventual replacement of skin (Bell et al., 1979). A collagen gel populated with fibroblasts was allowed to contract to give a more condensed state, which was then overgrown with KC to yield an immature epidermis yielding a "living skin equivalent;" the bilayer was then implanted in skin wounds. The result was a fully differentiated epidermis with a neodermal layer underneath (Bell et al., 1979, 1981a,b, 1983, 1984).

In an effort to synthesize a physiologically functioning liver, hepatocytes have been cultured on various matrices (Xu et al., 2000). A cartilaginous extracellular matrix has been synthesized in vitro following culture of chondrocytes on a synthetic polymeric substrate (Freed et al., 1994; Freed and Vunjak-Novakovic, 1995). The use of synthetic polymeric meshes for in vitro culture of fibroblasts and keratinocytes as a potential replacement for skin was studied extensively (Cooper et al., 1991; Hansbrough et al., 1992a, 1993) and the results of clinical studies with burn patients (Hansbrough et al., 1992b; Purdue et al., 1997; Dore et al., 1998) or diabetic foot ulcers (Naughton et al., 1997) have been reported. Efforts to synthesize in vitro several other tissues and organs using various synthetic polymers have been reviewed (Langer and Vacanti, 1993; Lanza et al., 1997b, 2000). One of the major directions being pursued consists in modification of the surface of synthetic polymeric substrates with specific functional groups that may control cell-substrate interactions, thereby dictating cell behavior in vitro (Griffith Cima, 1994; Peppas and Langer, 1994; Drumheller and Hubbell, 1997). The critical interactions between an organ cultured in vitro and the inevitable remodeling processes of the host, following implantation of the in vitro construct at the correct anatomical site, are expected to play a major role in the clinical future of such efforts.

1.11.6 Induced Organ Regeneration

The phenomenon of induced organ regeneration was discovered following development of methodology for synthesis of analogs of the extracellular matrix (ECM) with well-defined characteristics of the macromolecular network (Yannas et al., 1975a,b). These methods led to control of chemical composition, degradation rate, and specific surface of the highly porous networks (Yannas et al., 1975a,b, 1979, 1980; Dagalakis et al., 1980).

One of the ECM analogs showed unprecedented biological activity when used to graft full-thickness skin wounds in animals (Yannas et al., 1975a, 1977, 1981, 1982a; Yannas, 1981) and in humans (Burke et al., 1981). This analog was capable of inducing synthesis of dermis when grafted in a cell-free state; it induced nearly simultaneous synthesis of dermis, basement membrane, and epidermis in two weeks provided it had been seeded with autologous keratinocytes prior to grafting (Yannas et al., 1981, 1982a, 1989;

Murphy et al., 1990; Compton et al., 1998; Butler et al., 1999a). Although it was well known at that time that adults do not regenerate their organs spontaneously, the available data could only be explained by hypothesizing that these unexpected results were an instance of induced organ regeneration (Yannas et al., 1982b, 1984, 1989).

Since then, another ECM analog has shown regenerative activity in adult peripheral nerves, by facilitating formation of nerve trunk over an unprecedented distance across a tubulated gap in the rat sciatic nerve (Yannas et al., 1987a). The resulting regenerated nerve exhibited long-term physiological behavior at least equal to that of the autografted nerve (Chamberlain et al., 1998b, 2000b). The conjunctival stroma of the adult rabbit eye has also been induced to regenerate; the ECM analog used was identical to that which induced dermis regeneration (Hsu et al., 2000).

1.12 Synthesis of Tissues and Organs

From the point of view of the investigator, a process for in vitro synthesis of an organ differs remarkably from one conducted primarily in vivo (induced regeneration). Even though the two experimental approaches are quite different in protocol, they share an essential aspect: In the end, the product of each has to function inside the anatomy of the host as one of the host's own organs, over the lifetime of the host, without requiring special measures for its maintenance. Sooner or later, the outcome from either approach is tested under the same conditions: inside the tissues of the host. From the operational viewpoint, protocols in vitro and in vivo differ, therefore, primarily with respect to the relative amount of time that the investigator chooses to spend in vitro before the protocol moves to the obligatory stage in vivo.

Even the detailed processes themselves share an interesting aspect. In vitro synthesis and induced regeneration, even repair, can be viewed as highly complex processes of chemical synthesis. In particular, induced regeneration can be viewed as the synthesis of a physiological organ at the correct anatomical location (in situ synthesis). Let us pursue this analogy further.

The synthesis of tissues and organs is obviously a much more complicated exercise in building new matter than is synthesis of molecules, even of three-dimensional macromolecular networks. Cells, controlled by soluble and insoluble regulators, orchestrate elaborate reaction sequences. These sequences eventually lead to degradation of matrix components and polymerization of new ones to take their place, construction of tissues based mostly on cells that are joined to each other by newly synthesized proteins, and synthesis of adhesion proteins that maintain cells and new matrices tethered to each other. This activity takes place in the context of uniquely biological processes, such as mitosis and differentiation, that transform profoundly the cell population itself. The detailed mechanistic description of any one of these sequences that lead to a new tissue is still prohibitively difficult, even when the individual steps are reasonably well understood. Yet, it is possible to describe the beginning and the end of these elaborate pathways in a simple manner by employing elements of the systematic accounting approach used by chemists over the past two centuries.

Careful study of the literature of induced organ regeneration reveals that, with the exception of stoichiometric data, information of the type used to set up the equivalent of a chemical equation can be easily extracted from the detailed methodology described by an investigator. This information includes the three basic elements that are required to describe a regenerative process in the most elementary way: the identity of "reactants," a brief description of conditions inside the "reactor," and the identity of the "products." With the use of such data, it is possible to construct a "reaction diagram" for synthesis of a tissue or organ. The diagram is a qualitative summary of the experimental protocol and the tissues resulting from its use; it does not contain any stoichiometric data and it is not a chemical equation. The value of such a symbolic representation is that it provides an instant overview of a large number of complicated protocols studied by different investigators, all of which share the goal of synthesizing the same product. Analysis of the collective data by inspection is a winnowing process that yields the simplest, or "irreducible," conditions currently known for synthesis of a tissue or organ. This approach is simple and powerful.

In the following chapters, the discussion is first focused on the basic rules for the choice of reactor, the "anatomically well-defined defect" in which the synthetic process is induced (Chapters 2 and 3). This is followed by a discussion of the simple "defect closure rule," used in the standardized description of the products of regenerative or reparative processes (Chapter 4). These basic concepts are then used to classify and analyze, in a self-consistent manner, independent data from the literature on induced regeneration of skin and peripheral nerves by use of a large variety of reactants (Chapters 5 and 6). The analysis leads to identification of the irreducible reaction diagrams for synthesis of tissue components of skin and peripheral nerves, as well as of the organs themselves. The data encourage development of empirical rules relating the reactants and products of regenerative processes in skin and peripheral nerves. Hypothetical extension of these rules to other organs is briefly discussed (Chapter 7). Theoretical implications of the empirical data on the mechanism of induced regeneration is discussed in Chapter 8. This is followed by a detailed discussion of the data describing the kinetics and mechanism, including elementary cellular and molecular mechanistic steps, of the irreducible processes for synthesis of skin and peripheral nerves (Chapters 9 and 10).

1.13 Summary

Acute or chronic injury to any organ is followed by a spontaneous healing process. In the mammalian fetus and in certain amphibians, healing is a largely reversible process, leading to restoration of the original organ (regeneration). However, in the adult mammal, healing is typically irreversible and leads to formation of nonphysiological scar (repair). Every organ in the adult can be irreversibly injured, resulting in repair. In certain organs injury becomes irreversible when it is extensive enough, leading to a defect that exceeds a critical size, whereas in others the injury is irreversible when it leads to damage of specific tissues.

A number of theories have been proposed to explain the inability of the adult to regenerate its organs. Among these scar formation has been frequently cited as the cause for inhibition of regeneration.

Several approaches have been used to redress the loss of organ function that results from an extensive acute or chronic repair process in the adult. They include organ transplantation, autografting, implantation of permanent prostheses, use of stem cells, in vitro synthesis, and induced regeneration. The topic of this volume, induced regeneration, is a process in which physiological tissue, rather than scar, is deliberately synthesized at the anatomical site of the adult host that has been irreversibly injured. Conditions for synthesis of a tissue or organ will be summarized in the irreducible process, the simplest process known to yield a tissue or organ in its physiological structure.

In the following chapters, induced organ regeneration of skin and peripheral nerves, the two organs that have been studied most intensively in this respect, will be used as twin paradigms of such synthetic processes. The analysis will suggest, on occasion, development of trans-organ rules that could hypothetically be useful toward inducing regeneration of other organs in the adult mammal.

2
Nonregenerative Tissues

2.1 The Experimental Volume: In Vitro or In Vivo?

In the experimental study of induced tissue or organ regeneration, there is clear need to make an appropriate selection both of reactants and the assays that define the products. Less obvious, though equally important, is the need to make a rational choice of the experimental volume for the intended synthesis. Criteria for such a selection will be discussed in the present chapter as well as in the next. In this chapter we will discuss a fundamental characteristic of the tissues that need to be deleted in order to generate the experimental volume: their intrinsic inability to regenerate spontaneously.

An investigator who wishes to synthesize a tissue or organ has to make a basic choice very early: Is the study going to be carried on in vitro or in vivo? In the preceding chapter it was pointed out that, although the two approaches are remarkably different in the early part of the protocol, the final stage in both is implantation into the host's tissues (i.e., a process conducted in vivo). During that final step, an organ construct synthesized in vitro, or one about to be synthesized on location (in situ), has to become incorporated into the tissues of the host through a series of remodeling processes. In these processes, certain tissues, both of the implant and the host, will have to be resynthesized in order to reach a mutually compatible state that functions physiologically.

The advantages of a study in vitro are the ability to work with a reaction system that has fewer components and the opportunity to complete most of the synthetic work away from the occasional anatomical site that may be difficult to access experimentally. An example of the latter is an effort to replace a heart valve with an implant. A device that requires a long time to reach a functional state following implantation due to a lengthy ongoing synthetic process in situ is not an attractive prospect in this dynamic anatomical setting. On the other hand, in vivo synthesis holds the prospect of unprecedented results by harnessing the extraordinary amount of biological energy that is released following an injury.

A comparison of synthetic processes reported in the literature, carried on both in vitro and in vivo, is made in Chapter 7. Briefly, the comparison shows that, in studies of skin and peripheral nerves, protocols for in vitro synthesis have yielded so far epithelia and the associated basement membrane but not the physiological stroma. In contrast, a few of the protocols of induced regeneration, conducted mostly in vivo, have yielded not only the physiological epithelia with their basement membrane, but a near-physiological stroma as well. In the 20-year-old field of organ replacement the landscape is new and changing; new protocols are being developed rapidly. Future research may show that each of these two basic approaches holds an advantage in a given anatomical site.

2.2 Critical Presence of Exudate Inside the Defect

What kind of an experimental space is an injured anatomical site? Following injury, the tissues surrounding the defect respond by an inflammatory reaction that eventually leads to closure of the defect. A detailed discussion of mechanistic aspects of this response appears in a later chapter. We focus below on the nature of the fluid that fills the defect soon after injuring.

The initial events in the inflammatory response are the flow of blood and extravascular tissue fluid (collectively referred to here as "exudate") inside the defect, together with migration of cells from adjoining tissues. The exudate filling deep wounds, both in skin and nerve, contains a host of soluble regulators of cell function that orchestrate the inflammatory response; it is clearly one of the critical reactants in a study of induced regeneration. For example, following transection of the sciatic nerve in the rat, a cylindrical tissue about 1 mm in diameter, fluid exudate leaves the stumps at a rate estimated at about 1 µL per hour (Longo et al., 1983a,b; Williams and Varon, 1985). The exudate comprises primarily plasma that has leaked out of blood vessels, as a result of the increase in vascular permeability associated with trauma, as well as components synthesized by the injured neuron (Fu and Gordon, 1997). Axotomized neurons synthesize cytokines, including platelet-derived growth factor (PDGF) and acidic fibroblast growth factor (aFGF), which contribute to the inflammatory response of the transected nerve. They also synthesize neurotrophic factors, including nerve growth factor (NGF) (Lundborg et al., 1982b; Longo et al., 1983a,b; Fu and Gordon, 1997). These factors upregulate migration of non-neuronal cells and enhance angiogenesis (Fu and Gordon, 1997). Less is known about the composition of exudate is skin wounds; however, there is evidence that the exudate from a skin wound is endowed just as richly with soluble regulators (Regan and Barbul, 1991; Breuing et al., 1992).

In studies of spontaneous healing in the adult, the contents of the wound are simply allowed to be converted into scar. When the object is to attempt modification of the healing process, various experimental exogenous reactants (referred to simply as reactants) are supplied to the defect. These reactants, together with the exudate (endogenous reactant), induce synthesis of tissues that may, nevertheless, still consist of scar, if the reactants supplied happened to have been regeneratively inactive; or it may consist of physiological tissues, if the reactants are in fact regeneratively active.

The investigator who wishes to include the exudate as one of the reactants has to work inside the defect. The alternative is to conduct the study in a complex cell culture medium characterized by a time-dependent composition of solutes (e.g., cytokines, growth factors), as well as a program of cell expression (e.g., migration, synthesis, differentiation of appropriate cell types), that simulate the changing scenario inside the exudate during (say) the first several days of healing. The information currently available about the inflammatory response in the literature is too meager to allow construction of such a complicated experimental configuration. Instead, investigators who prefer to work in vitro have typically used a variety of culture media, each comprising an arbitrary selection from several of the components characterizing the inflammatory response. Obviously, the composition of these media is a very simple approximation of that in the exudate flowing into the defect during several days after injury. In Chapter 7 we will review the progress made in efforts to synthesize certain tissues and organs in culture media and will compare them to efforts made in the presence of exudate in vivo. In the meantime, all discussion will center on studies conducted in vivo (i.e., in the presence of physiological exudate).

2.3 Certain Tissues in an Organ Regenerate Spontaneously

Perhaps the most critical requirement for a defect that will be used to study the possible incidence of induced regeneration is the initial absence in it of the tissues that will eventually be synthesized. In the preceding chapter we found out that certain tissues sustain reversible injury whereas other tissues are injured irreversibly. Clearly, in studies of induced regeneration, the investigator seeks to synthesize tissues that do not regenerate spontaneously (nonregenerative tissues). These tissues must be carefully deleted from the defect; if not, their residual presence will lead to the erroneous conclusion that regeneration has been induced. On the other hand, tissues that regenerate spontaneously in the defect are expected to be present at the end of the healing process irrespective of whether the study has led to repair or regeneration.

The distinction between regenerative and nonregenerative tissues appears to be relatively sharp. It will be discussed in detail below using four well-known experimental paradigms, two each from the literature of defect healing in skin and peripheral nerves.

2.3.1 Epitheliocentric Viewpoint

The morphology of skin is illustrated in Figure 2.1. A more detailed description of structure and function of tissues comprising skin is presented in Chapter 5.

Briefly, skin is an organ with a two-dimensional geometry, consisting of a cellular epidermis attached to a basement membrane; the latter is attached to the dermis. Its main function is protection of the organism from injury originating in external energy sources. The epidermis is a specialized tissue consisting of several layers of epithelial cells (keratinocytes) that protects the organism from dehydration, bacteria, ultraviolet radiation, as well as insults of a chemical type. Protection is afforded principally by the outermost cell layer of the epidermis, the stratum corneum, consisting of dead, keratinized cells. In turn, the epidermis itself is supported by the dermis, a tough layer about 10 times the thickness of the epidermis, consisting primarily of collagen and elastin fibers. The dermis protects mechanically the thin, epidermal layer against shear and other mechanical insults. Itself highly vascularized, the dermis supplies the epidermis with metabolites through the basement membrane.

We consider the response of skin to different types of injury. In a large majority of such studies the emphasis of the investigators has favored measuring the outcome in terms of the rate of defect closure by the epidermis.

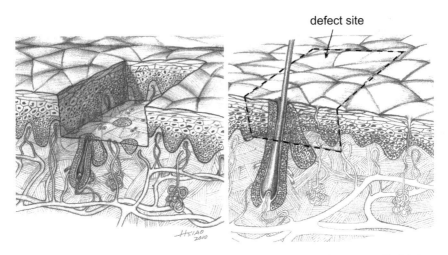

FIGURE 2.1. The epidermis is a regenerative tissue. Following controlled injury (stripping or blistering), which leaves the dermis intact (left), the epidermis recovers its structure completely at the site of the defect (right). Hair follicles are lined with epidermal tissue and participate in the regenerative process. (Adapted from Asmussen and Sollner, 1993.)

The highly focused emphasis on restoration of the epidermis is frequently motivated by the clinical urgency for defect closure. This experimental approach has been carried over in several experimental studies of induced skin regeneration; it suggests that a favorable outcome of the healing process is rapid completion of processes of keratinocyte proliferation, migration, and, finally, differentiation. This viewpoint of the healing response emphasizes, almost exclusively, the fate of the keratinocytes. We will refer to this as the epitheliocentric viewpoint.

The response of skin to two extreme types of injury, namely, a mild injury (blistering) and a very severe injury (full thickness skin excision), has been described extensively. A blister can be inflicted by abrasion or by a very mild burn. Shear forces or thermal injury cause failure at the interface between epidermis and dermis (dermal-epidermal junction), and exudation of lymph fluid into the separated space follows (Asmussen and Sollner, 1993). A similar model defect can be generated by repeated stripping of the epidermis with tape (Nanney and King, 1996). The blister typically separates the dermis and the epidermis at the level of the basement membrane; if the experiment is conducted carefully enough, the basement membrane remains partly intact. The underlying dermis reddens, swells, and forms a small amount of exudate but remains, otherwise, relatively intact. Since the injury does not extend into the dermis, blood vessels are not injured and there is no bleeding. Soon, the necrotic epidermis forming the blister is sloughed off, leaving behind an epidermis-free surface. Keratinocytes migrate from the injured edges and reattach themselves onto the inner layer (lamina densa) of the relatively intact basement membrane (Krawczyk and Wilgram, 1973; Beerens et al., 1975). Keratinocyte migration also originates in the appendages of skin (hair follicles, sweat glands, sebaceous glands) that are located in the dermis, below the lower surface of the blister. Migration of keratinocytes finally leads to formation of a continuous cell layer (confluence) over the basement membrane and the migration stops; the cells undergo mitosis and differentiation to a multilayered, mature, and keratinized epidermis (Figure 2.1). No sign of the blister can be detected on the regenerated epidermis, indicating that the ruptured dermo-epidermal junction has been restored (Briggaman et al., 1971; Marks et al., 1975; Konig and Bruckner-Tuderman, 1991; Stenn and Malhotra, 1992).

A much more severe injury is excision of the epidermis and the entire layer of dermis to generate a dermis-free defect (full-thickness skin wound). In a well-known example, involving a clinical trial of human volunteers, a dermis-free defect in the forearm was studied and a richly vascularized connective tissue (granulation tissue) soon formed inside the defect. Two different processes of defect closure, epithelialization and contraction of the dermal edges, were monitored. After the seventeenth day, contraction of the dermal edges had led to closure of somewhat less than half of the original defect area (Figure 2.2). The balance of defect closure, somewhat over 50% of the original area, was contributed by epithelialization

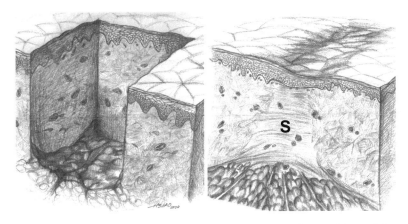

FIGURE 2.2. The dermis is a nonregenerative tissue. Following excision of the epidermis and of the dermis to its full thickness (left), the wound edges contract and close with simultaneous formation of scar tissue (S) in place of a physiological dermis (right). Adipose tissue (fat) shown underneath dermis or scar. The epidermis that forms over scar is thinner and lacks undulations (rete ridge).

(Ramirez et al., 1969). A simple analysis of the data in this study shows that the keratinocytes from the edges migrated and proliferated over distances at least as long as 15 mm and covered an area totaling more than 5 cm².

The two familiar examples of skin defect healing described above span the range from complete recovery of physiological skin function (regeneration), following careful blistering, all the way to formation of scar without recovery of physiological function (repair), following excision of the dermis through its full thickness. The functional outcomes of these healing models are as different as they can be. Nevertheless, in both cases, keratinocytes migrated and proliferated extensively from their original location at the edge of the injured tissue, eventually forming a regenerated epidermis over a large area. The evidence clearly suggests that extensive epithelialization that leads to formation of a new epidermis is an intrinsic property of migrating keratinocytes rather than being a property of the type of injury. We conclude that in studies of induced regeneration of skin the regenerative activity of an experimental reactant cannot be judged by success in recovering the epidermis.

2.3.2 Axonocentric Viewpoint

There is a profound topographic difference between the organization of tissues in skin and in a peripheral nerve trunk. Whereas tissues in skin are layered in a largely planar configuration, in a nerve trunk, the tissues are wrapped around each other concentrically to give a cylindrical arrangement. Briefly, a nerve trunk comprises one or more bundles (fascicles), each consisting of many elementary conducting units (nerve fibers). Its main function is transmission of electrical signals from the spinal cord to the periphery. Many mature nerve fibers comprise an axon surrounded by a sheath of the protein myelin (myelinated axon), provided by the wrappings of many Schwann cells around the axon perimeter, and a tubular basement membrane that lines the external surface of the Schwann cells. Other nerve fibers are, however, nonmyelinated. The axon is a long, cylindrical extension (cytoplasmic process) of a nerve cell (neuron). Individual nerve fibers are surrounded and supported by "nonneuronal" tissues arranged cylindrically around the fibers. Proceeding from a nerve fiber radially toward the periphery of the nerve trunk, we encounter the following nonneuronal tissues: the endoneurium, comprising a loose stroma (endoneurial stroma) and specialized blood vessels that establish a blood-nerve barrier; a tight, multilayered, and highly specialized tissue that provides a diffusion barrier, the perineurium; and, when the nerve trunk comprises more than one fascicle, a strong sheath that surrounds all fascicles, the epineurium. The permeability barriers provided by the endoneurium and the perineurium protect the space immediately outside the nerve fibers from changes in chemical composition, thereby preserving the electrical conductivity of the fibers. A detailed description of the structure and function of a nerve trunk is presented in Chapter 6.

Investigators have treated injured peripheral nerves with a variety of agents that are hypothetical reactants for inducing regeneration. In these studies, outcome measurements are collected by studying cross sections of regenerated nerves and typically consist of counts of myelinated and unmyelinated axons, measurements of the average thickness of the myelin sheath that surrounds an axon, as well as data on the distribution of the axon diameter. This is a decidedly axonocentric view. It is based on the well-known fact that interruption of axon continuity causes loss of the ability to conduct electrical signals that nerves uniquely possess. In studies of peripheral nerve regeneration very little attention has been traditionally paid in the literature to nonneuronal tissues. Does the number and morphology of axons merit being the single, exclusive, set of structural outcomes to be considered in a study of induced nerve regeneration?

Consider the response of axons and Schwann cells in a peripheral nerve following two types of injury: a mild injury (crushing of nerve trunk) and a severe injury (complete cutting of nerve or transection; also referred to as resection or division). In detailed studies of rat peroneal and sural nerves that had been crushed using smooth-tipped forceps, observations were made at the crush site and adjacent to it. It was reported that the tubular basement membrane (BM tube) that surrounded a crushed nerve fiber persisted at the crush site; the tube diameter became shrunken but the tube wall did not rupture. Axon cytoplasm (axoplasm), myelin, and Schwann cell cytoplasm inside the BM tubes were all displaced out of the crushed site. Even though separated by a clear gap at the crush site, however, the displaced tissues were retained inside the intact tubes. In the regions adjacent to the crush site, the BM tubes accommodated this displaced material by becoming distended but not rupturing. Following release of the crushing force, the shrunk BM tubes rapidly filled once more at the crush site with the tissues that had been displaced, and structural recovery across the defect followed (Haftek and Thomas, 1968). Not only the axoplasm, but the myelin sheath as well recovered its structure following a carefully administered crush. By two weeks, the myelin sheath had degenerated to the point where very little myelin could be detected; however, by four to ten weeks, regeneration of the myelin sheath was complete (Goodrum et al., 1995, 2000). It has been shown that normal function was eventually restored following mild crushing (Madison et al., 1992). We conclude that, following this mild injury that severed the axons and induced degeneration of the myelin sheath, but left the BM tubes intact, axons recovered the continuity of their structure and the nerve fiber functioned physiologically once more (Figure 2.3).

We now review the response of axons and Schwann cells in a peripheral nerve to transection; clearly, this is a much more severe injury than mild crushing. Since we are concerned with the potential for spontaneous (unaided) regeneration, we focus on the response of a transected nerve in which the stumps were not ensheathed in a tubular prosthesis (tubulation); the response of the more common tubulated configuration is a clear case of

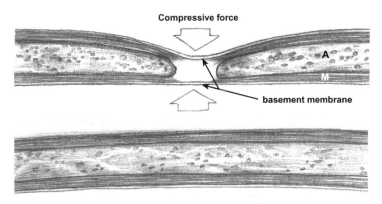

FIGURE 2.3. Axons and their myelin sheath inside a nerve fiber are regenerative tissues. After a mild crushing injury, the axoplasm (A) separates and the myelin sheath (M) degenerates on either side of the crushed, but not transected, nerve fiber. The basement membrane has remained intact throughout (top). Regeneration of the nerve fiber occurs after a few weeks (bottom).

induced, rather than spontaneous, regeneration and is discussed in detail in Chapter 6. Of the two nerve stumps resulting from transection, only the proximal one was still connected to the cell body (neuron). When the gap separating the stumps was sufficiently long, the proximal stump bulged out, forming a semispherical mass (neuroma); however, a neuroma-like structure also formed at the distal stump (Chamberlain et al., 2000a). A neuroma is the product of a repair process in a peripheral nerve. It comprises highly disorganized and poorly vascularized connective tissue. Embedded in it are Schwann cells and a large number of tangled axons, some of which are myelinated; most axons are reported to end blindly, or to be nonmyelinated and to be oriented in a highly irregular manner (Cajal, 1928; Denny-Brown, 1946; Young, 1948; Aguayo et al., 1973; Wall and Gutnick, 1974; Jenq and Coggeshall, 1985b; Olsson, 1990; Sunderland, 1990; Zochodne and Nguyen, 1997; Chamberlain et al., 2000a). Certain authors reserve the use of the term "neuroma" for the outgrowth of the proximal stump alone; the two stumps differ in the presence of elongating axons and of a proliferating perineurium in the proximal, but not the distal, stump (Thomas, 1988) (Figure 2.4).

Axons and associated Schwann cells have been observed to have elongated or migrated into and through the tissues of a growing neuroma over

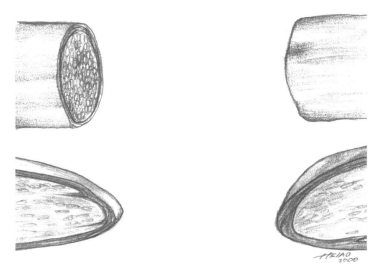

FIGURE 2.4. Most of the supporting tissues (stroma) surrounding nerve fibers are not regenerative. Although nerve fibers are regenerative following complete transection of the nerve trunk, the rest of the tissues in the nerve trunk are not. Following transection (top), each of the stumps that are formed becomes a neuroma, a clump of scarred tissue that has closed largely by contraction (bottom).

distances at least as long as a few mm. Considering that the diameter of most myelinated axons in the rat sciatic nerve, a popular model for studies of regeneration, is about 1 to 5 μm, a distance of a few millimeters corresponds to an axon elongation of about 1000 times its diameter. Reports of axonal elongation through a neuroma, over a distance of about 1 to 2 mm, have appeared on several occasions (Cajal, 1928; Denny-Brown, 1946; Wall and Gutnick, 1974). In other studies, axons managed to cross an untubulated 4-mm gap in the rat sciatic nerve (Archibald et al., 1991) or an untubulated 2-mm gap in the mouse sciatic nerve (Butí et al., 1996) and to establish substantial recovery of nerve function. In a more striking report, axons were observed to pass through the proximal neuroma, along the sling stitch surgically uniting the untubulated stumps, and finally to enter the distal stump, a distance of about 10 mm (Noback et al., 1958). Following a detailed study of this phenomenon, it was concluded that "nerve fibers can certainly grow in neuromas" (Denny-Brown, 1946).

The two healing outcomes described above are extreme examples of spontaneous response of the nerve fiber to injury: restoration of a physiological nerve fiber (regeneration) following mild crushing (Figure 2.3) and formation of nonphysiological neuroma (repair) following transection (Figure 2.4). Axons appear to have the intrinsic ability to elongate over substantial distances, though not necessarily in a straight line, independently of whether other tissues, such as the endoneurium or perineurium, are undergoing regeneration or repair. Schwann cells are also capable of proliferation and myelination of axons independently of the extent of injury to the nerve trunk. Neither the incidence of axon elongation nor that of axon myelination appear to be, by themselves, either sensitive or conclusive evidence of recovery of overall physiological function in an injured peripheral nerve.

2.3.3 Spontaneously Regenerative Tissues

Let us summarize the results of the four well-documented experiments described above with models of skin and peripheral nerve injury. The combined evidence showed that an increase in the severity of injury did not suppress the incidence of spontaneous proliferation and migration of keratinocytes in skin; nor was the spontaneous elongation of axons and the myelinating activity of Schwann cells suppressed in nerves. We conclude that keratinocytes and axons, as well as Schwann cells, are intrinsically capable of restoration of the original specialized functional tissues (epidermis and myelinated axons, respectively) and that they exhibit this property after a wide range of injuries. Even when the injured organ as a whole does not recover its structure, these individual tissue components show a remarkable ability to migrate and proliferate (skin), or elongate and become myelinated (nerve).

2.4 Other Tissues Are Nonregenerative

A reactant cannot be pronounced to have regenerative activity unless it leads to synthesis of a tissue that does not regenerate spontaneously. Preparation of an experimental defect for the study of induced regeneration should, therefore, be based on thorough excision of nonregenerative tissues and critical assays of induced regeneration should be focused on their identification. In this section we will identify these tissues.

2.4.1 The Dermis Is Nonregenerative

The structure of the dermis was described briefly above; a more detailed description of it appears in Chapter 5. The structure and functional properties of dermal scar are described in detail in Chapter 4.

The adult mammalian dermis does not regenerate spontaneously. This can be observed most clearly in the response to a severe injury, such as the excision of the epidermis and of the dermis down to its full thickness (dermis-free defect). The resulting defect closes spontaneously by contraction of edges and synthesis of epithelialized scar (Figure 2.2). The epidermis of scar is thinner and there are few, if any, undulations (rete ridges) in its dermal-epidermal junction; in the subepidermal region of scar, skin appendages, as well as collagen fibers with their axes oriented in a relatively random array, are absent. The connective tissue layer of scar (dermal scar) is largely avascular, rarely has nerve endings, and the collagen fibers are packed tightly with their axes oriented largely in the plane of the epidermis. When only part of the thickness of the dermis has been excised (partial-thickness skin wound), as in a donor site used in harvesting a split-thickness graft, the skin appendages in the residual dermal layer form centers from which epithelial cells proliferate and eventually reepithelialize the thin scar tissue that forms over the entire donor site. The inability of dermis to regenerate has been documented abundantly in animal studies (Billingham and Reynolds, 1952; Billingham and Medawar, 1955; Billingham and Russell, 1956; Ross and Benditt, 1961; Luccioli et al., 1964; Peacock and Van Winkle, 1976; Goss, 1992) and in studies with humans (Ross and Odland, 1968; Peacock, 1971, 1984; Madden, 1972; Boykin and Molnar, 1992). Very few exceptions to this rule have been reported: Unlike the ear of sheep and dogs, the rabbit ear has been reported to regenerate after a full thickness hole has been punched through it (Goss and Grimes, 1972, 1975; Goss 1992).

Neither do the appendages of skin regenerate spontaneously (Martin, 1997). It might have been expected that the epidermal origin of these appendages (Burkitt et al., 1993) would have prevailed and that, like the epidermis itself, hair follicles, sebaceous glands, and sweat glands would be capable of spontaneous regeneration; but such is not the case.

2.4.2 The Endoneurial Stroma Is Nonregenerative

The structure of the endoneurium has been outlined briefly above; it is described in greater detail in Chapter 6.

Following peripheral nerve transection and, provided that the untubulated stumps were initially separated by a few mm, each stump heals individually by formation of a capsule of neural scar around the edge of the stump (capping) (Cajal, 1928; Denny-Brown, 1946; Chamberlain et al., 2000a) (Figure 2.4). A neuroma was formed both when the nerve was transected by scalpel as well as by use of a laser (Fischer et al., 1983).

Clear and irreversible changes have been observed in the connective tissue of the intrafascicular space (endoneurial stroma), both in the distal and proximal stumps, following nerve transection. In the distal stump, by four weeks after transection, collagen accumulation (endoneurial fibrosis) had occurred; the average diameter of the new collagen fibrils was 25 to 30 nm (i.e., about 50% of the value in normal endoneurial stroma). Collagen fibrils surrounded columns of Schwann cells (Büngner bands), leftovers from degeneration of nerve fibers (Wallerian degeneration) (Salonen et al., 1985, 1987a). By 20 to 30 weeks after transection, the Schwann cell columns had become shrunken, showed decrease in laminin content, and occasionally had become fragmented, with dispersion of fragments inside the intrafascicular space and replacement of fragmented Schwann cells by collagen fibrils (Salonen et al., 1987b; Röyttä and Salonen, 1988; Giannini and Dyck, 1990). Finally, as long as 26 months after transection, the site of previous nerve fibers was indicated by sharply demarcated domains of approximately circular outline consisting of densely packed longitudinally oriented collagen fibrils, with diameters that were smaller than those in the uninjured endoneurium (Bradley et al., 1998) (Figure 2.5).

In the proximal stump, some of the morphological changes following repair were very similar to those observed in the distal stump; others were unique to the proximal stump. The following changes were common to both stumps: Following transection, continuous extrusion of intrafascicular contents was observed (endoneurial bulge) (Archibald and Fisher, 1987) and a significant mass of collagen was deposited in the stump (fibrosis) (Eather et al., 1986). The collagen fibrils that were deposited immediately outside Schwann cells in the proximal stump had an average diameter of 30 nm, compared with 50 nm in normal endoneurial stroma (Morris et al., 1972b). In the repaired proximal stump, the original uni- or difascicular structure of the normal nerve trunk disappeared and was replaced by a collection of small fascicles, filled with small-diameter axons, each fascicle surrounded by its own multilaminate perineurium (compartmentation) (Morris et al., 1972d). Compartmentation (also referred to as micro- or minifasciculation) was not observed in the distal stump; nor was formation of Schwann cell columns observed in the proximal stump (Morris et al., 1972d). Subdivision of a single facicle into many was accompanied by significant loss in cross-sectional area occupied by endoneurial stroma (Morris et al., 1972d). The subdivision of the injured nerve trunk into many fascicles has been observed in early studies (Cajal, 1928). Compartmentation, typically accompanied by decrease in axon diameter compared with the intact nerve, has been firmly associated with the abnormally low conduction velocity that is frequently observed with incompletely regenerated nerve trunks under a

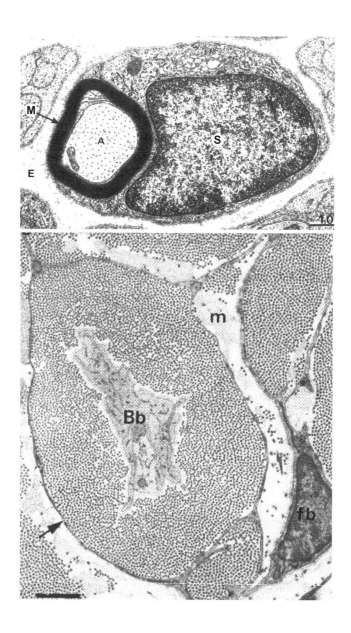

large variety of conditions (Fields and Ellisman, 1986a,b; Chamberlain et al., 1998b, 2000a).

The evidence shows that, both in the proximal and the distal stump, the endoneurial stroma is not spontaneously regenerated. In the distal stump, the original nerve fibers are replaced by a dense sheath of collagen fibrils (Figure 2.5); in the proximal stump, stroma characterized by nonphysiological morphology is synthesized next to Schwann cells and axons, while the repaired nerve fibers are confined within a remarkably small intrafascicular space. The conclusion that the endoneurial stroma is nonregenerative is based entirely on the morphological evidence, and is consistent with the finding that the vascular endoneurial permeability barrier is not recovered even under conditions in which another nonneuronal tissue, the perineurium, is regenerated in a physiologically functioning state (Azzam et al., 1991).

2.4.3 Evidence for and Against Regeneration of Other Nonneuronal Tissues

A detailed description of the structure of the perineurium and the epineurium appears in Chapter 6. A brief characterization of the morphology of these tissues appeared above.

There is conflicting evidence in the literature concerning the spontaneous regenerative potential of the perineurium. In the study described above, in which compartmentation of the original fascicle was observed in the proximal stump following its transection, a collection of small fascicles, each surrounded by a multilaminate perineurium, was observed at the stump by six weeks (Morris et al., 1972d). As with cells in the intact perineurium, the cells comprising the new perineurium were each ensheathed in its own

---

FIGURE 2.5. The endoneurial stroma is nonregenerative. *Top*: A nerve fiber before transection, showing the axoplasm (A), myelin sheath (M), the associated Schwann cell (S) to the right of the axon, as well as a very thin basement membrane surrounding M and S. The entire nerve fiber is surrounded by the endoneurium (E), a loosely structured stroma (not clearly visible in this photo; a clearer image of collagen fibers in intact endoneurial stroma fibers is shown in Figure 6.2). Bar: One-half of the 1-μm bar in the original photo is shown. *Bottom*: Twenty-six months after transection, the domain previously occupied by a nerve fiber in the distal stump is now filled with a sheaf of collagen fibers, shown mostly as dots, that enclose groups of Schwann cell processes (Büngner bands, Bb) encircled by a basement membrane. The entire sheaf of fibers is enclosed in a thin fibroblast process (arrow). The fibroblast (fb) in the lower right has been partly transformed to a perineurial cell. Microfibrils (m) are observed outside the sheaf. Bar: 1 μm. (Top photo from Burkitt et al., 1993. Copyright 1993. Harcourt Publishers Ltd. Bottom photo from Bradley et al., 1998.)

basement membrane. However, the original perineurial structure, at the perimeter of the single large fascicle that surrounded the uninjured nerve trunk, had not been recovered; the authors had difficulty distinguishing any characteristic perineurial laminae at all at this boundary (Morris et al., 1972d). In another study, the sural nerve of adult rats was transected, leaving a gap of 5 mm that was not closed by tubulation; tissue, synthesized between the stumps and bridging the gap, was studied at eight weeks. In a number of sites inside the tissue bridge it was observed that groups of myelinated and unmyelinated axons as well as Schwann cells were surrounded, in a manner resembling fascicular sheaths, by perineurial cells, each possessing its own basement membrane. Adjacent perineurial cells were closely associated with one another, in multilaminate fashion, displaying multiple tight junctions. Spontaneous regeneration of perineurial sheaths was clearly observed in this study (Thomas and Jones, 1967).

In another investigation, specifically directed toward study of the regenerative potential of the perineurium, the transected stumps of a single fascicle in the rat sciatic nerve were joined by suturing together the perineurial sheaths across the gap. Care was taken to pass the needle through the perineurium, damaging the underlying axons in the intrafascicular space to a depth not greater than 50 μm. It was observed that, irrespective of whether the endoneurial bulge from both stumps had been trimmed before suturing, the changes observed after the surgery were very similar. The normally compact layers of the perineurium separated considerably from each other and lost part of their basement membrane. Axons and Schwann cells were observed between the layers of perineurial cells, a clear departure from the structure of an intact perineurium. Myelinated axons penetrated through the scar that had formed at the repair site and were observed to enter and leave the suture line, bridging the short gap between the stumps; however, no bridging of the gap between the ends of the divided perineurium in each stump with any tissue resembling perineurium was observed, even after 42 days (Behrman and Acland, 1981).

The dependence of regenerative potential of the perineurium on the type of injury it had sustained was shown in a study in which the perineurial sheath was stripped off the sciatic nerves of rats over a 5-mm length, at a segment along the length where the nerve consists of a single fascicle. Care was taken not to injure the axons inside the intrafascicular space immediately underneath the stripped perineurial sheath, and a record of specimens that had inadvertently suffered such damage was carefully maintained. In several undamaged specimens, in which no degenerative changes were observed in axons present immediately underneath, it was reported that an apparently normal perineurial sheath had been formed as early as 10 days, extending along the length that had been injured. It was hypothesized that the new perineurium had been synthesized by endoneurial fibroblasts migrating from within the fascicle (Nesbitt and Acland, 1980). Consideration of this data with other related data described above (Behrman and

Acland, 1981) leads to the intriguing conclusion that the regenerative potential of the perineurium is very high provided that the injury is entirely confined to it; when the injury extends deeply to the intrafascicular space (endoneurium) underneath it, the injury becomes irreversible.

We recall that careful blistering (Asmussen and Sollner, 1993) or stripping of the epidermis (Nanney and King, 1996) with no injury to the underlying dermis, described above, was followed by regeneration of the epidermis; in contrast, a deeper injury extending to the dermis led to irreversible healing. We conclude that the regenerative potential of these two tissues, the perineurium in a peripheral nerve and the epidermis in skin, depends critically on the type of injury sustained. In particular, we note that, in both cases, the injury became irreversible only after it had crossed into the neighboring tissue (stroma). Further comparison between the epidermis and the perineurium is, however, complicated by the fact that, unlike keratinocytes, the cells comprising the perineurium are each encased in its own basement membrane.

The available evidence shows that the transected perineurium does not regenerate either in its original structure or at the original anatomical site; new perineurium-like tissue is, however, synthesized around the minifascicles in the new, compartmented nerve trunk that results from healing. Synthesis of a new perineurium with altered structure outside its original anatomical site does not constitute regeneration, at least in the sense in which the term was defined in Chapter 1; yet, the morphology of the new tissue is approximately physiological. In view of this evidence, I will refer to the perineurium below as being a partly regenerative tissue.

Very little evidence has been collected specifically about the regenerative potential of the epineurium. Especially lacking are data following well-defined traumatic injury, such as transection. Although several authors have reported the presence of "neural scar" at each stump, following transection, a clear association of such tissue with scarring of the epineurium (epineurial fibrosis) was not made. Several investigators have reported epineurial fibrosis following a variety of insults on peripheral nerves, including chronic compression (Mackinnon et al., 1986), exposure to anesthetics (Barsa et al., 1982), and saline neurolysis (Frykmann et al., 1981).

We conclude that, following complete transection of a peripheral nerve, the endoneurial stroma, and to some extent the perineurium as well, is not spontaneously regenerated.

2.4.4 The Supporting Tissue (Stroma) of Several Organs Is Nonregenerative

In organs other than skin or peripheral nerves a clear distinction between regenerative and nonregenerative tissues can be made only tentatively due to the paucity of data from well-defined models of defect healing. In the large majority of studies reviewed in Chapter 1, the experimental injury inflicted was not designed to differentiate between regenerative and non-regenerative tissues in an organ. A few studies have, however, been conducted in a manner that provides useful preliminary information on this important property of tissues.

Among the organs that have been studied in a way leading to clear observations on regenerative activity of individual tissues are blood vessels and certain internal organs. In the preceding chapter reference was made to the observation that traumatic removal of the endothelial lining of blood vessels (intima) led to spontaneous reendothelialization provided that the injury did not extend through the basement membrane deeply into the adjacent layer (media); if the injury was deep, the blood vessel wall suffered irreversible fibrotic changes (Stemerman and Ross, 1972; Schwartz et al., 1975; Stemerman et al., 1977). Similarly, it was observed that the gastric epithelium responded to superficial injury (erosion) by reepithelialization; however, a deeper injury that extended to the submucosa and muscularis propria led to formation of ulcers (Graham et al., 1992). Likewise, injury of the epithelia in the urinary bladder and the gall bladder was followed by reepithelialization but injury to the underlying stroma was not regenerated (Goss, 1964).

Extensive data on the healing response of several organs have been reviewed (Vracko, 1974). The data were derived from studies on skeletal muscle fibers (Allbrook, 1962; Vracko and Benditt, 1972), the lung (Vracko, 1972), the kidney (Oliver, 1953), and the pancreas (Tiscornia et al., 1965; Fitzgerald et al., 1968; Lehv and Fitzgerald, 1968). In some of these studies, the injuries inflicted were relatively slight and caused the epithelia in each of these organs to die without disrupting the basement membrane; these methods included freezing, ischemia, and use of pharmacological agents that caused cell necrosis. In other studies, however, the injury protocols were more severe, occasionally involving severe crushing, cauterization with heat or treatment with strong acids, or large-scale surgical excision of organ tissues. These severe injuries were designed to rupture the basement membrane in the various organs.

Provided that the injury was slight and limited to the epithelia of these internal organs, the response invariably was regeneration of the epithelia. Deeper injuries (i.e., those in which the basement membrane was penetrated) resulted in irreversible damage, consisting of scar formation and loss of function. The conclusion that emerged was that an injury that is limited to epithelia leads to healing with spontaneous regeneration whereas extension of the injury through the basement membrane leads to irreversible healing (repair) (Vracko, 1974).

In this review, the emphasis throughout was on the effect of the injury on the approximately 100-nm thin basement membrane; the integrity of the underlying stroma following injury was typically not explicitly discussed (Vracko, 1974). Considering that the basement membrane is closely attached to the underlying stroma, it can be safely concluded that the protocols that led to the reported penetration of the basement membrane also led to significant injury to the stroma. The persistent observation of scar formation in the organs in which the basement membrane had been penetrated (Vracko, 1974) can, therefore, alternatively be explained entirely by reference to the injury inflicted to the stroma.

The collective evidence strongly suggests that the basement membrane is the limiting boundary that separates regenerative from nonregenerative tissues in several organs. This generalization is not applicable to all organs since a basement membrane is missing from several parts of the mammalian organism.

2.5 Are Basement Membranes Regenerative?

Independent data of greatly improved structural resolution have shown that healing processes inside the basement membrane can be separated from those going on in the tissues immediately over and underneath it. Improved experimental approaches have provided intriguing information on the limiting surface inside the basement membrane that separates regenerative from nonregenerative tissues.

In studies of epidermolysis bullosa (EB), an inheritable disease that leads to compromised defect healing in skin, formation of suction blisters was used as the method for generating defects (Uitto et al., 1996). The blister pulled and separated the epidermis away from the dermis, splitting the dermo-epidermal junction at the mechanically weakest tissue layer. In skin, hemidesmosomes line the interior of the basal cell membrane (the interface between epithelia and basement membrane) and the basement membrane comprises three specialized structures: lamina lucida, lamina densa, and the fibroreticular layer; the latter is closest to the stroma. The location of the plane of tissue separation was identified in this study by transmission electron microscopy, and the extent of scarring resulting at the end of the healing process was recorded separately.

Although as many as 10 different forms of EB have been tabulated (Lever and Schaumburg-Lever, 1990), the results of this study (Uitto et al., 1996) were grouped according to three major categories of inherited defects. In the first (EB simplex), blister formation occurred through the epidermis and healing proceeded without significant scarring. In the second type of defect (junctional EB), tissue separation occurred through the basement membrane, specifically within the lamina lucida, while the lamina densa remained intact; in this case also, no scarring was observed (Haber et al., 1985). Finally, in the third type of defect (dystrophic EB), tissue separation occurred below the basement membrane, within the papillary dermis, at the level of anchoring fibrils; here, healing resulted in extensive scarring (Uitto et al., 1996). The data suggest that the basement membrane itself is regenerative (Figure 2.6).

Similarly detailed evidence on the basement membrane tubes ensheathing nerve fibers is not available. However, following severe injury, Schwann cells in peripheral nerves have been shown to spontaneously synthesize a basement membrane (Fu and Gordon, 1997) even in the absence of axons (Ikeda et al., 1989). The available evidence favors viewing basement membranes both in skin and peripheral nerves as if they were, at least in part, regenerative tissues.

2.6 Regenerative Similarity of Tissues in Different Organs

It will be useful directly to compare the tissues in skin and peripheral nerves that are spontaneously regenerative as well as those that are nonregenerative.

In skin, the epidermis is spontaneously regenerative following injury. During epidermal regeneration over a dermal layer, epithelial cells at the edge of the defect lose their firm attachment to the laminin-rich layer (lamina lucida) of the basement membrane and become migratory (Stenn and Malhotra, 1992). They migrate over the dermal surface and synthesize a basement membrane; eventually, epithelial cells stop migrating when laminin (a major component of lamina lucida), the so-called "laminin brake," has been synthesized underneath (Woodley et al., 1988b; Woodley, 1996). After stopping, the cells begin the program of differentiation that leads to synthesis of a highly specialized tissue, the keratinized epidermis, the only tissue in the organism that acts as an efficient barrier to a large variety of substances.

In peripheral nerves, the myelin sheath, synthesized by Schwann cells, is also a spontaneously regenerative tissue. Following injury, Schwann cells switch their function (phenotype) from myelination of electrically active axons to a phenotype of support for survival and growth of the injured tissues (nonmyelinating Schwann cells). During that sequence, myelinating Schwann cells lose their attachment to the axon surface, proliferate, and start migrating. They synthesize several factors, such as cell-adhesion molecules, as well as neurotrophic factors and their receptors; they also synthesize a tubular basement membrane. Eventually, Schwann cells become reattached to the surface of the elongating axon and resynthesize a myelin sheath, even in a neuroma. The extensive evidence for this reversible conversion from the myelinating to the nonmyelinating phenotype of the Schwann cell phenotype following nerve transection has been reviewed (Fu and Gordon, 1997).

The evidence presented in the preceding sections showed that, both in skin and peripheral nerve, basement membrane was synthesized by

a typical blister

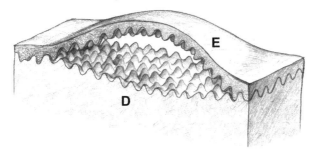

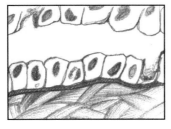

blister through epidermis: regeneration

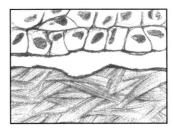

blister through basement membrane: regeneration

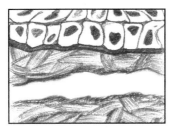

blister through dermis: repair (scar)

FIGURE 2.6. The basement membrane in skin is regenerative. Following blistering, skin separates at its mechanically weakest layer. *Top*: A blister in physiological skin separates the epidermis (E) from the dermis (D) at a level determined by the extent of injury (abrasion or burn); the sketch shows the egg-carton topography of the dermo-epidermal junction. (From Burkitt et al., 1993. Copyright 1993. Harcourt Publishers Ltd.) *Bottom three sketches*: Epidermolysis bullosa (EB) is a series of genetic diseases that are characterized by fragility and easy blistering of specific layers of the junction. In EB simplex, the separation occurs at the basal keratinocytes of the epidermis; healing occurs without scarring. In junctional forms of EB, the blister occurs at the level of lamina lucida of the basement membrane and also leads to healing without scarring. In dystrophic forms of EB, cleavage occurs within the subepidermal region of the dermis (papillary dermis) and leads to scarring. (From Uitto et al., 1996.)

TABLE 2.1. Regeneratively similar tissues in skin and peripheral nerves.

Skin	Peripheral nerves
A. Regenerative tissues	
epidermis	myelin sheath
basement membrane	basement membrane (perineurium, in part only)
B. Nonregenerative tissues	
dermis	endoneurial stroma

keratinocytes and Schwann cells, respectively, irrespective of whether the outcome of the healing process was regeneration or repair. It was concluded that the basement membrane in skin and peripheral nerves is a regenerative tissue.

In clear contrast, the dermis in skin and the endoneurial stroma did not spontaneously regenerate. Following injury, the new tissues that were synthesized at the same anatomical site were quite different from those originally present in the intact organ.

"Regenerative similarity" of two tissues in different organs will be defined as the resemblance in their long-term response to injury, i.e., healing either by regeneration or repair. Since both the epidermis in skin and the myelin sheath in a peripheral nerve fiber are spontaneously regenerated they will be referred to as regeneratively similar tissues. Basement membranes in skin and nerve are both regenerative and will also be classified as being regeneratively similar. Neither the dermis in skin nor the endoneurial stroma in peripheral nerves regenerate; since they share the same response to injury (repair), they will also be referred to as being regeneratively similar. The perineurium appears to be regenerative in part only. These distinctions are summarized in Table 2.1.

2.7 The Tissue Triad

As mentioned earlier, a useful approach for classifying tissues in an organ is to focus on three tissue layers grouped together in all organs: epithelia, basement membrane, and stroma (Martinez-Hernandez, 1988; Burkitt et al., 1993). We will refer to this ubiquitous configuration as the "tissue triad" and will briefly review its structure (Figure 2.7). We will then compare the response to injury in different organs in terms of the tissues in the triad.

Epithelia cover all body surfaces, cavities, and tubes. All epithelia, whether epidermal, endocrine, genitourinary, respiratory, or gastrointestinal, are separated from stroma by continuous basement membranes. An exception is the liver: hepatocytes lack a basement membrane. In the central

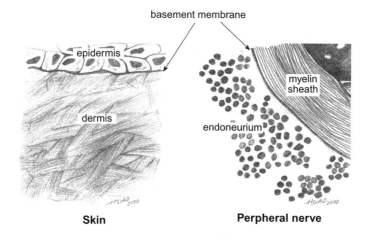

Skin   **Perpheral nerve**

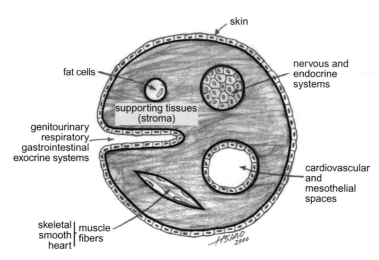

FIGURE 2.7. Basement membranes are strategically located in the organism. *Top*: A triad of tissues present in skin and peripheral nerves, as well as in most organs. The basement membrane is a very thin extracellular matrix (ECM) flanked on one side by epithelia, a cellular and nonvascular tissue that lacks ECM, and by stroma, a supporting tissue comprising primarily ECM and blood vessels, on the other side. *Bottom*: Diagram of anatomic distribution of basement membrane (shown as heavy black line) in its typical location between epithelia and stroma. Epithelia (also called parenchyma) include tissues comprising all epithelial cells in skin, as well as in the genitourinary, respiratory, and gastrointestinal tracts; exocrine glands; endothelial cells of cardiovascular system; mesothelial cells of body cavities; cells comprising central and peripheral nervous systems; muscle fibers; and fat cells. The space occupied by stroma (shaded area) contains bone, cartilage, and their associated cells; also collagen, elastin, and fibroblasts. (Bottom figure from Vracko, 1974.)

nervous system, only blood vessels have a basement membrane. Cardiac, skeletal, and smooth muscle cells are individually surrounded by a basement membrane; however, most other cell types, including fibroblasts, histiocytes, synovial cells, and blood cells, lack a basement membrane (Martinez-Hernandez, 1988). The diagram in Figure 2.7 provides a simplified view of the anatomic distribution of basement membranes in the organism (Vracko, 1974). Following standard treatments (Martinez-Hernandez, 1988; Burkitt et al., 1993), we will use the term "basement membrane" consistently in this volume in preference to "basal lamina" or other terms.

The basement membrane is totally acellular and is not penetrated by blood vessels; for this reason, epithelia generally depend on diffusion of oxygen and metabolites from the stroma. Stroma typically contains blood vessels and other supporting tissues, often referred to as connective tissues; it mediates the exchange of nutrients, metabolites, and waste products between tissues and the circulatory system. Of the three tissues, the epithelia is the only one that does not contain extracellular matrix.

Using the tissue triad as a reference, we can identify certain similarities between two organs. Both in skin and peripheral nerves, the tissue triad includes on either side of the basement membrane a tissue that spontaneously regenerates (epithelia) and one that does not (stroma). Additional similarities between the keratinocytes in skin and Schwann cells in peripheral nerves are expressed in a developmental context (Bunge and Bunge, 1983). Schwann cells that ensheath axons resemble epithelial cells in their ability to form a specialized, totally cellular, tissue that has a foothold on a basement membrane. The latter separates the Schwann cell-axon units from the endoneurial stroma, an extracellular matrix (ECM). In addition, Schwann cells have been shown, like epithelial cells, capable of synthesizing ECM components, including a basement membrane. As keratinocytes are "polarized," exhibiting a side that is attached to the basement membrane and another that is part of the maturation gradient that characterizes the epidermis, so are Schwann cells polarized, with one surface directed toward the basement membrane (abaxonal side) and the other devoted to axonal contact (adaxonal side) (Bunge and Bunge, 1983).

A further interesting similarity exists between migrating epithelial cells in skin, i.e., keratinocytes which have lost their stationary character (phenotype) and are migrating toward the center of a wound, and nonmyelinating Schwann cells in a nerve, i.e., Schwann cells which have left the myelin sheath. In neuron-Schwann cell culture, myelin synthesis and synthesis of basement membrane by Schwann cells were both initiated in the presence of laminin but not in the presence of type IV collagen or heparan sulfate (both are components of the basement membrane) (Eldridge et al., 1989). Nonmyelinating Schwann cells apparently require interaction with a specific component of the basement membrane before changing phenotype and participating in myelin sheath formation (myelination). The data suggest, somewhat speculatively, that, like migrating keratinocytes, which require a "laminin-brake" to initiate keratinization, nonmyelinating Schwann cells may also utilize laminin as a "Schwann-cell brake." Interaction with laminin hypothetically arrests Schwann cell migration and sets the stage for the highly specialized differentiation program at the surface of the axon that leads to formation of the myelin sheath. The similarity between the two cell types is hypothetically observed, therefore, both with the stationary and the migratory phenotypes.

A profound change in response to injury in both organs occurs when the basement membrane is crossed, a span of a mere 100 nm. The stroma in both organs is remarkably nonregenerative. This fact suggests hypothetically that the mechanism for the irreversibility of injury in these two organs is independent of the epithelia and is instead embedded entirely inside the stroma. An alternative hypothesis suggests, however, that rupture of the basement membrane is critical not only because it presumes injury of the stroma, but because it exposes the stroma to the injured epithelia that change their phenotype from stationary to migratory as a result of the interaction with stroma.

We conclude that keratinocytes in skin and Schwann cells in peripheral nerves display a stationary phenotype in the absence of injury and a migratory phenotype following injury. Cells displaying the stationary phenotype in the uninjured organ comprise the highly specialized epithelia (epidermis in skin, myelin sheath in peripheral nerves) that is attached to the basement membrane. The migratory phenotype features mobility which is, however, arrested following synthesis of a key ECM component (probably laminin). The arrested cell proceeds to complete the program of synthesis that leads to formation of the specialized epithelia that characterizes the organ and acquires once more the stationary phenotype.

2.8 Summary

In response to injury, the epidermis in skin and the myelin sheath in peripheral nerves are spontaneously regenerated. In contrast, the dermis in skin and nonneuronal tissues in nerve (such as the endoneurial stroma) are not spontaneously regenerated. In an experimental study of induced regeneration, the experimental injury must, therefore, be extended to delete these nonregenerative tissues thoroughly. It also follows that outcome assays should focus as intensely, preferably even more so, on the evidence for synthesis of these nonregenerative tissues as on synthesis of the epidermis or myelinated axons.

Regenerative similarity characterizes tissues that, even though components of different organs, respond in like manner following injury, i.e., they both heal by regeneration or both heal by repair. The epidermis in skin and the myelin sheath in peripheral nerves spontaneously regenerate and are regeneratively similar. The basement membranes in both organs also regenerate spontaneously. The dermis in skin and certain nonneuronal tissues (e.g., endoneurial stroma) in a peripheral nerve do not spontaneously regenerate; they both heal by repair and are also considered to be regeneratively similar.

Observations made in several organs other than skin and peripheral nerves, such as blood vessels, intestine, gall and urinary bladder, and the kidney, suggest that the response of other organs to injury as well can be fruitfully discussed in terms of the tissue triad, consisting of the basement membrane with epithelia and stroma located on either side.

Injury to skin, to peripheral nerves, and to several other organs is reversible, leading to spontaneous regeneration, whenever it is confined to the epithelia covering or lining the organ and does not injure the basement membrane. Injury becomes irreversible, leading to repair, whenever it penetrates the basement membrane and enters into the stroma closely attached to the basement membrane.

3
Anatomically Well-Defined Defects

3.1 Spatial Parameters of an Experiment in Induced Regeneration

In this chapter we describe the detailed characteristics of the defect in the host organ where the study is conducted. Such an experimental defect should provide the conditions required to reach an unambiguous conclusion about the regenerative activity of a large variety of reactants. The most important questions to answer are: What kind of a space is required for the study? How long should the study last? What is going to be measured at the end? In this chapter we focus on the spatial features of the experiment. The remaining two experimental parameters are discussed in the next chapter.

In Chapter 2 we identified the nonregenerative tissues that must be deleted from the experimental volume. In this chapter we describe an additional three experimental parameters that must be adjusted in order to obtain an anatomically well-defined defect. But why is it so important to adjust all these experimental variables?

An example will provide an idea about what happens when a large variety of apparently similar experimental conditions are used by different investigators. In the field of peripheral nerve regeneration, the adult rat sciatic nerve, completely transected in the femoral region, where it measures about 20 mm in length, is a popular model for a screening study. Investigators ensheathe the stumps inside a silicone tube, and the gap separating the stumps becomes an isolated space in which investigators can insert various candidate reactants to find out whether regeneration will be enhanced. It has been established that, when other factors are kept constant, the probability of a successful reconnection by elongation of axons across the gap depends critically on the gap length (Lundborg et al., 1982a,c; Williams et al., 1987; Yannas et al., 1987a; Madison et al., 1988). Investigators in this field are aware of this effect, discussed in detail in Chapter 6. Accordingly, the gap length has been carefully controlled in each investigation, typically within no more than ±0.5 mm, somewhere inside the experimental range 0 to 20 mm. In the real-life example considered here, a library search yielded some 58 studies published in the period 1982 to 2000, all based on the transected and tubulated rat sciatic nerve. The pool of independent investigators studied as many as 14 different gap lengths. Since the gap length was varied apparently randomly from one investigation to the next, the collective results of these studies were essentially uncontrolled with respect to this critical experimental parameter. Regretfully, these extensive results cannot be pooled together and analyzed to elicit conclusions on the regenerative activity of various reactants. Clearly, there is need to identify experimental conditions such that results from one laboratory can be compared directly with those from another.

3.2 Generation of the Experimental Volume

Using an analogy with synthetic chemistry, we will refer to the defect as a laboratory reactor, kept under carefully controlled conditions. The reactor must accommodate occasionally bulky reagents as well as the product. The reagents may include any combination of cell cultures, cytokine solutions, or matrix components. The product eventually will be separated from residual reagents as well as from the tissues that comprise the reactor itself and will be identified by suitable analytical techniques.

The most direct surgical procedure that can be used to generate space is the controlled deletion of tissues by a surgical instrument (excision). Injuries such as those inflicted by freezing tissue, by abrading skin superficially, and even by simply incising skin, or by crushing nerve, do not generate the desired unoccupied volume. Excision is typically carried out by mechanical instruments, such as a scalpel, fine scissors, or a dermatome. Methods of tissue deletion using other forms of energy, such as a laser, could also accomplish the same end result. A direct comparison of three methods for producing a skin defect, namely, excision with a dermatome, use of a laser to inflict burn injuries, and use of a heated brass template to burn the skin in the swine by direct contact, showed unambiguously that generation of partial-thickness skin wounds by use of burns significantly delayed the reepithelialization process compared to wounds produced by surgical excision (Schaffer et al., 1997). The delay in healing in wounds produced by burns was interpreted as a direct result of thermal tissue destruction extending considerably beyond the boundaries of the nominal defects, which were of equal depth (Schaffer et al., 1997). In another study, a delay in reepithelialization was observed in wounds produced by laser ablation relative to wounds produced by dermatome (Green et al., 1992).

In a comparative study of neuroma formation in the rat sciatic nerve after neurectomy by laser and scalpel it was observed that neuromas were formed in both types of injuries; however, neuromas produced by laser showed a foreign body reaction with multinucleated giant cells surrounding carbonaceous debris that was not present in scalpel neuromas (Fischer et al., 1983). It appears that generation of a defect by laser treatment, at least as currently practiced, introduces certain artifacts that should complicate the interpretation of data relative to a defect produced by excision; for this reason, the discussion below is limited to defects in peripheral nerves produced by excision.

It can be argued that reagents do not require excision of tissue in order to be inserted; for example, a skin incision could be hypothetically considered to be a suitable defect. This approach is countered by two experimental problems. First, there is very little space to insert and retain relatively bulky reactants (e.g., a solution of cytokines) in an incision. Second, there is a problem of measurement of the outcome. At the completion of a wound healing process, and irrespective of whether it leads to regeneration or repair, the mass of newly synthesized tissue is roughly equal to the mass of injured tissue. The mass of new tissue formed following an incision is clearly much smaller than that following an excision. It is usually quite difficult, using current marker methodology, to conclusively demonstrate the presence of a finite mass of newly synthesized tissue in an organ environment replete with nearly identical, uninjured tissue (the "needle in a haystack" analogy). Excision of a substantial organ mass simply leads to a much higher experimental signal-to-noise ratio and a much less ambiguous result. The experimental disadvantage associated with obtaining quantitative data in incisional wounds relative to full-thickness wounds prepared by excision has been pointed out (Beck et al., 1990a,b; Pierce et al., 1991). A choice between incision and excision can change the quality of outcome in important ways; for example, incisional defects in a fetal lamb model healed without scar while excisional defects, produced by deleting a piece of skin, healed with synthesis of scar (Lovvorn et al., 1998).

The nerve trunk has been subjected to crushing with a smooth-tipped forceps (compression injury) or has been injured by excision of part of the cross section of the trunk (hemisection) or else has been completely transected (neurotmesis). Studies of transected nerves have been conducted at different magnitudes of the length separating the two stumps, including a length of approximately zero resulting from transection followed by immediate apposition, either by suturing or by tubulation, of the stumps. Of these methods for injuring nerves, crushing does not lead to generation of an experimental volume; nor does transection followed by apposition of stumps. The other protocols will be considered further below.

3.3 Deletion of Nonregenerative Tissues

The discussion in the preceding chapter leaves little doubt that, in a study of induced regeneration, the tissue that must be excised is precisely the nonregenerative one that the investigator is attempting to synthesize at that site. Clearly, the tissues to be deleted are the dermis in studies of skin and endoneurial stroma, as well as possibly other nonneuronal tissues as well, such as the perineurium, in peripheral nerve studies. In practice, in a skin defect, it may be experimentally awkward to delete the dermis without affecting the epidermis attached to it, or in a nerve defect, to delete the endoneurial stroma without deleting the axons with which they are so intimately arrayed. As a result, the experimental defect is typically prepared by excising both regenerative and nonregenerative tissues that are intimately associated (Figures 3.1 and 3.2). The experimental volume has to be demonstrably free at the beginning of the study from the nonregenerative tissue that one tries to synthesize. The investigator simply wishes to eliminate the possibility that residual nonregenerative tissue inside the defect, dermis in skin or the endoneurium in nerve, will be erroneously concluded to be regenerated tissue, thereby yielding a false positive.

Two examples that illustrate the violation of this rule in studies with skin are the study of partial-thickness wounds and the use of dermal grafts; in either case, the presence of dermis inside the defect introduces a critical ambiguity. The experimental problem that results from the presence of undegraded nonregenerative tissues has been discussed (Carver et al., 1993b). In another study, it has been pointed out that residual epidermal appendages in partial-thickness skin defects participate in healing, and confuse the interpretation of results (Figure 3.1, bottom left) (Carver et al., 1993a). Neither studies based on partial-thickness defects nor those based on application of dermal grafts are reviewed in this volume. Such an omission is clearly unrelated to the clinical value of these procedures.

An example of a defect to be avoided in studies of peripheral nerves is transection of a fraction of the cross section of a peripheral nerve (hemisection), a defect that allows the presence of residual nerve trunk at the site of partial transection (Figure 3.2, top). This configuration is unsuitable for assay by electrophysiological methods, conducted by passing an electrical signal along the regenerate. The amplitude of an electrical signal conducted through the nerve depends on the precise mass of conducting tissue in the cross section; when the latter includes residual conducting tissue, the interpretation of data becomes very difficult. In contrast, the completely transected nerve conducts no signal unless a regenerate is present.

3.4 Anatomical Boundaries

The experimental volume requires boundaries that clearly mark the surfaces separating the experimental volume from the rest of the organism. These boundaries will ensure that the reactants are in intimate contact only with tissues of the reference organ or with the intact external surface of a nearest-neighbor organ. If this condition is observed, the healing process going on inside the experimental volume will be isolated from conflicting

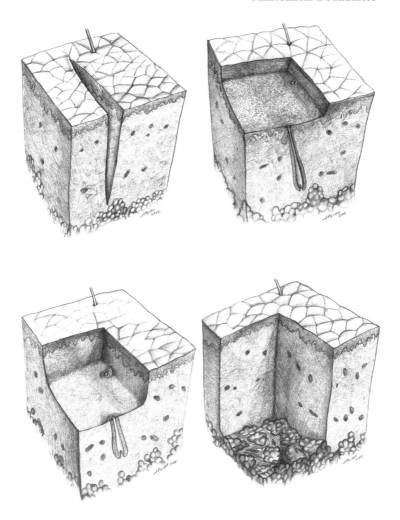

FIGURE 3.1. Selection of an anatomically well-defined defect for study of induced skin regeneration. *Top left:* Incision through entire dermis. *Top right:* Epidermis has been removed but dermis remains intact. *Bottom left:* Partial-thickness skin excision. *Bottom right:* Full-thickness skin excision. Of the four, only the last is an appropriate defect (dermis-free defect).

healing processes going on in another organ, usually due to collateral damage during the surgical procedure. An additional reason for insisting on clear boundaries is the need to reproduce the experimental volume at the same anatomical site from one animal to the next as well as in the laboratories of independent investigators. Reproducibility of the surgical protocol from one defect to the next is a critical factor in an area of research in which statistical power is gained by studying several defects either in the

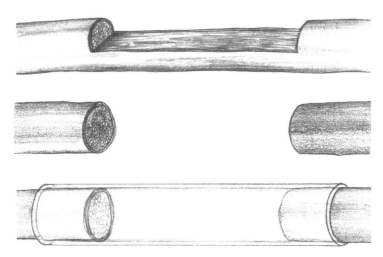

FIGURE 3.2. Three options for a defect suitable for study of induced peripheral nerve regeneration. *Top:* Hemisection. *Middle:* Transection. *Bottom:* Stumps have been inserted into tube (tubulation). A transected nerve is an anatomically well-defined defect; however, the majority of regeneration studies in the peripheral nervous system have been conducted with a tubulated nerve. In these studies, the tube serves as a device for containment of exudate but also contributes strongly to regeneration across the gap and must be controlled appropriately. In a typical experimental configuration, the gap length is about 10 mm (about 10 nerve diameters) while the stumps are inserted about 5 mm inside the tube at each end.

same animal or in different animals. In skin, the organ is bounded distally by the atmosphere (in terrestrial mammals) and proximally by subcutaneous muscle. Exceptionally, in the rabbit ear, the skin is bounded distally to cartilage (Goss and Grimes, 1972; Mustoe et al., 1991). The epineurial sheath (epineurium) of a multifascicular peripheral nerve marks the outside boundary of the nerve trunk; the boundary of a unifascicular trunk is the perineurium while a multifascicular nerve trunk is bounded by the epineurium.

   If the experimental volume is unintentionally extended to include a variable mass of tissues of a nearest-neighbor organ, or to include an uncontrolled mass of the nonregenerative tissue of the reference organ, the variance in the data becomes very high. For example, excision of the complete dermis down to the clearly defined layer of muscle fascia yields distinct surgical end points at either side of the thickness axis (muscle-covering fascia at one end, the atmosphere at the other). In contrast, in a partial-thickness skin wound, the fractionally excised dermal bed lacks a clear anatomical boundary (Figure 3.1, bottom left). The difficulty of reproducing the partial-thickness skin defect from one animal to another relative to that of the full-thickness defect has been discussed (Beck et al., 1990a). This problem has significant consequences in a study of skin wound healing since it has been shown that variation in the depth of the wound significantly affects the healing response, including contraction (Rudolph and Klein, 1973). We conclude that, in an experimental volume without clearly defined anatomical boundaries, the mass of residual nonregenerative tissue can easily rise to the level of a major uncontrolled experimental variable. On the other hand, accidental extension of the boundary to the nearest-neighbor organ inflicts an injury to it, setting off a healing response that confuses the interpretation of healing in the reference organ.

An example of a poorly bounded defect in the nerve is the hemisection, a defect without clear anatomical boundaries and, therefore, difficult to reproduce readily from one animal to the next (Figure 3.2, top). When the progress of regeneration is assayed in a hemisection by electrophysiological measurements, measurements of the amplitude of the signal, the value of which depends on the mass of conducting tissue in the cross section of the nerve trunk, should suffer from excessively high variance.

3.5 Magnitude of Experimental Volume

Having considered the identity of tissues that must be deleted from the experimental volume, we now focus on the quantity of tissue that requires deletion. An important upper limit of defect size is usually set by the need to maintain the experimental animal model as free of morbidity as possible in order to maximize the amount of information obtained in the experiment.

In an effort to identify the lower limit one may well ask if there is a flaw of irreducible size, a critically sized defect (CSD), above which the response to injury changes rather suddenly from spontaneous regeneration to repair. If a limit of that type exists, it makes sense to make sure that it is exceeded in order to study a wound that is as free of spontaneous regeneration as possible. In the literature of skin wound healing, it is known that the kinetics of contraction of a spontaneously healing full-thickness dorsal wound in the rabbit are not significantly affected as the wound area is reduced to 50% or even to 25% of its initial value (Billingham and Russell, 1956). In another study, the kinetics of skin wound contraction in the rat model were not affected when the size of the wound was increased by a factor of 1.8 (Kennedy and Cliff, 1979); nor, in another study, was the incidence of induced regeneration affected by a change in wound size by a factor of 3.6 (Orgill, 1983). If the range in wound size studied is increased considerably more, however, one should expect to observe quantitative effects potentially arising from heterogeneity in skin tethering and perhaps in skin thickness in different anatomical locations. Additional detail on the effect of wound size and related parameters on the healing process is presented in Chapter 4. There is no report, however, in which wound size alone has been shown to affect the qualitative outcome of the healing process in skin (i.e., repair versus regeneration).

In contrast to the skin wound literature, the CSD concept appears persistently in the literature of peripheral nerve regeneration. For example, in the absence of tubulation, it was observed that a 2-mm gap in the mouse sciatic nerve led to a 20 percent frequency of spontaneous reinnervation while a gap of 4 mm or larger consistently yielded a reinnervation frequency of zero (Butí et al., 1996). In the rat sciatic nerve, it was observed that an untubulated 5-mm gap was bridged spontaneously by a nerve trunk (Thomas and Jones, 1967) while a 15-mm gap resulted in no regeneration at all (Lundborg et al., 1982a). The CSD concept also appears in the literature of bone healing. There is evidence that defects in bone that exceed several millimeters in characteristic size do not spontaneously heal to form a mechanically stable, osseous tissue but result, instead, in formation of a "nonunion" (Wornom and Buchman, 1992). For example, an increase in size of the defect in the rat skull (calvaria) from 4 to 8 mm led to a sharp drop in the bone content of the newly formed tissue that bridged the defect (Schmitz et al., 1990).

The evidence presented in the preceding two chapters points quite convincingly to an interruption of the basement membrane, a scale of injury as small as 50 to 100 nm, as a critical defect in several organs. This conclusion was found applicable to several organs, including the lung, kidney, pancreas, and muscle. In the preceding chapter, it was shown that crossing of this threshold was sufficient to dramatically change the response of skin and peripheral nerves to injury. These data clearly show that most organs are strongly heterogeneous in their spontaneous response to injury; certain tissues in an organ spontaneously regenerate while others, in very intimate contact with the regenerative tissues, do not. Small-scale heterogeneity in organ morphology shows up as a response to injury that changes quite suddenly (e.g., from regeneration to repair), with very small changes in location inside the organ.

In spite of such a consideration, the concept of a critically sized defect is nevertheless useful in describing changes in response to injury that depend on size of tissue alone, without reference to a particular location inside the tissue. The CSD appears to become meaningful principally in reference to a tissue structure that is sufficiently homogeneous with respect to response to injury along a characteristic dimension, such as cortical bone or peripheral nerve along the major axis of each organ. In such cases, the scale of the wound must be carefully designed, based on data from control studies, in order to empirically identify the size that needs to be exceeded in order to eliminate, or at least maintain constant throughout the study, the incidence of spontaneous regeneration of tissues of interest. The topic of a critically sized defect in a transected nerve will be discussed in detail in Chapter 6.

3.6 Physical Containment

The discussion about the flow of exudate inside a defect in the preceding chapter led to the conclusion that the exudate is a critical contributor to the healing process, both in skin and peripheral nerves. Following the reasoning presented in Chapter 2, it was concluded that a characteristic of working in vivo is the opportunity to convert the exudate into a physiological tissue or organ. In studies of induced regeneration, the exudate must therefore be contained inside. Unchecked escape of exudate from a defect, or even a significant alteration in concentration of its soluble regulators, significantly modifies the outcome both of a spontaneous and an induced healing process. For example, the rate of epithelialization in dehydrated skin wounds, in which the soluble regulators were presumably unable to exist in a diffusible state, was significantly inhibited and the time for wound closure was increased compared with wounds that were maintained moist by use of an occlusive dressing (Winter, 1972). In another example, a transected nerve that was allowed to lose a significant mass of exudate before the two stumps were sutured directly together had a markedly diminished expectation for regeneration (de Medinacelli et al., 1983; Terzis, 1987).

Additional need for containment arises due to extraneous processes that take place in nearest-neighbor organs. If injured in the process of forming the experimental volume, a nearest-neighbor organ undergoes a healing process that may yield cells and related connective tissues. Extraneous cells invading the experimental volume will likely alter the healing response taking place inside it. A common example of such an extraneous process in a skin is bacterial invasion from the atmosphere, a process that strongly inhibits both regeneration and repair. In a peripheral nerve study, migration of cells into the tubulated gap may lead to synthesis of extraneous connective tissue inside the experimental volume.

All of the interfering processes mentioned above originate in transfer of mass, either into or out of the experimental volume. Accordingly, the desired containment is achieved most simply by a device that acts as a physical barrier. In this idealized approach, the device contributes only a biologically inert presence (i.e., it does not modify the spontaneous healing response). This ideal is reached in studies of skin regeneration, where a film of a synthetic polymer (e.g., a thin silicone sheet) placed on top of the wound (dressing) is used both to contain the exudate and control moisture loss from the defect, while behaving as if it were a reactant with relatively negligible activity to induce or suppress wound contraction. In the study of induced regeneration across a peripheral nerve gap, containment is achieved most simply by a tubular device that encloses the entire gap; however, in this case, a silicone tube turns out to be both a reactant significantly favoring regeneration as well as a device for containment (Fields and Ellisman, 1986a,b). When the silicone tube is replaced by a collagen tube, a large additional increase in regenerative activity takes place (Chamberlain et al., 1998b). These results clearly suggest that the device chosen for containment must be carefully controlled in each case for its own potential activity as a reactant for inducing regeneration.

3.7 The Anatomically Well-Defined Defect

We summarize the discussion in this chapter by describing the appropriate experimental volume as a space generated by excision of tissue, particularly free of nonregenerative tissue, located in an anatomically well-bounded site inside the reference organ, large enough to limit the incidence of significant spontaneous regeneration and contained by a physical barrier that modifies the outcome to a known extent.

Systematic use of all criteria described above leads to description of an anatomically well-defined defect, suitable for study of induced regeneration in the adult. A suitable defect in the study of skin regeneration is the dermis-free defect (full-thickness skin wound) (Figure 3.1, bottom right); in the peripheral nerve, it is the completely transected nerve trunk (Figure 3.2, middle). Although they have occasional uses in the clinical setting, neither the incised or partial-thickness skin wound nor the hemisectioned nerve trunk are appropriate defects for such an experimental study; they will not be discussed further.

In the rest of this volume, the term "defect" will be used in place of "wound" to specifically indicate an anatomically well-defined defect in an organ of choice. Furthermore, in Chapters 5 and 6, in which the data on induced regeneration are presented, the discussion will be limited to studies conducted with anatomically well-defined defects in skin and peripheral nerves. This choice has the effect of sparing the reader from the need to understand and factor in the effect of differences in anatomical details among experimental wounds used by various investigators; instead, attention can be focused almost entirely on the reactants used and the outcome obtained.

3.8 Widely Used Animal Models

We identified above the dermis-free defect and the fully transected nerve trunk as appropriate defects for study of induced regeneration. We now describe the most frequently used animal models for study of these defects.

Several individual efforts toward identification and standardization of an animal species have been made in studies of skin or nerve. Studies on skin have focused on rectangular full-thickness skin defects in rodents since the pioneering studies of Carrel and Hartmann (Carrel and Hartmann, 1916) as well as those of Billingham and Medawar (Billingham and Medawar,

1951, 1955). Other authors, especially since the 1970s, have favored the swine (porcine) model over rodent models as being more similar to the human in skin anatomy and wound-healing behavior (Hartwell, 1955; Rudolph, 1979; Breuing et al., 1992; Carver et al., 1993a; Kangesu et al., 1993a; Orgill et al., 1996). Studies on peripheral nerves have clustered on the use of the rat sciatic nerve (Williams et al., 1983, 1984, 1987; Jenq and Coggeshall, 1985b; Williams and Varon, 1985; Fields and Ellisman, 1986a,b; Madison et al., 1988; Ohbayashi et al., 1996). The mouse sciatic nerve has been a close second in popularity (Henry et al., 1985; Madison et al., 1985; Butí et al., 1996). However, behavioral outcomes can be studied in much greater detail using nonhuman primates (Archibald et al., 1991, 1995).

Porcine skin approximates human skin more closely than does rodent skin in thickness, hair follicle density, and firm attachment to the underlying tissues (Hartwell, 1955; Kangesu et al., 1993a). The latter feature accounts for the significantly smaller extent of wound contraction in full-thickness porcine wounds compared to rodents' wounds of the same depth. In addition, as many as 30 wounds (Breuing et al., 1992) can be studied on the extensive surface of the Yorkshire pig ("mini pig"). Comparisons between the two models, rodent and swine, have been drawn (Hartwell, 1955; Rudolph, 1979; Kangesu et al., 1993a; Compton, 1994; Orgill et al., 1996). A major structural difference between human and porcine skin is lack of eccrine sweat glands and an abundance of apocrine glands (Winter, 1972; Compton, 1994) as well as a paucity of elastin fibers and vasculature in the swine (Kangesu et al., 1993a). Furthermore, unlike human skin, porcine skin has an elastic membrane in the hypodermis and an underlying panniculus carnosus (Kangesu et al., 1993a). The small size and the relatively slow growth rate of the guinea pig, and of other small rodents, make it preferable in long-term studies or in tests of the average response of a population of animals to a wound-healing treatment (Orgill et al., 1996). In contrast, the larger Yorkshire pig offers an advantage in detailed studies of wound fluid composition, especially when wound chambers are used (Eriksson et al., 1989; Breuing et al., 1992). Another advantage of the swine model is the relatively small importance of contraction in wound closure relative to the rodent models, making the swine wound-healing behavior similar in this respect to the human (Rudolph, 1979). Reviews of wound-healing models in different species have been presented (Cohen, 1991; Hayward and Robson, 1991).

The skin wound that is perhaps most free of contraction in the adult mammal is the dermis-free defect in the rabbit ear, discovered during a search for a model that could be used to study epidermal migration in the absence of contraction (Vorontsova and Liosner, 1960; Joseph and Dyson, 1966; Goss, 1992). The rabbit ear model of wound healing has been described in great detail (Mustoe et al., 1991). Briefly, the dermis and epidermis are excised down to the depth of bare cartilage, an avascular tissue, and the perichondrium is also removed; new granulation tissue arises, therefore, entirely from the periphery of the wound rather than from the tissue below, as in dermis-free defects in other anatomical sites (Mustoe et al., 1991).

In studies of peripheral nerves, the most commonly used defect has been the transected, and typically tubulated, nerve. It has been pointed out above that tubulation of the transected nerve has a significant regenerative effect. A limitation of the rat sciatic nerve is the length available for tubulation, about 15 to 20 mm; it suffices to test most tubulated devices but is insufficiently long when the regenerative activity of the device is unusually high (Spilker, 2000). A relationship exists between regenerative activity of reactants in the rat and mouse sciatic nerves, as discussed in Chapter 6. Studies with monkeys have been also conducted; in these cases, nerves of the arm have been studied in order to extract neurological information of a more complex nature that is more closely applicable to the injured human (Archibald et al., 1991, 1995).

3.9 Summary

The experimental space that is most suitable for a study of induced organ regeneration consists of a volume free of nonregenerative tissue that is generated by excising a mass of the organ, marked by unambiguous anatomical boundaries, physically contained to prevent loss of exudate flow and entry of extraneous tissues or bacteria, and large enough to limit the extent of spontaneous regeneration. The full-thickness skin wound (dermis-free defect) in the rodent or the swine and the fully transected peripheral nerve, typically tubulated, in the rat or mouse are widely used defects that satisfy these criteria.

Whereas sheet-like covers for skin defects appear to have negligibly small regenerative activity, tubulation of transected nerves introduces significant activity that must be appropriately controlled. The partial-thickness skin wound and the hemisectioned nerve trunk do not meet the criteria for an anatomically well-defined defect and will not be discussed further.

4
The Defect Closure Rule

4.1 Measuring the Outcome of a Regenerative Process

In the preceding chapter we discussed the experimental space required for a study of induced regeneration. The next questions to settle are: How long should the study last? And, what exactly is one going to measure at the end?

Once more, an example will illustrate the need to pay very close attention to these questions of experimental protocol. A researcher who wishes to find out the consensus on the effectiveness of basic fibroblast growth factor (bFGF or FGF-2) in modifying healing of skin wounds may wish to consult a thoroughly detailed review on the topic (Abraham and Klagsbrun, 1996). The reviewers have concisely summarized the conditions and results of studies of bFGF in animal models of unimpaired healing. One of their tables consists of results from studies published by 24 investigator groups during the period 1984 to 1995. In these studies, observations of the effects of bFGF application (outcome data) were generally made during the period from 3 to 10 days after wounding, with apparently arbitrary choice of timing for the observations made by the investigators. Furthermore, the outcome was reported by use of over 15 different assays, including the following: reepithelialization; kinetics of wound closure by contraction; time for wound closure; neovascularization; content of DNA, or collagen, or glycosaminoglycan (GAG) and fibronectin; fibroplasia; collagenase activity; new granulation tissue formation; wound cellularity; breaking strength; morphology of basement membrane zone; dermal and epidermal thickness of healed wound.

This is certainly an extensive database. Yet, the researcher who wishes to extract even the simplest qualitative cause-effect relations on bFGF activity from this data pool will be frustrated. Wound healing is a very complex process and it is understood that clear-cut relations are quite elusive; nevertheless, much could have been deduced about bFGF activity if the timing of observations and the choice of assay experiments by the investigators were made in a more uniform and controlled format. An attempt at standardization of the timing of observations and choice of assays to measure the outcome of studies in induced regeneration is made in this chapter.

4.2 Mechanism of Healing versus Total Resulting Change

It has been pointed out that biology is intrinsically different from physics in that it is impossible to understand a living organism without knowing its evolutionary history; in contrast, a system in physics can be adequately defined in terms of its current state, without necessary knowledge of the path that led to this state (Mayr, 1996). This distinction faithfully repeats the main theme in Darwin's seminal text. The pioneering author made it clear that he was not interested in adding his own voice to the polyphony of contemporary authors who were advancing their views about the location of a species to others in the architecture of natural order; instead, he was simply interested to establish a model about the pathway that led to the current physiological status of a species (Darwin, 1872).

The argument made above is that a biological process, such as evolution, cannot be understood completely without clear knowledge of its detailed mechanism. Obviously, this argument applies to the healing process of a defect as well. Just as the organism cannot be understood in detail without reference to the forces of natural selection that led to its existence, so it is that the structure of the healed tissue cannot be completely appreciated without knowledge of the mechanism by which healing occurred.

Advances in understanding of the mechanism of spontaneous regeneration (e.g., amphibian limb regeneration) have been reviewed (Hay, 1966; Wallace, 1981; Goss, 1992; Tsonis, 1996; Brockes, 1997); however, the detailed molecular pathways for this process are still not well understood. Even the repair of adult mammalian wounds, a phenomenon that has been observed, in one way or another, at least as early as about 10,000 B.C. (when trepanation of the skull, an operation to remove a portion of the bone, was reportedly performed; see Majno, 1982), can still not be described definitively (Martin, 1997). A 600-page volume of the skin wound repair process (Clark, 1996a) is a very valuable treatise on this topic; yet, the reader who pores over this thesaurus in order to identify an agent for reversing the process of repair is beset with many unanswered basic questions such as: which among the many pathways of the healing process should be tampered with in order to influence the outcome in the direction of regeneration? Should the investigator focus on the soluble regulators (cytokines and growth factors) that appear to control cell function during the inflammatory response? Or is it more expedient to focus on description of cell surface receptors for cell-matrix interactions? And, since these processes are closely coupled, what is the best place to start in an effort to describe the entire system?

As it happens, a tremendous amount of information becomes available when each of a series of related biological processes have been described consistently by just two clear snapshots, both taken at the same time for each process. Very simply, description of a process by two snapshots separates the problem of measuring the total extent of change from that of understanding just how the change occurred in detail. A measure of the total change is a simple measure of the effect resulting from a known cause. Once the total change has been recorded consistently in a large variety of investigations, by reporting just two observations made at the same time with each investigation, an empirical database of cause-effect relationships between the nature of reactant used and the outcome of the healing process can be constructed. This information can now be used empirically to modify the outcome, either regeneration or repair, even without knowing anything about the basic mechanism.

There is no doubt that discussions of mechanism inspire and motivate investigators. Nevertheless, and while the specific mechanism by which regeneration is induced is being debated, there is need for reliable quantitative relationships between specific manipulations of the healing process of a defect and the resulting changes in outcome. Such empirical data are required quite beyond the need for development of improved clinical treatments of organ healing: If solidly supported by the evidence, these cause-effect relationships are the reliable benchmarks that will be used to measure the relative value of competing hypothetical mechanisms of regeneration. Simply put, the correct mechanistic pathway starts at the time of injury but then has to go through the well-defined final state that has been empirically established.

In this volume, the empirical data that describe the effect of several reactants on the final state of a defect are presented first (Chapters 5 through 8); the evidence supporting a hypothetical mechanism for the activity of selected reactants is presented later (Chapters 9 and 10). Since the empirical data included in the discussion are based exclusively on investigations in which anatomically well-defined defects were employed, it is relatively easy to reach conclusions about which reactant supports regeneration and which does not. These empirical cause-effect relations eventually become the focus of a detailed inquiry on mechanism.

4.3 Initial and Final States of a Healing Process

Before we can start constructing a reliable database of cause-effect relationships about healing processes in various defects, we need to define the time at which the hypothetically causative agent will be introduced as well as the time at which its effect will be determined. In other words, we need to isolate the healing process inside a reasonable time segment. The two snapshots that describe the extent of change will be consistently taken at the beginning and end of this segment.

Investigators enjoy great freedom in selecting the temporal conditions of their experiments. Usually, this choice follows their hypotheses of what is going on in the process. Often, a hypothesis suggests that a particular event among the many that comprise the entire healing process is the critical one. If the preselected event takes place early during healing, the investigation focuses the relevant assays on that early time interval while the rest of the process is typically neglected. Another investigation may focus on a much later time interval. Although both sets of data, those that were recorded early and those observed much later, are part of a single healing process that takes place inside a nominally identical experimental volume, they are spaced in time so far apart that they reflect events taking place inside two defects that are biologically distinct. The two studies have nominally focused on the same healing process; yet, the two investigators have been observing two quite different phenomena. Inevitably, the results of assays in these two investigations are largely unrelated to each other.

It can be seen that a series of such studies, each focusing on a different temporal segment of the strongly time-dependent healing process, can result in an almost random collection of data, collectively signifying very little to anybody. In our search for cause-effect relations based on independent data from several laboratories, or in the design of new experiments, we wish to focus on data that have been collected inside a time period that has been employed consistently by a large number of investigators.

This reasoning leads to the concept of an "initial" and a "final" state of the healing process in a defect. A state is described by the information contained in each of the snapshots of the example used above. Obviously, these are not equilibrium or stationary states in the sense used in thermodynamics since a great deal of change takes place in the biological system long after each snapshot has been taken.

The initial state is defined as the recently generated defect, described by the recent interruption in structural continuity of one or more tissues. This event coincides with the beginning of loss of tissue fluid (exudate), as well as general loss of physiological homeostatic control by the organ.

The final state will be taken to coincide with recent closure of the defect. Closure corresponds to definitive stemming of the flow of tissue fluid and reestablishment of substantial homeostatic control at the injured site. With few exceptions, such as the rupture of a major blood vessel or the healing of a skin defect in a diabetic patient, defects in organs close spontaneously both in regeneration and repair processes. The initial and final states of healing in any organ, selected here, are therefore experimentally well-defined, since they can be described unambiguously in terms of appropriate anatomical structures and physiological functions of the reference organ.

A well-known defect in skin can be used to simply illustrate these two states in the healing process. The open skin defect allows rapid escape of tissue fluid, leading to potential water and electrolyte imbalances in the organism, while also permitting ready access of infectious organisms to the interior of the organism, as well as causing other disturbances (Woodley, 1989). Of these, the potential for massive infection appears to represent the clearest threat to survival of the organism (Greenhalgh et al., 1990; Boykin and Molnar, 1992; Goss, 1992; Mast, 1992; Rudolph et al., 1992). This fact becomes urgently clear in the well-studied case of a person who has sustained a massive burn, losing in the process a large fraction of total skin mass and ending up with a very deep skin defect over a large area of the body. If the defect is untreated, the patient suffers rapid, substantial loss of water and electrolytes that leads to loss of blood volume, severe acceleration of the metabolic rate, and, eventually, shock; furthermore, the extensive trauma induces considerable depression of immune function, which places the patient at risk for life-threatening sepsis (Burke et al., 1974; Boykin and Molnar, 1992). These risks to survival of the organism are eliminated, and vital homeostatic control is restored, after the defect has been closed either by spontaneous healing or by grafting (Peacock, 1984). This description is consistent with the strong emphasis placed by independent investigators on the rate of reepithelialization of a wound, as well as on the time to closure by reepithelialization, a process which stems loss of fluids and protects against bacterial invasion (Brown et al., 1986; Greenhalgh et al., 1990; Nanney et al., 1990; Tsuboi and Rifkin, 1990; Mustoe et al., 1991; Pierce et al., 1992; Staiano-Coico et al., 1993). Wound closure in skin is usually identified with little ambiguity either noninvasively, by gross observation of the disappearance of light-reflecting granulation tissue and its replacement by a nonreflecting confluent epithelialized surface (Greenhalgh et al., 1990), by a relatively sudden drop in flow of exudate or in moisture permeability measured by evaporimetry (Yannas and Burke, 1980; Orgill, 1983), or by invasive procedures, such as histological observation of the appearance of a continuous epidermis (Staiano-Coico et al., 1993).

Injured peripheral nerves also lose tissue fluid and stray significantly from their state of physiological homeostasis. A transected peripheral nerve continuously loses a very large volume of fluid exudate from both stumps (Williams and Varon, 1985). The process is arrested when a tissue capsule, associated with neuroma, is spontaneously formed around each stump, stemming the flow of exudate from the nerve stumps (Weiss, 1944; Wall and Gutnick, 1974; Chamberlain et al., 1998b). Significant restoration of the homeostatic control characteristic of an intact peripheral nerve returns after closure of the defect by neuroma formation, however, there is no restoration of physiological electrical excitability in axons inside the neuroma (Wall and Gutnick, 1974). Both in skin and peripheral nerves defect closure partly restores organ homeostasis, even though it does not necessarily restore physiological function.

Far from being systems at static equilibrium, the freshly opened and the freshly closed defect in a living organism are both time-dependent states. Immediately after being opened, a defect immediately undergoes a host of changes (e.g., bleeding, platelet degranulation, flow of exudate, and so on). In spite of such complexity, however, the investigator knows with great accuracy the time at which an experimental injury has been inflicted. Neither is the closed defect an anatomically static system. Early reports (Carrel and Hartmann, 1916; Clark, 1919), as well as more recent accounts, have described extensive tissue modifications that continue for a long time after closure (scar "remodeling") (Peacock and Van Winkle, 1976; Mast, 1992). Such continuing activity partly reflects continuing contraction of granulation tissue underneath the epidermis, long after closure of the skin defect by epidermal confluence had been completed (see Chapter 9 for detailed discussion). Severe defects in peripheral nerves also continue to undergo structural and functional changes over at least one to two years after the defect has closed (Le Beau et al., 1988; Archibald et al., 1991, 1995; Chamberlain et al., 1998b).

In addition to the remodeling processes in scar or in a regenerate, another process that is going on before injury has been inflicted as well as continuing after a defect has closed is the normal development of the organism. The effect of development on the outcome of a healing process becomes evident in two quite different ways. First, development modifies the outcome of the healing process quantitatively; for example, a change in the area of a defect during healing generally reflects both the effect of contraction (area decrease) as well as that of growth of the organism (area increase). In this case, raw data showing, for example, a net decrease in area with time must be corrected for growth before they can be used to describe the kinetics of contraction. Second, the outcome of healing of a defect is profoundly affected by the developmental stage of an organism at the time of injury, reflected in the typically sharp difference between the outcomes of fetal and adult healing in the same species. This important developmental transition from fetal to adult healing, discussed later in this chapter, affects the data qualitatively and becomes a major experimental variable in its own right rather than being a simple quantitative correction, as with simple growth data.

Remodeling and development alter, each in its own way, the raw data that describe the healing process. With the exception of the major developmental transition in healing behavior discussed above, however, these alterations are typically small and do not affect the outcome of the healing process qualitatively (i.e., repair vs. regeneration). The occurrence of scar remodeling after a skin defect has closed does not change the fact that scar, rather than physiological skin, has formed as a result of the injury. Whether these general rules apply in a given situation needs to be carefully examined. An example is the relation between the time constant (a reciprocal measure of rate) for metamorphosis from a larva (tadpole) to a young adult frog, t_{meta}, a transition analogous to that from fetal to adult healing, and the time constant for healing of a full-thickness skin defect, t_{heal}, in the same species (Yannas et al., 1996):

$$t_{\text{meta}}/t_{\text{heal}} = 25$$

In this example, the large value of the ratio of time constants suggests that the two processes (i.e., the developmental transition in healing outcome and the healing process itself) probably unfold separately and can likely be studied largely independently of each other. In contrast, a healing process that hypothetically straddles across the developmental transition will probably reflect two or more different responses depending on whether the injury was inflicted just before, during or just after the transition.

4.4 Configuration of the Final State

Having isolated the healing process within a time segment, extending from injury to defect closure, we now wish to select a suitable method for studying its progress during that period.

The strikingly time-dependent nature of the healing process immediately suggests a study of its kinetics. Most investigators have taken this approach in devising a large number of assays that describe the unfolding of the healing process. Examples of such assays include measurement of the rate of various processes expressed in terms of morphological changes, such as reepithelialization, granulation tissue formation, capillary formation, basement membrane formation, collagen synthesis, glycosaminoglycan synthesis, upregulation of a given growth factor receptor, and so on. Other investigators have considered several assays of physiological function.

Although continuous kinetic data are very valuable, a few isolated observations frequently are not because they are typically reported at just two or three time points randomly selected by independent investigators. The proliferation of unrelated observations is compounded by the practice of employing a large number of assays, as discussed above. The result is that overlap of assay results observed at the same time during the healing process is a rare event in studies conducted in different laboratories. It is not surprising that neither confirmation nor rejection of hypotheses occurs frequently in studies of healing.

Information obtained at the time of closure is particularly valuable compared with any other single time point during healing. Such information is obtained at a relatively well-defined time point, characterized by a sharp drop in the velocity of the healing process, that can be readily identified experimentally (e.g., rapid decrease in moisture evaporation rate following completion of reepithelialization). A useful measure of the extent of total change during healing can then be expressed in terms of the configuration of the final state (i.e., the relative incidence of regeneration or repair) using a small number of variables. In the absence of continuous kinetic data describing the healing process, a comparison of the configuration of the final and the initial states could become a valuable benchmark. Since the initial state is identical when investigators study anatomically well-defined defects, the configuration of the final state suffices to measure the effectiveness of a reactant to induce regeneration.

4.5 Three Modes of Defect Closure in Organs

A survey of the literature of skin wound healing shows that no more than three processes (modes) are used to close a defect: contraction of the dermal edges of the defect, formation of epithelialized scar, and regeneration (for example, see Martinez-Hernandez, 1988). The evidence shows that these three modes of closure are also responsible for closure of severe nerve defects, such as transection, with the exception that the second mode is described in studies of peripheral nerves as a neuroma rather than epithelialized scar, as in skin. Additional, but much less extensive, evidence with other organs throughout the anatomy of the adult, similar so that presented in Chapter 1, generally supports the conclusion that no mode of defect closure other them contraction, scar formation and regeneration is observed throughout the anatomy during healing of injuries.

4.5.1 Closure of Defects in Organs by Contraction

Contraction has been historically defined in extensive studies of skin wounds. Contraction of defects in other organs also has been observed but has not been studied systematically, as in skin.

Contraction of a skin defect is the reduction in defect surface area by inward (centripetal) movement of skin from the margins of the defect (perilesional skin) (Figure 4.1). This process originates in fibroblasts inside the defect and largely comprises the sliding, and secondarily stretching, of perilesional skin over the open defect (Peacock and Van Winkle, 1976; Rudolph et al., 1992). A detailed description of the hypothetical mechanism of contraction during spontaneous healing is presented in Chapter 9. Even though it has been observed that the surface area of the skin defect decreases by processes which intrinsically differ from the model of contraction (Troxel, 1994; Gross et al., 1995), the term has strong historical value and will be retained throughout this volume.

Authors have generally assumed that the difference in extent of contraction of skin defects in different species reflects variation in skin mobility, itself the result of a difference in firmness of attachment of the skin to the subdermal tissues (tethering). For example, the skin of rodents has been described as a "fully mobile integument" (Billingham and Medawar, 1951, 1955). Some authors have additionally emphasized the stiffness of the fascia that is attached to major musculature underneath skin (Peacock and Van Winkle, 1976). In the sheep (Horne et al., 1992), the rabbit, as well as in rodents (Billingham and Medawar, 1951, 1955), the skin is attached rela-

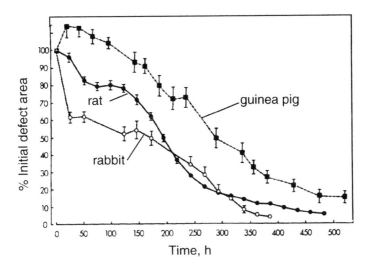

FIGURE 4.1. Contraction kinetics of the dermis-free defect observed with three rodent models. Data for the guinea pig, rat, and mouse are shown. (From Kennedy and Cliff, 1979.)

tively loosely to the *panniculus carnosus*, a layer of involuntary muscle underneath the dermis. In contrast, in the rabbit ear, the dermis is very firmly attached to a relatively rigid sheet of cartilage and is considered to be essentially immobile (Joseph and Dyson, 1966; Goss and Grimes, 1972).

The quantitative importance of contraction as a mode of defect closure has been established in several species by use of kinetic studies (Figures 4.2 and 4.3). In species with mobile skin, such as the rabbit and several rodents, closure takes place almost entirely by movement of perilesional skin until its edges are opposed and separated by a thin layer of scar ("stellate" scar) (Billingham and Medawar, 1951, 1955) (Figure 4.2, left). In the human, and to some extent in the swine, there is only modest movement of perilesional skin; full closure of the defect therefore depends to a large extent on formation of an epithelialized scar layer over the newly synthesized connective tissue (granulation tissue) (Figure 4.2, right) (Peacock and Van Winkle, 1976; Hayward and Robson, 1991). In the rabbit ear, contraction is prevented and defect closure takes place entirely by regeneration (Joseph and Dyson, 1966; Grimes and Goss, 1972). Kinetic data show clear differences in the asymptotic extent to which contraction closes up a defect in different species (Figure 4.3).

The detailed study of contraction of nerve stumps has seriously lagged behind similar studies in skin defects. However, contraction of transected peripheral nerves has been reported on several occasions. In earlier studies, it was observed that the distal nerve stump eventually shrunk. It was hypothesized that the constricted distal stump would lack the cross-

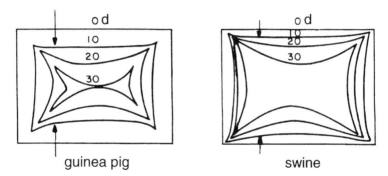

FIGURE 4.2. Closure of dermis-free defects mostly or partly by contraction in various species. *Left*: Guinea pig. *Right*: Swine. Data in the two diagrams represent the change in defect area as viewed directly on the indicated day after excision. The defect area decreases much more rapidly in the guinea pig; it also approaches a lower asymptotic level, indicative of a larger extent of contraction in this species. (Guinea pig data from Billingham and Reynolds, 1952; swine data from Rudolph, 1979.)

sectional area required for elongation into it of axons from the proximal stump (Holmes and Young, 1942; Weiss, 1944; Weiss and Taylor, 1944a). In another study, reduction of the cross-sectional area of the distal nerve trunk by 30 to 50% was reported and was found to be less significant than fascicular contraction, which reached 50 to 60%; also, the cross-sectional area of the proximal stump was observed to be about twice as large as that of the distal stump (Sunderland, 1990).

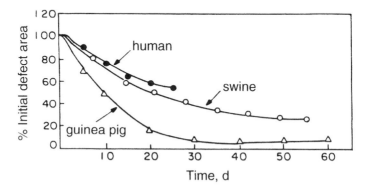

FIGURE 4.3. Extent of defect closure by contraction. Contraction kinetics for dermis-free defects in the human (from Ramirez et al., 1969), swine (Rudolph, 1979), and guinea pig (Yannas, 1981). The percentage of initial defect area eventually closed by contraction was highest in the guinea pig and lowest in the human. The remainder closed by formation of epithelialized scar.

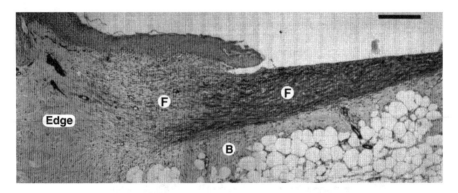

FIGURE 4.4. Contractile cells (F) extend across the entire area of the dermis-free defect in the guinea pig. Day 9 postinjury. Contractile cells were stained with a monoclonal antibody to α-smooth muscle actin, characteristic of myofibroblasts. In the photo, the defect edge (Edge) intersects the base (B) of the defect. Bar: 200 μm. (From Troxel, 1994.)

Contractile fibroblasts (myofibroblasts) have been credited with generation of most of the contractile forces in skin wounds (Gabbiani et al., 1971; Rudolph, 1979; Rudolph et al., 1992; Gabbiani, 1998) (Figure 4.4) and have been also observed in transected peripheral nerve stumps. Identification of myofibroblasts in a transected nerve was made in early studies, although the role of the cells in the healing process was not investigated (Badalamente et al., 1985). The hypothetical mechanism by which contractile cells induce closure of skin and peripheral nerve defects is described in Chapters 9 and 10.

Contractile cells have been also identified in the uninjured perineurium (Ross and Reith, 1969). Spontaneous closure (capping) of each of the two nerve stumps by a thick tissue capsule, about 15 to 20 cell layers in thickness, comprising primarily connective tissue and covered with elongated cells that were fibroblast-like in appearance, was observed (Chamberlain, 1998; Chamberlain et al., 1998a, 2000a). The cells forming the capsule around each stump stained for α-smooth muscle actin, a positive identification of myofibroblasts (Figure 4.5), as well as displaying densely bundled actin microfilaments at the perimeter of the highly elongated cells. The thickness of the outer layer (capsule) was observed to become diminished to a single layer of myofibroblasts when the silicone tube was exchanged with a collagen tube (Chamberlain et al., 2000a). Longitudinal sections of nerves regenerated through silicone tubes showed thick bundles of contractile cells in the regions where the proximal and distal stumps were originally formed by transection (Figure 4.6).

The identification of myofibroblasts in healing nerve defects (Chamberlain et al., 1998a, 2000a) provided an interpretation for persistent indepen-

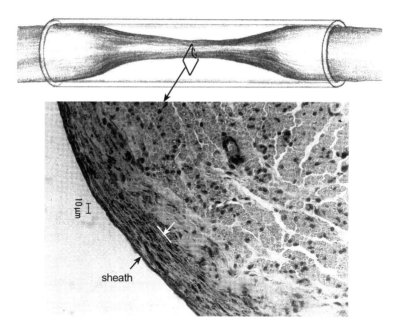

FIGURE 4.5. Contractile cells ensheath the entire perimeter of the nerve trunk regenerated across a gap bridged with a silicone tube. *Top*: Schematic diagram showing the cable that forms across the tubulated gap. *Bottom*: Cross-sectional view of regenerated trunk at the gap center at 60 d. The sheath of contractile cells (arrows), about 50 μm thick, comprised 15 to 20 layers of cells that stained with a monoclonal antibody to α-smooth muscle actin (myofibroblasts). *Bar*: 10 μm. (Copyright 2000. Wiley-Liss, Inc. From Chamberlain et al., 2000a. Connective tissue response to tubular implants for peripheral nerve regeneration: The role of myofibroblasts. *Journal of Comparative Neurology* 417:415–430. Reprinted with permission of Wiley-Liss, Inc., a subsidiary of John Wiley & Sons, Inc.)

dent reports of concentric sheaths of fibroblast-like cells around the fibrin cable that forms spontaneously inside the tubulated gap of the rat sciatic nerve (Lundborg et al., 1982a; Williams et al., 1983; Jenq and Coggeshall, 1985a,b; Williams and Varon, 1985; Hurtado et al., 1987; Madison et al., 1988; Kljavin and Madison, 1991). It now appears that these cell structures should be designated as myofibroblasts and their role in defect healing in the peripheral nervous system assessed accordingly. Hypotheses describing the mechanism of nerve stump closure by contractile cells are described in Chapters 9 and 10.

Defect contraction has been frequently reported following injury of several organs other than skin and peripheral nerves. It has been occasionally reported as reduction in length of a slender organ (shortening), the constriction of a hollow organ (stricture), or the warping of a thin sheet-like organ. Examples of organ deformation following trauma in experimental animal models are the observation of contraction of the ureter following resection of a portion of the circumference (Oppenheimer and Hinman,

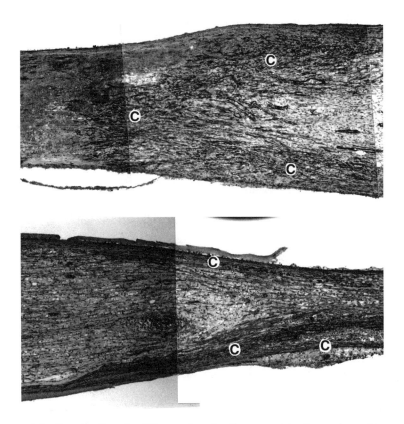

FIGURE 4.6. Contractile cells (C) are abundantly present in the region of transection of the peripheral nerve at 11 d and have been identified by immunostaining for
α-smooth muscle actin (myofibroblasts). They appear as bundles of long fibers
oriented along the axis of the regenerate. The photos show segments of a nerve
trunk regenerated across a 10-mm gap in the rat sciatic nerve that was bridged with
a silicone tube. The diameter of the intact nerve is about 1 mm. *Top*: Near location
of original proximal stump. *Bottom*: Near original distal stump. (Yannas, unpublished data.)

1955; Kiviat et al., 1973) and the contraction of the transected ligament
(Dahners et al., 1986; Wilson and Dahners, 1988). In humans, the stricture
of the urethra that follows trauma (Rudolph et al., 1992), narrowing of
the esophagus (esophageal stenosis) after swallowing a corrosive agent
(Peacock, 1984), and contraction of a defect in the upper eyelid (ectropion),
have been attributed to the same mechanism that leads to closure of skin
defects. Biologically inert implants, inserted inside an organ in a space that
has been prepared by tissue excision, are typically covered by a capsule of
contractile tissue; examples are silicone breast implants and cardiac pacemakers (Rudolph et al., 1992). The detailed structure of the contractile
capsule surrounding breast implants has been described in great detail

(Rudolph et al., 1978; Ginsbach et al., 1979; Brodsky and Ramshaw, 1994; Tarpila et al., 1997).

Furthermore, contraction has been reported not only in defects resulting from acute injury but also as a result of a disease process that leads to formation of chronic lesions. Among the examples in humans are the narrowing and sometimes complete obstruction of the duodenum following repeated ulceration (Billingham and Russell, 1956) and the shrinking of heart valves in rheumatic heart disease (Peacock, 1984; Rudolph et al., 1992). A striking decrease in liver size, attributed to contraction, is a feature of terminal cases of liver cirrhosis (Rudolph et al., 1979a; Rudolph, 1980; Nimni, 1983).

4.5.2 Measurement of Contraction in Skin and Nerve Defects

Quantitative studies of contraction of skin defects owe much to the methods devised by Spallanzani (Carrel and Hartmann, 1916). In these early studies the methods of tattooing spots at the edges of the defect with India ink and of planimetry to measure defect area, as well as the mathematical representation of the kinetics of contraction, had already been in place. The most important changes made in later studies included the systematic practice of measuring the defect area lying between the dermal edges rather than the edge of advancing epithelium (Billingham and Medawar, 1955), the use of tattooed grids (rather than isolated spots) around contracting defects (Straile, 1959; Alvarez et al., 1987) in order to locate the original defect perimeter without ambiguity, and the use of computerized morphometric image analysis of standardized photographic slides of the defect (Staiano-Coico et al., 1993).

There is evidence, obtained with the rabbit, rat, and guinea pig models, that defect size and the sex of the animal have no effect on contraction kinetics (Carrel and Hartmann, 1916; Billingham and Russell, 1956; Peacock and Van Winkle, 1976; Kennedy and Cliff, 1979). Excessive reliance on the assumed independence of contraction from defect size should, however, be guarded against; a defect large enough to extend to a quite different anatomical location inside its perimeter would be expected to show a substantially different rate, and possibly major direction, of contraction. For example, in a mid-dorsal full-thickness skin defect in the rat, the lateral edges moved closer together than the anterior and posterior edges; in contrast, in a flank wound, the anterior and posterior edges moved closer than the lateral edges, suggesting that the contraction pattern was not uniform over the entire anatomy (Kennedy and Cliff, 1979). Controversial data have been obtained relating the effect of wound shape on contraction rate. Although there is early evidence that circular wounds contract slower than rectangular wounds in the rabbit (Billingham and Russell, 1956) and in the rat (Cuthbertson, 1959), a later study showed no significant difference between the kinetics of contraction of rectangular and of circular wounds in the rat (Kennedy and Cliff, 1979).

Measurements of the extent of defect closure by contraction depend on direct observation of the surface of the defect rather than of tissues underneath. This description omits reference to the total mass of scar formed inside the volume of the defect that consists of two parts, visible and underlying scar. In the process of contraction, skin slides over newly synthesized connective tissue (granulation tissue) inside the defect. When the contraction process has stopped, the sliding skin has covered the underlying mass of granulation tissue, which eventually becomes modified to underlying scar. Histological observations on rodents have revealed the presence of a significant volume of scar, lying underneath the mobile contracted integument and presenting itself at the surface of the defect only as a thin stellate scar (Figure 4.2, left) (Luccioli et al., 1964; Peacock and Van Winkle, 1976; Horne et al., 1992; Troxel, 1994).

A transected peripheral nerve that has not been tubulated heals with contraction and neuroma formation provided that the stumps have been separated by a few mm immediately after transection. The evidence has suggested that the transected cross section of the proximal nerve stump closes by contraction to an extent of about 95% of initial cross section area of the uninjured nerve; the remainder of the cross-section area of the stump was occupied by very dense connective tissue that was quite different from supporting tissues in uninjured nerve and was classified as neural scar (Chamberlain et al., 2000a). When the nerve was tubulated, the extent of contraction changed dramatically. For example, when the stumps had been inserted in a silicone tube and were separated by a 10-mm gap, the area of the nerve trunk contracted only to about 47% of the original cross section area. The remainder 53% had closed by contraction, a much smaller value than that observed when the transected nerve had not been tubulated. Much lower values of extent of contraction, close to 0%, were observed when collagen tubes were used.

4.5.3 Closure by Epithelialized Scar (Skin) and by Neuroma (Nerve)

In the adult mammal, the injured dermis does not spontaneously regenerate; scar forms instead (Billingham and Medawar, 1955; Ross and Benditt, 1961; Dunphy and Van Winkle, 1968; Ross and Odland, 1968; Peacock, 1971, 1984; Madden, 1972; Boykin and Molnar, 1992; Goss, 1992). Provided that the depth of the injury extends well into the dermis, a layer of granulation tissue forms over the entire defect area. Eventually, the defect area that has not been closed by contraction becomes epithelialized by migration of keratinocyte sheets from the edges toward the interior of the defect and over the granulation tissue layer. The result is closure of the skin defect by epithelialized scar. In contrast with rodents, where contraction provides almost all of the closure, in the human, as much as roughly one-half of the original defect area closes by formation of epithelialized scar. Skin appendages, such as hair follicles, sweat glands, and sebaceous glands, also do not spontaneously regenerate in the adult (Martin, 1997).

Scar is not dermis in a variety of ways. The quantitative distinction between the two can, in principle, be made by several methods. In mechanical tests, scar is both less extensible than dermis and fractures at a lower tensile stress (Dunn et al., 1985). Morphologically, the normal dermo-epidermal junction in scar appears abnormally smooth, typically lacking the complex rete ridge configuration of normal skin (Figure 2.2) (Kiistala, 1972). The connective tissue layer of scar contains no hair follicles or sebaceous or sweat glands. Optical microscopic views of scar typically show collagen fibers preferentially aligned in the plane of the epidermis, packed more tightly and possessing an average diameter that is smaller than that of intact dermis. Scanning electron microscopic views have confirmed the planarity of orientation of collagen fibers in scar (Hunter and Finlay, 1976; Knapp et al., 1977). In contrast to scar, the dermis has been described as a sheet of collagen fibers aligned almost randomly; however, there is evidence of a modest amount of orientation of the axes of dermal collagen fibers in the plane of the epidermis (Gibson et al., 1965; Dawber and Shuster, 1971; Brown, 1972; Holbrook et al., 1982; Ferdman and Yannas, 1993). Differences in chemical composition between normal dermis and scar also have been demonstrated; for example, type III collagen makes up 20% of collagen fibers in the dermis, 30% in granulation tissue, and 10% in scar (Bailey et al., 1975). No difference was observed between the axial periodicity of collagen fibrils, $D = 65.5 \pm 0.15\,nm$, in a granuloma (i.e., essentially scar tissue forming around an implant) and the value of D in normal skin (Brodsky and Ramshaw, 1994).

Laser light scattering has been used to provide a quantitative measure of the degree of orientation of collagen fibers in dermis (Kronick and Buechler, 1986) as well as in scar (Ferdman and Yannas, 1986, 1987, 1993; Ferdman, 1987). In this method, laser light is passed through a histological tissue section and the characteristics of the resulting scattering pattern depend on both the orientation and the average diameter of the collagen fibers (Figure 4.7). Analysis of the azimuthal intensity distribution of scattered light yields numerical average values of the degree of fiber alignment in the plane of the epidermis, expressed in terms of an orientation index, S, a simple trigonometric function that varies between 0 for randomly oriented fibers and 1 for a perfectly aligned arrangement. The average diameter of the collagen fibers is calculated from the scattering angle at which the intensity reaches its first minimum (Ferdman and Yannas, 1986, 1993; Ferdman, 1987). The results of a light-scattering study, in which data from guinea pig scar were compared with intact skin adjacent to it, are presented in Table 4.1. The data show the presence of a small amount of orientation in sections of intact dermis cut either parallel to or perpendicular to the major contraction direction, which is perpendicular to the long axis of the scar in Figure 4.7 (top). In contrast, fibers in scar are highly, though not perfectly, oriented in the plane in sections cut parallel to the direction of contraction, though not perpendicular to it. Data in Table 4.1 also show that the collagen fibers in intact dermis are thicker than those in scar.

Methods for quantitative differentiation between dermis and scar can, in principle, also be based on the noncollagenous components of these tissues. The proteoglycan content in scar differs significantly from that in the dermis, amounting, in essence, to a 16% higher content of dermatan sulfate and a 35% lower content of hyaluronic acid in scar (Swann et al., 1988; Garg et al., 1989, 1990, 2000). Scar also differs from dermis in the size of the glycosaminoglycan (GAG) side chains, the degree and location of sulfation of GAGs, the size of the protein core of the proteoglycans, the degree of D-glucuronic acid to L-iduronic acid epimerization and the ratio of biglycan to decorin (Garg et al., 2000). The presence of elastin fibers has been confirmed in skin scars in the human and in rodents (Davidson et al., 1992); however, scar from skin wounds has been reported to contain a smaller proportion of elastic fibers (elastin) than in normal dermis (Peacock and Van Winkle, 1976). The paucity of elastic fibers and the orientation of collagen fibers preferentially along lines of tension during wound healing have been cited as the structural basis for the observation that scar is stiffer (less extensible) than skin adjacent to it (Peacock and Van Winkle, 1976).

Neuroma formation characterizes the spontaneous closure of stumps generated by transecting a peripheral nerve. Closure of a stump by capping prevents the reconnection of the severed axons and leads to total loss of electrophysiological function along the transected nerve. However, capping of stumps stems the flow of exudate and restores much of the homeostatic balance that was lost after transection. As with the spontaneous healing of a skin defect that leads to formation of mechanically inferior dermal scar, the price of spontaneous healing of a nerve wound is loss of specialized organ function.

The tissue mass that caps the proximal nerve stump at the end of the healing process comprises, as described in Chapter 2, disorganized connective tissue that is poorly vascularized and interspersed with Schwann cells together with a large number of tangled axons that have very small diameters and are mostly unmyelinated (Cajal, 1928; Denny-Brown, 1946; Wall and Gutnick, 1974; Olsson, 1990; Sunderland, 1990; Zochodne and Nguyen, 1997; Chamberlain et al., 2000a). A morphological report of neuroma structure has shown that the transected cross section of the proximal stump closed to an extent of about 5% by formation of very dense connective tissue that was morphologically quite different from the nonneuronal tissues in uninjured nerve (Chamberlain, 1998; Chamberlain et al., 2000a). Histological study of the connective tissue in the proximal neuroma showed that it consisted of dense and fibrous collagenous tissue, somewhat

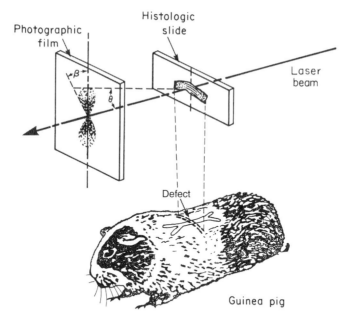

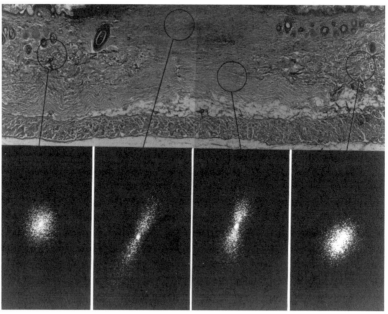

FIGURE 4.7. Quantitative distinction between scar and physiological dermis using laser light scattering from tissue sections. *Top*: The laser beam passes through a histologic tissue section, shown above as a tissue slice perpendicular to the long axis of the closed defect. The major direction of contraction is perpendicular to the long axis of the scar. The resulting scattering pattern is viewed on the photographic plane; it is characterized by the scattering angle θ and the azimuthal (or rotation) angle β. Tissue sections can be cut either parallel or perpendicular to the major direction of contraction; values of the orientation index for such tissue sections are shown in Table 4.1. *Bottom*: Four areas (shown as circles in photograph of histologic section, top) in a tissue section were sampled by the light beam. The resulting scattering patterns are shown below; they contain information on the average orientation and diameter of the collagen fibers in each of the areas. Patterns from physiological dermis (extreme left and extreme right) deviate from being perfectly circular, indicative of a very small amount of normal fiber orientation in the plane of the epidermis. Patterns from scar tissue (inside left and inside right) show strong fiber orientation in the plane. (From Ferdman and Yannas, 1993.)

◄————————————————————————————

TABLE 4.1. Quantitative distinction between dermis and scar. Orientation index and fiber diameter of normal guinea pig dermis[1] and adjacent scar.[2,3]

	Orientation Index[4]	
Tissue	Tissue section cut parallel to major contraction direction	Tissue section cut perpendicular to major contraction direction
Normal dermis	0.20 ± 0.11	0.13 ± 0.05
Scar	0.75 ± 0.10	0.18 ± 0.08

	Average Fiber Diameter, μm	
Tissue	Light scattering	Light microscopy
Normal dermis	20 ± 7	26 ± 13
Scar	13 ± 5	11 ± 8

[1] Sections of dermis used in this study were sampled from the reticular dermis of white, female Hartley guinea pigs. These sections, about 4μm in thickness, were obtained from tissue adjacent to the scar.

[2] Sections of scar were obtained between 189 and 389 days after excision of a dermis-free wound down to, but not including, the *panniculus carnosus* muscle. Defects were rectangular, $1.5 \times 3.0\,cm^2$, or square, $3.0 \times 3.0\,cm^2$. Sections were fixed in 10% buffered formalin for 24 hours and processed using standard histological methods prior to study by laser light scattering.

[3] Data from Ferdman, 1987; Ferdman and Yannas, 1993.

[4] The orientation index varies from 0 (randomly oriented fiber axes) to 1 (perfect alignment of fiber axes in plane of epidermis).

resembling dermal scar. The surface of this tissue was capped with a thick collagen capsule, approximately 20 to 50 μm in thickness. In the distal neuroma, less evidence of a dense collagenous tissue was observed than in the proximal stump; however, a similar collagenous tissue capsule, about 50 μm in thickness, capped off the distal stump as well (Chamberlain et al., 2000a).

The long-term changes in the distal stump following transection have been described in Chapter 2. Briefly, they include degenerative loss of axons and the associated myelin sheath (Wallerian degeneration) and the formation of linear arrays of Schwann cells (bands of Büngner) encased inside the empty tubular basement membranes (Weiss, 1944; Fu and Gordon, 1997).

4.5.4 Closure by Regeneration

Spontaneous regeneration of skin in adults has been observed to spontaneously occur in the perforated ear of the rabbit and other lagomorphs, including hares and pikas; it included recovery of hair follicles and sebaceous glands (Joseph and Dyson, 1966; Goss and Grimes, 1972, 1975). Furthermore, deer antlers, shed and regrown annually, are also spontaneously regenerated (Goss, 1980, 1987). Spontaneous regeneration of transected peripheral nerves across a distance of very few mm has been observed in the mouse (Butí et al., 1996).

Induced regeneration of skin in adults has been observed in a number of instances that are described in detail in Chapter 5. Conducting peripheral nerve trunks have been induced to regenerate in several instances; these are reviewed in Chapter 6. Regeneration of the conjunctival stroma has also been induced (Hsu et al., 2000) and is described further in Chapter 8.

The basic assay in studies of induced regeneration comprises determination of the extent of regeneration, typically consisting of measurement of one or more morphological or functional properties, followed by comparison with the corresponding value in the normal organ. Several examples of such assays are described in detail in Chapter 5 (skin) and Chapter 6 (peripheral nerve). Especially simple is the fidelity of regeneration, a measure of the fractional extent to which a selected morphological or functional property of the regenerate approaches the value of the property in normal tissue.

4.6 Defect Closure Rule

The preceding sections included descriptions of the three modes by which a defect in skin and peripheral nerves closes during healing, as well as the methodology employed to measure the contribution of each mode. The configuration of the final state can be described now simply in terms of the relative contribution made by each closure mode. This approach reduces the description of configuration of a healed defect to just three numbers.

Each mode has participated in closure by covering a fraction of the initial surface area of the defect. Using percentage values for contributions from contraction (C), scar formation (S), and regeneration (R), respectively, and summing up to 100, we get the "defect closure rule":

$$C + S + R = 100 \qquad [1]$$

Equation 1 simply states that the final state of the healing process (defect closure) in any organ can be described by just three outcomes: contraction, scar formation (neuroma or fibrosis), and regeneration (partial or total). For example, the result of spontaneous healing of a full-thickness skin wound in the dorsal region of the rabbit can be described in the final state by $C = 96 \pm 1\%$, $S = 4 \pm 1\%$, and $R = 0$ (estimated from data by Kennedy and Cliff, 1979). In contrast, spontaneous healing of a full-thickness skin defect (actually, a perforation) of the rabbit ear can be described as $C = 3 \pm 3\%$ (males), $S = 0$, and $R = 97 \pm 3\%$ (Joseph and Dyson, 1966).

For simplicity of presentation, the three numbers describing the configuration are enclosed in brackets; furthermore, the percentage symbol and error limits are generally omitted, leading to $[C, S, R]$. For example, the data from the study of the rabbit dorsal region described above are presented as [96, 4, 0] whereas the data from the rabbit ear study are [3, 0, 97]. This compact representation provides an immediate glimpse at the effect of anatomical site in the rabbit on the pattern of skin defect healing: Clearly, the defect in the rabbit dorsal region closed mostly by contraction, and to a small extent by scar formation with no evidence of regeneration; in contrast, the defect in the rabbit ear closed by contraction to a very minor extent, while no scar was formed and the defect closed mostly by regeneration. The order of the terms inside the brackets is a convention that will be preserved though this volume. Each term inside the brackets is defined in a strictly operational manner and can be experimentally measured independently of other terms, as described in the sections above. In one sense, the defect closure rule is a statement of conservation. If the magnitude of a given mode of closure is unknown but data on the other two modes are known, the rule can be used to predict the unknown magnitude.

Special cases of this rule can be used to classify various well-known patterns of defect healing. For example, in spontaneously healing defects in the adult mammal, where regeneration is typically absent, it has been observed that $R = 0$. Whenever defects close exclusively by repair (i.e., by contraction and scar formation), we find:

$$C + S = 100 \text{ (repair)} \qquad [2]$$

Equation 2 is a simple definition of repair. Alternately, repair can be described as $[C, S, 0]$. Examples of final state configurations for several representative cases of spontaneous defect healing in the fetus and in adults are presented in Table 4.2. Adult healing is represented well by Equation 2.

TABLE 4.2. Approximate[1] data on configuration of the final state following spontaneous healing of an organ defect.

Defect	Configuration of final state[1]
General case of organ defect healing	[C, S, R]
Ideal fetal healing of dermis-free defect (complete regeneration model)	[0, 0, 100]
Spontaneous healing of dermis-free skin defect in several adult rodents and lagomorphs	[96, 4, 0]
Spontaneous healing of dermis-free skin defect in the adult human	[37, 63, 0]
Spontaneous healing of transected adult peripheral nerve (rat)	[96, 4, 0]
Spontaneous healing of stroma-free defect in adult conjunctiva (rabbit)	[45, 55, 0]

[1] See Table 4.3 for references to the detailed data.

4.7 Relative Importance of the Three Modes of Defect Closure in Different Species

Detailed data on the contribution of contraction, scar formation, and regeneration in spontaneous healing of defects in skin, peripheral nerves and the conjunctiva in adults are presented in Table 4.3.

Data in Table 4.3 have been collected from studies of full-thickness excision of the epidermis and the dermis to its full depth; in peripheral nerves, by full transection; and, in the conjunctiva, by excision of the conjunctival stroma down to bare sclera. All data have therefore been obtained with anatomically well-defined defects. Table entries of percent contraction, C, were observed directly. Scar formation inside the defect was identified by observing distinct histological and functional differences between the subepidermal connective tissue inside and directly outside the defect boundary. The percentage of initial defect area that was closed by epithelialized scar was calculated as $(100 - C)$, after ensuring, based on authors' direct or indirect reports, that no significant fraction of the initial defect area had closed by regeneration $(R = 0)$. Error of each table entry was assumed identical to that of the corresponding entry for C. All entries in the table other than contraction data were calculated or estimated by the author based on contraction data and qualitative evidence reported by the investigators. Remodeling effects were neglected in Table 4.3.

Inspection of the data in Table 4.3 shows that the relative contributions of scar and contraction vary extensively with the species. The data quantitatively state the well-known fact that contraction makes a larger contribution to defect closure in adult rodents than in the human or the swine. In the rodent (rat, mouse), as well as in the rabbit, classified as a lagomorph rather than a rodent (Goss, 1980), the contraction term is about nine times as large as the scar formation term. If we take $C \gg S$, we get a rough approximation for the closure rule in the rodent and the rabbit:

$$C \approx 100 \text{ (several adult rodents; adult rabbit)} \qquad [3]$$

It follows that, to the rough approximation of Equation 3, the configuration of the final state in the rodents and lagomorphs is [100, 0, 0]. There are no comparable data on mammalian fetal healing in the literature. However, the available evidence with skin defects in certain fetal models has led authors to the qualitative conclusion that scar formation and contraction make negligible contributions to defect closure in certain mammalian fetal models (see reviews by Mast et al., 1992b; McCallion and Ferguson, 1996), referred to below as the "idealized" fetal model. This suggests that $C = S = 0$, and, therefore, the simple approximate result follows:

$$R = 100 \text{ (idealized fetal model)} \qquad [4]$$

The final state configuration for this model is [0, 0, 100]. In an adult human, where the evidence (Ramirez et al., 1969) shows that $R = 0$, we have the approximation represented by Equation 5:

$$C \approx S/2 \qquad [5]$$

Certain very useful quantitative conclusions, most of them well known as qualitative statements, emerge from the defect contraction data of Table 4.3. The dermis-free defect in the guinea pig, rabbit, rat, and mouse closes largely by contraction of a "fully mobile integument" (Billingham and Medawar, 1951, 1955). Contraction contributes less to closure in adult porcine skin than in rodents (Rudolph, 1979). In the rabbit, the tissue immediately underneath the dermis consists of several thin layers of connective tissue (superficial fasciae). In the guinea pig, the layer of tissue immediately underneath the dermis is fatty tissue (*panniculus adiposus*). Located even deeper underneath the dermis there is, in both rabbit and guinea pig, but in the sheep as well (Horne et al., 1992), a layer of striped muscle (*panniculus carnosus*) that is responsible for skin-twitching movements. The striped muscle layer is absent in the human except in the muscles of the jaw and of facial expression (Billingham and Medawar, 1951). The dominant role of contraction ensures a minimal contribution of epithelialized scar formation to defect closure, as indicated in Table 4.3. Porcine skin is more firmly attached to subdermal tissues than is true in rodents; in that respect, porcine skin resembles human skin more closely (Kangesu et al., 1993a).

In adult human skin defects, contraction appears to contribute no more than about 40% to closure (Ramirez et al., 1969). This experimental result is in qualitative agreement with the generally accepted clinical reality that contraction plays a much smaller role in the human than in the rodent. In the human, skin is attached relatively firmly to nondeformable fascia and the latter is tethered to major musculature or bone; the *panniculus carnosus*

TABLE 4.3. Spontaneous defect closure in adults. Relative magnitudes of percent contraction, scar formation, and regeneration in the final state.

Species[1]	% Contraction[2]	% Scar[2]	% Regeneration[2]	Reference
A. Skin (dermis-free defect)				
Rabbit (agouti; 57 d)	96	4	0	Billingham and Russell, 1956
Rabbit (male; 16d)	96 ± 1	4 ± 1	0	Kennedy and Cliff, 1979
Rabbit ear (49 d)[3]	3 ± 3 (males); 1 ± 5 (females)	0	97 ± 3 (males); 99 ± 5 (females)	Joseph and Dyson, 1966
Guinea pig (white male; 25 d)[4]	83.7 ± 3	16.3 ± 3	0	Grillo et al., 1958
Guinea pig (male; 12d)	95	5	0	Zahir, 1964
Guinea pig (male; 22d)	84 ± 3	16 ± 3	0	Kennedy and Cliff, 1979
Guinea pig (Hartley; 50d)	90 ± 4	10 ± 4	0	Yannas, 1981
Guinea pig (Hartley; 40d)	92 ± 5	8 ± 5	0	Yannas et al., 1989
Guinea pig (Hartley; 21d)	87 ± 6	13 ± 6	0	Orgill et al., 1996
Rat (Wistar; 12d)	approx. 98	approx. 2	0	Cuthbertson, 1959
Rat (Wistar; 20d)	93 ± 1	7 ± 1	0	Kennedy and Cliff, 1979
Rat (Fischer; 21d)	87.7 ± 10.5	12.3 ± 10.5	0	Rudolph, 1979
Rat (Sprague Dawley; 40d)	96 ± 2	4 ± 2	0	McGrath, 1982
Mouse (Jackson Labs.; day 21)	90	10	0	Greenhalgh et al., 1990
Mouse (Charles River; 10d)	93	7	0	Mellin et al., 1992
Swine (Pitman-Moore minipig; 126d)	75 ± 7	25 ± 7	0	Rudolph et al., 1977
Swine (Pitman-Moore minipig; 140d)	72 ± 7	28 ± 7	0	Rudolph, 1979
Swine (domestic pig; 35d)	90[5]	10	0	Leipziger et al., 1985

	Contraction	Scar	Regeneration	Reference
Swine (domestic pig; 45d)	89[5]	11	0	Alvarez et al., 1987
Swine (24d)	89.2 ± 2.3	10.8 ± 2.3	0	Carver et al., 1993a
Swine (domestic pig) (>17d)	91	9	0	Gross et al., 1995
Human (day 21)	37 ± 2	63 ± 2	0	Ramirez et al., 1969
B. Peripheral nerve (transection of nerve trunk)				
Rat (Sprague-Dawley; 42d)	95[6]	5	0	Chamberlain et al., 2000a
C. Conjunctiva (full-thickness excision of stroma)				
Rabbit (N. Zealand, albino; 28d)	45[7]	55	0	Hsu et al., 2000

[1] The strain of the animal and the number of days after injury on which the observation was made is also reported, when available.

[2] Table entries are percentages of total initial defect surface area covered by a given mode of defect closure (contraction, scar formation, or regeneration). Contraction data were usually reported directly by the investigators while values for scar or regeneration were often estimated by the author. Error limits applied to scar data were usually those used by the investigators when reporting contraction data. See text for additional discussion of methodology used to report entries in the table.

[3] In studies with the rabbit's ear, the dermis-free defect was a hole passing completely through the ear. Percent contraction was observed to be zero. Skin was regenerated in a morphological state that was apparently completely physiological, including elastic fibers in the dermis, hair follicles, and sebaceous glands. Accordingly, percent scar was assumed to be 0 and percent regeneration was calculated as [100 − % contraction], using the directly observed value of % contraction = 0.

[4] In this study, the panniculus carnosus muscle, underneath the dermis, was also excised. The base of the defect consisted of deep fascia and its overlying loose connective tissue (Grillo et al., 1958).

[5] Rough estimate by author based on published photographs of healing defects.

[6] Rough estimate by author based on published photographs of neuroma histology from Chamberlain et al., 2000a.

[7] Rough estimate by author of change in area of excised conjunctival stroma based on data for shortening of adjacent fornix: from Hsu et al., 2000.

is largely missing (Billingham and Medawar, 1951, 1955; Peacock and Van Winkle, 1976). Low skin mobility in the human has unfortunate clinical consequences since scar is quite firmly fixed to tissues underneath and largely prevents the motion of skeletal components or joints to which it is attached. Added to the cosmetic deformity, itself limiting the quality of human life significantly, the effect of a large scar on motion can be occasionally crippling. Examples are cases where contracting skin edges cause a healed chin to be pulled down to the chest or where a joint is dislocated from the traction acting on it by the combined processes of contraction and scar formation (Rudolph et al., 1992). These are the long-term consequences for the adult human of spontaneous repair of a large skin defect.

Even though closure of a defect in the peripheral nerve has not been studied as extensively as in skin, histological observations appear sufficient to describe approximately each term in the defect closure rule for this organ. For example, following transection of the peripheral nerve, the initial area of the defect is the cross section of one of the stumps. In a spontaneously healed nerve, contraction induces a reduction in this area down to approximately 5% of initial cross-section area while formation of a neuroma closes up the remaining 95% (Chamberlain et al., 2000a) (Table 4.3). The absence of direct quantitative observations is stressed.

The conjunctiva and the underlying stroma form the smooth tissue layer that covers the internal surface of the eyelid (Burkitt et al., 1993). Excision of the conjunctiva and the complete stroma down to the bare sclera is an anatomically well-defined defect that spontaneously leads to contraction and synthesis of scar (Hsu et al., 2000). Direct observation of the excised area was not convenient during the study; accordingly, contraction was monitored by measuring changes in depth of the conjunctival fornix at the location of the defect, and assuming that to be a measure of deformation of the adjacent conjunctiva (Hsu et al., 2000). Measurements of fornix shortening in this study were converted by the author to a rough estimate of the extent to which the area of the excised conjunctival defect closed by contraction and scar, leading to the values 45% and 55%, respectively, as presented in Table 4.3. It is stressed that these values are rough estimates.

4.8 A Transition in Healing Behavior with Development

In the embryo and, to a lesser extent, in the fetus, excisional dermal defects often close by spontaneous regeneration; healing appears scarless (Longaker and Adzick, 1991; Mast et al., 1992; Lorenz and Adzick, 1993; Adzick and Lorenz, 1994; McCallion and Ferguson, 1996; Martin, 1997). Contraction, a well-known characteristic of excisional skin defects in the adult (Rudolph et al., 1992), is suppressed in certain fetal defect healing models, such as the fetal rabbit (Somasundaram and Prathrap, 1970; Krummel et al., 1989, 1993; Mast et al., 1992b). Occasionally, however, fetal healing behavior resembles that in the adult. For example, a study of healing of exisional skin defects in fetal sheep showed clear evidence of contraction and scar formation at 75-d, 90-d, and 120-d gestation stages (term = 145 d), as well as in newborn lambs and adult ewes (Horne et al., 1992). Similar results were obtained in independent studies of the fetal sheep model (Burrington, 1971; Longaker et al., 1991a). There is a general shortage of numerical observations, primarily due to the experimental difficulty in studying the kinetics of fetal defect contraction quantitatively.

For most species studied so far, including the human, there is evidence that a developmental transition exists, sometime in late gestational age, from healing by regeneration to healing by repair (McCallion and Ferguson, 1996; Martin, 1997). A basic question that needs to be answered is the nature of the biological switch. It has been suggested that the observed lack of spontaneous regeneration in adult mammals reflects the inhibition of a latent capacity to regenerate rather than an intrinsic and irrevocable change at the genetic level (Goss, 1987).

Only a modest amount of information appears to be currently available on the genetic basis of regeneration and its expression during development, even in the relatively mature field of study of limb regeneration in amphibians (Stocum, 1995; Tsonis, 1996).

Studies of nerve regeneration have also provided evidence that the contribution of regeneration to healing drops rather suddenly with development in this organ as well. For example, the axons of the hamster optic tract are known to regenerate only if the tract is transected on or before postnatal day 3. After that day, transection results in a small amount of sprouting proximal to the lesion but axons fail to regrow across the lesion site (Carman et al., 1988). Axon regeneration in vitro was observed to decline as the nervous system matured (Bjorklund and Stenevi, 1984). In another study, neurite outgrowth by embryonic retinal cells on laminin was shown to be integrin-mediated and to decrease as the neurons matured (Cohen et al., 1986). In the absence of data, it is not clear whether the developmental transition in modes of defect closure observed with skin defects coincides with the transition in closure of nerve defects.

There is some evidence that not all organs in a given species go through the transition from fetal to adult healing at the same developmental stage. For example, although the human fetal intestine was always densely adherent to the diaphragmatic defect (evidence of scar formation in injured skeletal muscle), no scar was evident on the previously made thoracic skin excision (Longaker and Adzick, 1991). Furthermore, while 1-cm radial full-thickness diaphragmatic defects in the fetal lamb, at the 100-d gestation stage, healed with scar formation (Longaker et al., 1991b), an excisional defect in a bone in the forelimb (ulna) in a fetal lamb model of the same

TABLE 4.4. Modes of closure at different developmental stages. Dermis-free defects in an amphibian.[1]

Developmental stage[2]	% Contraction[3]	% Scar[4]	% Regeneration[5]
Larva, premetamorphic stage	40.8 ± 6.8	0	59.2 ± 6.8
Larva, early prometamorphic stage	62.1 ± 3.0	0	37.9 ± 3.0
Larva, mid-prometamorphic stage	66.3 ± 8.1	0	33.7 ± 8.1
Larva, late prometamorphic stage	90.1 ± 2.3	0	9.9 ± 2.3
Adult frog	94 ± 4	6 ± 4	0

[1] North American bullfrog (*Rana catesbeiana*). Data from Yannas et al., 1996.
[2] Developmental staging was based on classic staging criteria for *Rana pipiens* relating chronological age and total body length (Taylor and Kolross, 1946).
[3] Percentage of original defect area closed by contraction. Measured by direct photography of defect after contraction had stopped. Defect boundaries were directly observed and values were confirmed by matching with histologically identified discontinuities in morphological features at the defect edges. Original defect area was generated by excising down to muscle (full-thickness dermis-free defect) an area measuring 5 mm × 5 mm, approximately 1 cm caudal to the eyes. Error was determined directly from data.
[4] Percentage of original defect area closed by epithelialized scar. Scar inside the defect was identified by observing distinct histological and functional differences between the subepidermal connective tissue inside and directly outside the defect boundary. Table entry calculated as [100 − % contraction], after ensuring, by histological observation, that no significant fraction of the initial defect area had closed by regeneration. Error of each table entry assumed identical to that of corresponding entry for % contraction.
[5] Percentage of original defect area closed by regenerated skin. Regenerate inside defect boundary was identified by observing lack of significant difference in histological and functional features inside and directly outside defect boundary (intact skin). Table entry calculated as [100 − % contraction], after ensuring, by histological observation, that no significant fraction of the initial defect area had closed by scar. Error of table entry assumed identical to that of corresponding entry for % contraction.

gestation time showed complete morphological recovery even though the defect was greater than three times the width of the bony cortex (Longaker et al., 1992).

The experimental difficulties associated with collecting kinetic and other data with mammalian fetal models were absent in a study of an anuran model (North American bullfrog) (Yannas et al., 1996). In this study, the anatomically well-defined dermis-free defect in the skin was accessible to direct observation at different stages of development, both before and after metamorphosis of the larva (tadpole) to the froglet (adult frog). Each of the three modes of closure of the dermis-free defects (contraction, scar formation, and regeneration) was measured directly. The data, presented in Table 4.4, suggest that contraction is generally the dominant mode of defect closure, both before and after metamorphosis. In contrast, regeneration continuously declines during tadpole development; just beyond metamorphosis, regeneration is replaced by scar (Yannas et al., 1996). The mechanistic consequences of the data in Table 4.4 will be discussed in Chapters 8 to 10.

4.9 Summary

Two basic questions of methodology were discussed in this chapter: (1) How can the healing process be consistently confined within a time period so that investigators can extract firm cause-effect relations based on the total change in tissue configuration during that fixed period? (2) Which assays will provide an unambiguous measure of the regenerative activity of an unknown reactant? Although continuous kinetic data are very valuable in that respect, the literature of defect healing has very few such data. Furthermore, investigators have used a very large number of assays, making it very difficult to reach valid conclusions on the regenerative activity of reactants. The approach presented in this chapter attempts to circumvent this methodological problem.

In the absence of continuous kinetic data, it was proposed to study the regenerative activity of an unknown reactant by the total change that is caused during a fixed period confined between two states in the healing process. An initial state (newly generated defect) and a final state (recently closed defect) of the experimental healing process were defined. The final state of the healing process is not a biologically static state but instead undergoes quantitative changes over a long time due to the underlying processes of growth and remodeling. The qualitative outcome of healing (repair or regeneration) is not affected by such time dependent changes unless healing coincides with the developmental transition from fetal healing (by regeneration) to adult healing (by repair). The results of assays can be corrected to quantitatively account for the effect of remodeling and growth processes on the observed outcome. In this approach, the regenerative activity of unknown reactants can be simply deduced from knowledge of the structure and function of the injured organ site at its final state (configuration of final state).

Defects in organs close by three modes: contraction, scar (or neuroma) formation, and regeneration. Methodology for quantitative determination of the contribution of each closure mode was described. The experimental evidence was concisely summarized by the defect closure rule, which simply states that the percentages of initial defect area closed by each of three modes add up to 100. The rule describes the configuration of the final state of defect healing by just three numbers, each corresponding to the relative contribution of a closure mode. It can be used to analyze in a self-consistent manner a large variety of data obtained by independent investigators.

Systematic use of the defect closure rule has led to a quantitative description of spontaneous outcomes following injury of skin in different species as well as at different developmental stages of a species. The data presented were limited to dermis-free defects. They provided a quantitative expression of the well-known generalization that contraction dominates closure in rodents whereas closure in humans is shared both by scar formation and contraction. Changes in the configuration of the final state of healing were also used to describe the major developmental transition from fetal to an adult mode of healing in an amphibian species; following the transition healing primarily by regeneration was replaced by scar formation. Rough estimates of contraction extent in peripheral nerves and in the conjunctiva were used in the application of the closure rule to these organs.

The methodological guidelines developed in this chapter will be used in later chapters as filters for sifting through the extensive literature on skin and peripheral nerves. Such sifting will lead to identification of reactants that induce regeneration in these two organs. Because these guidelines have been defined in a general way, it is suggested that they are not specific to skin and peripheral nerves but are applicable to other organs (trans-organ).

5
Regeneration of Skin

5.1 Parameters for Study of Healing Skin Defects

In the preceding two chapters the focus was on identification of the basic experimental parameters that must be controlled in a quantitative study of induced organ regeneration. These parameters are the experimental defect space, the timescale for observation of the outcome, and the specific assays of outcome. Substantial evidence has been marshaled in earlier chapters to show that the conclusions from an experiment in induced regeneration are profoundly affected by the investigator's choice of the levels at which these parameters are set. The detailed set points vary from one organ to another; they will be selected below specifically for the study of skin defects.

We seek to empirically identify the reactants that induce regeneration of skin and will rely heavily on the literature for the necessary evidence. These reactants are added to the skin defect in the form of solutions of macromolecules, cell suspensions, insoluble substrates, or a combination of these states of matter. If insoluble, the reactant has been commonly referred to as a "graft" that is applied on the skin defect. In its simplest form, a graft may have been prepared without incorporating any cells; at the other extreme of complexity, two or more different cell types may have been cultured inside a graft over extended periods of time.

The data in this chapter will be used to answer several questions: Can an epidermis, a basement membrane or a dermis be induced to regenerate, even partly? If so, which reactants can induce regeneration of individual tissues or of the entire organ? Does regenerated skin function physiologically? Which are the simplest conditions for induced regeneration? As pointed out earlier, the answers to these questions will go a long way toward providing a solid basis on which to construct, later in this volume, a reasonably complete hypothesis for the mechanism of induced regeneration of skin in adults.

5.1.1 Anatomically Well-Defined Skin Defects

The selection of an experimental volume was previously based on four criteria that will be briefly reviewed and specifically applied to the study of induced skin regeneration.

First, it is necessary to designate a volume in which reactants with presumptive regenerative activity can be inserted reproducibly as well as one in which the outcome of the experiment will be correctly recognized. A second criterion that must be met is thorough deletion of the non-regenerative tissue that the investigator wishes to synthesize. The third criterion is the requirement for an anatomically well-bounded defect. Fourth, the exudate diffusing away from the defect must be contained by use of a physical barrier that prevents transfer of matter to or from the atmosphere. This barrier should have, if possible, a negligible effect on the outcome of an experiment in induced regeneration of the dermis (biologically inert cover).

All four of the above criteria for an anatomically well-defined skin defect are adequately met by the dermis-free defect, also known as the full-thickness skin wound, prepared by excision of the epidermis, the dermis with all its appendages, and fat down to muscle fascia, and covered with a silicone film or another cover that is biologically inert. This defect has been described in anatomical detail in the rodent (Billingham and Medawar, 1951; Billingham and Reynolds, 1952; Billingham and Russell, 1956) and in the swine (Carver et al., 1993b). Only data obtained with the dermis-free defect by various investigators will be presented in this chapter.

5.1.2 Timescale of Observations

Investigators of healing skin defects have had widely divergent objectives. This has led to a variety of morphological and functional observations over a very broad range of timescales, extending from about 8 d to 720 d (two yr). As discussed in Chapter 4, the core of the healing process is contained between the time that the defect has been generated (initial state) and closed (final state). The time for closure is typically about two to four weeks for a large number of the experimental protocols reported in the literature. Data reported at the final state, rather than before, will be presented in this chapter.

Since remodeling of newly synthesized connective tissue, whether scar (Peacock and Van Winkle, 1976; Mast, 1992) or regenerated dermis (Yannas et al., 1989), continues for several months, investigators occasionally have reported data much beyond the time of defect closure. Such data should be indispensable in establishing the fidelity of the regeneration process in the long term. However, the available evidence suggests that the outcome of the healing process of skin defects has been largely determined, at least with respect to the incidence of repair or regeneration, by the time that the defect has fully closed (final state). It follows that data on the configuration of the final state are not qualitatively affected by the incidence of extensive remodeling events in the post-closure period. Nevertheless, outcome data that are reported at the time of defect closure (e.g., the fraction of initial defect area that has closed by scar synthesis) undergo a small but often significant quantitative change long after closure. These quantitative changes in the configuration of the final state after closure is complete must be taken into account in future studies, as long-term data become available.

5.1.3 Assays of Configuration of the Final State

Many of the studies of skin defect healing were not at all designed as experiments in induced regeneration but as efforts to understand or modify (typically accelerate) the healing process. A very wide variety of experimental outcomes have been measured, including the time for defect closure by epithelialization, percent "take" of experimental grafts, ability to cross over major histocompatibility barriers and regeneration of a dermo-epidermal junction. Most of these observations do not allow the reader to draw a firm conclusion on whether the dermis, the key nonregenerative tissue in skin, has been even partly synthesized or whether spontaneous scar formation has been at all inhibited. In spite of such divergence in objectives, studies were included in the review of this chapter provided that they were conducted under the same initial conditions (i.e., in a dermis-free defect).

The major questions that must be answered in order to provide a complete description of the outcome of an experiment in induced regeneration are: Which tissue(s) were synthesized? What fraction of the initial defect area eventually closed by regeneration? The first question is qualitative; it is answered by reference to the morphological characterization of the tissues inside the defect in the final state and the degree of their resemblance to intact skin, the physiological "standard". The second question is quantitative; it is answered by data that are expressed in terms of the defect closure rule.

5.2 Synthesis of an Epidermis and a Basement Membrane

A skin defect can be considered to have closed when its initial surface area has been fully covered by confluent, mature epithelium (epidermis). Let us describe in some detail the epidermis, the critical marker of closure in a skin defect. Such a detailed description is an indispensable aid in following the outcomes of various protocols.

5.2.1 Morphology and Function of the Epidermis

The epidermis is the external tissue layer of skin. It protects the organism against dehydration and acts as a physical barrier against invasion by microorganisms; it also protects against diverse insults, including those of mechanical, thermal, chemical, and ultraviolet origin. Approximately 0.1 mm in thickness, it consists of five morphological layers (strata), as follows: Basal cell layer (stratum germinativum or stratum malpighii), the germinal layer; prickle cell layer (stratum spinosum), named for the prickly appearance of cells at high magnification; granular layer (stratum granulosum), consisting of intracellular granules (keratohyalin granules) that contribute to the process of keratinization; stratum lucidum, present only in extremely thick skin found in fingertips, palms, and soles of the feet; and the cornified or horny layer (stratum corneum) that comprises flattened, fused cell remnants full of the fibrous protein keratin (Burkitt et al., 1993).

The epidermis can be represented as a cell maturation gradient along which cells move continuously, while becoming increasingly filled with keratin in the process. Cells in the basal cell layer are relatively immature and undergo mitosis; they gradually move along the layers toward the outside, becoming progressively more keratinized, and eventually they die and are sloughed off (desquamated). Cells of this lineage are referred to as keratinocytes. A steady-state process of cell movement with a period of 25 to 50d is established along the maturation gradient. The collection of epithelial cells comprising the epidermis is bound into a coherent tissue by junctions, that is, spots at which cells adhere to each other (desmosomes). Further stabilization of the epidermal layers is afforded by a meshwork of filaments inside the cytoplasm (tonofilaments) that serves to anchor neighboring cells to each other. The result is a mechanically stable, stratified, squamous (comprising flattened cells), keratinizing epithelium that withstands the constant abrasion, desiccation and the variety of biological and physicochemical assaults to which the body is continuously exposed. Additional, quite substantial mechanical stabilization is supplied to the epidermis by the underlying thick, tough dermis, described below. The epidermis is attached to the dermis by a thin basement membrane. The latter is attached to the epidermis by hemidesmosomes, which are located inside the membrane of basal cells and attach to junctions outside the cell membrane (sub-basal plates) (Burkitt et al., 1993).

5.2.2 Synthesis of an Epidermis In Vitro

It makes intuitive sense to attempt covering a skin defect with an epidermis that has been synthesized in vitro. A great deal of research activity has been expended toward preparation of such an epidermal graft. Grafts based on cultured keratinocytes (KC) have been referred to in the literature as KC sheets, cultured epithelia (CE), cultured epithelial autografts (CEA), or cultured autologous keratinocytes (CAK). The generic acronym, KC sheets, will be used consistently below. Major questions addressed in this section are: How are KC sheets synthesized? What happens when KC sheets are grafted on a dermis-free defect?

Approximately 90% of the epidermal cells in mammals are keratinocytes. Three sources of KC for eventual cultivation have been employed as follows: (1) KC sheets formed from epidermal explants, (2) suspensions or pellets of disaggregated KC, and (3) KC sheets formed from dissociated cells. A comprehensive review of the evolution of methodology for preparation of KC sheets has been compiled (Compton, 1994).

During early studies it had been established that suspensions of epithelial cells could be isolated from skin by trypsinization (Billingham and Reynolds, 1952; Billingham and Russell, 1956). Epithelial cells isolated from the skin of chick and mouse embryos were shown to be capable of spontaneous reaggregation and reconstruction of epidermal structures when placed directly on the chorioallantoic membrane of the chick. Reaggregation also took place in flasks or in roller tube cultures. When transplanted to a graft site on an autologous rabbit host, cell cultures multiplied, differentiated, and formed an epidermis.

Some of the experimental problems facing workers who cultivated keratinocytes were contamination of potential grafts with dermal cells (Billingham and Reynolds, 1952; Cruickshank et al., 1960; Delecluse et al., 1974; Prunieras et al., 1976, 1979), cell viability following grafting (Billingham and Medawar, 1950, 1951; Karasek, 1968; Prunieras, 1975), and relatively low cell expansion factors (Karasek, 1968; Igel et al., 1974; Regnier and Prunieras, 1974). Expansion of epithelial cells on a dermal substrate or a plastic film by a factor of 50 over a three-week period provided for complete cover of full-thickness skin defects in rabbits (Igel et al., 1974). In an early clinical application of this concept, autologous epithelial cells were cultured in vitro on an irradiated porcine dermis substrate; the resulting epidermis was detached from the substrate and placed on burn wounds in direct contact with the wound bed. Although the technique was reported to be successful, it could not generate large amounts of epithelium; nor could the epithelial sheet be separated from the culture dish without being damaged.

Many of these problems were overcome with the development of in vitro methods for the rapid, serial subcultivation of keratinocytes from disaggregated cell suspensions, resulting in expansion factors of over 10,000 within three to four weeks (Rheinwald and Green, 1975a,b). Methods for culturing KC have been developed in several animal models (mice, Yuspa et al., 1970; rats, Bell et al., 1981a,b; dogs, Eisinger et al., 1980; guinea pigs, Hefton et al., 1983; rabbits, Lui and Karasek, 1978; pigs, Eisinger et al., 1984) as well as in humans (Rheinwald and Green, 1975a,b; Freeman et al., 1976; Eisinger et al., 1979; Peehl and Ham, 1980; Boyce and Ham, 1983, 1985).

Keratinocytes are typically isolated from skin biopsies by enzymatic treatment that removes the dermal components and dissociates the coherent epidermal cell mass. They have been cultured in media that have typically comprised a combination of fetal bovine serum and defined media, including hormones and growth factors (Eisinger et al., 1979; Boyce and Hansbrough et al., 1988; Cooper et al., 1993). Other media have also been employed, including medium incorporating lethally irradiated fibroblasts (Rheinwald and Green, 1975a,b; Barrandon et al., 1988; Carver et al., 1993b), medium harvested from fibroblast cultures (Green and Rheinwald, 1977), or medium completely free of dermal components (Eisinger et al., 1979). The availability of oxygen has also been recognized as an important factor in the synthesis of an epidermis (Prunieras, 1975).

Synthesis of a coherent, intact sheet of stratified epithelium, typically four to six cell layers thick, kept together by desmosomal attachments has been readily achieved without many restrictions. The level of maturity of the epidermis synthesized in vitro has typically been moderately high; however, keratinization has not always been achieved. Epidermal maturity obtained in vitro has significantly increased when the keratinocyte sheet was grafted on a dermis-free defect. For example, in a well-known study (Carver et al., 1993b), the epidermis cultured in vitro consisted of five to six layers of flattened, undifferentiated cells joined by desmosomes, with sparse keratin filaments running parallel to the long axis of the flattened cells. The plasma membrane of the basal cell layer was in some regions closely apposed to the synthetic polymeric substrate supporting the structure mechanically and formed attachment structures, including hemidesmosomes with sub-basal plates underneath. Use of the enzyme dispase to detach the KC sheets from the culture flasks resulted in the disappearance of these attachment structures. However, following grafting on a dermis-free defect, the epidermis continued maturing, as evidenced by the time-dependent increase in number of hemidesmosomes, average length of a desmosome and of a sub-basal plate (Carver et al., 1993b). The grafted epidermis induced synthesis of a basement membrane as described in the next section. Similar observations have been made by others (Aihara, 1989; Cooper et al., 1993).

Although the maturity of the neoepidermis has been discussed so far with emphasis on keratinization, at least one study has shown that maturation of epidermal attachment structures also depends critically on the identity of the substrate. When stratified epithelium was grown on collagen gels, hemidesmosomes were not synthesized; however, use of a surface consisting of a reconstituted basement membrane led to synthesis of hemidesmosomes (Lillie et al., 1988).

The evidence clearly shows that a partly mature epidermis is synthesized in vitro by condensation of disaggregated keratinocytes. There is no requirement for the presence of fibroblasts or of any dermal component in order to form a partly differentiated, relatively immature epidermis; however, there is a temporary requirement for a nondiffusible substrate on which cells are plated, eventually becoming stratified and keratinized. Contact with surfaces of certain connective tissues or their analogs induces maturation of a stratified epidermis very effectively in vitro; however, significant, though not complete, epidermal maturation occurs even on glass or plastic surfaces.

5.2.3 Structure of Basement Membranes

Below we briefly review the structure of the basement membrane region in skin in order to follow the details of the relevant synthetic processes. The terms "basal lamina" and "basement membrane" were used interchangeably in the literature, leading to considerable confusion, until it was realized that all three layers seen with the electron microscope represent the single layer (lamina densa or basal lamina) seen with the light microscope (Figure 5.1) (Burkitt et al., 1993). It has been recommended that the term *basal lamina* should be confined to its meaning as just one of the layers, lamina densa, as originally employed (Martinez-Hernandez, 1988; Burkitt et al., 1993).

As mentioned in an earlier chapter, the basement membrane (BM) of an organ is generally an avascular, cell-free tissue layer interspersed between a layer of avascular epithelia (tissues that cover or line all body surfaces, cavities, and tubes) and a layer of stroma (vascularized connective tissue, or "supporting" tissue). Several roles of basement membranes have been identified in different organs. These include functions such as that of a boundary that restricts transfer of cells and molecules (Farquhar, 1981), an anchorage matrix for epithelial cells and a mechanically competent adhesive-like layer that binds the epithelia to the stroma (Furthmayr, 1988; Uitto et al., 1996), a scaffold that facilitates tissue repair after injury (Vracko, 1974; Woodley and Briggaman, 1988), as well as several specialized roles during differentiation and growth (Hay, 1981). Although subtle variations in both composition and assembly of components have been observed in basement membranes of different organs and species (Kefalides and Alper, 1988), there are strong similarities that appear to overshadow the differences (Burkitt et al., 1993). For example, there are significant thickness differences depending on anatomical site or species (Furthmayr, 1988). Also, the mature glomerular BM in the kidney, as well as segments of the alveolar BM in the lung are three-layered (trilaminar) (Martinez-Hernandez, 1988). However, there are strong similarities in composition between basement membranes of species as different as Drosophila and mouse (Fessler et al., 1984). The basement membranes in skin and peripheral nerves, the two organs that are treated in detail in this volume, are very similar in composition and structure.

The first layer of the BM, 20 to 40nm in thickness, is next to the cell membrane of the innermost (basal cell) layer of the epithelia and is the

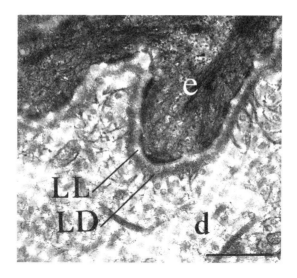

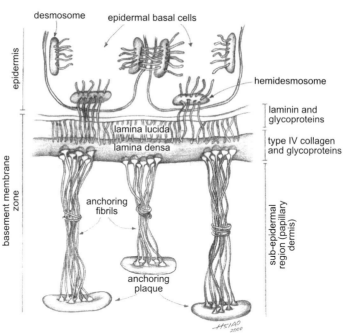

FIGURE 5.1. Structure of the intact basement membrane in skin. *Top*: Electron micrograph showing the two major layers comprising the basement membrane, lamina lucida (LL), and lamina densa (LD), that separate the epidermis (e) from the dermis (d). Bar: 0.5 μm. (From Uitto et al., 1996.) *Bottom*: Schematic diagram defining various tissues in the zone of the basement membrane.

electron-lucent lamina lucida that consists primarily of the glycoprotein laminin (Figure 5.1, bottom). The intermediate layer is electron-dense, about 40 to 50 nm in thickness (lamina densa); it consists primarily of type IV collagen. Adjacent to it is an electron-lucent reticular (fibroreticularis) layer that merges with the fibers of the underlying stroma; in skin, this layer comprises fibers of type VII collagen (anchoring fibrils) that are connected to the dermis by specific structures (anchoring plaques) (Briggaman and Wheeler, 1975; Carver et al., 1993b). Hemidesmosomes are discrete plaques inside the layer of epithelial cells closest to the BM (basal cells); they serve to anchor the basal cells to the BM by means of keratin filaments (tonofilaments) and by connections to junctions in the BM (sub-basal plates) (Burkitt et al., 1993). Although the basement membrane is frequently described as consisting of three zones (lamina lucida, lamina densa, and reticular layer), authors have occasionally described the hemidesmososmes with their tonofilaments, a zone about 20 to 40 nm in thickness, as a fourth zone (Woodley and Briggaman, 1988; Carver et al., 1993b). In addition to types IV and VII collagen, BMs contain fibronectin, heparan sulfate proteoglycan, chondroitin sulfate proteoglycan, nidogen/entactin, α1-microglobulin, thrombospondin, and tenascin (Rigal et al., 1991). The total thickness of the BM is only about 100 nm, typically one-tenth the thickness of the epidermis (Briggaman and Wheeler, 1975). In skin, the BM surface is topologically similar to the surface of a filled egg carton; viewed in planar cross section, the BM appears as an undulating line (rete ridges) (Figure 5.1, top).

5.2.4 Synthesis of a Skin Basement Membrane

An early in vitro synthesis of the BM of skin has been reported (Briggaman et al., 1971). In this study, a partial-thickness skin graft (epidermis attached to a partial-thickness dermis) was treated with trypsin at low temperature (4°C), leading to separation of epidermis from dermis. Separation appeared to have occurred sharply and uniformly at the lamina lucida, as shown by ultrastructural observations of the isolated tissues. The outer surface (basal cell membrane) of the isolated epidermis was lined with hemidesmosomes containing tonofilaments; no lamina densa or anchoring fibrils were seen. The isolated dermis showed an intact lamina densa and anchoring fibrils. Recombination of the isolated epidermis and dermis, followed by incubation, was then pursued in an effort to find out whether a BM would form at the new interface of the two tissues. In order to eliminate the possibility of contamination of the new interface by residual BM from the previous interface, the freshly cut dermal layer was turned around from its normal position (inverted dermis) so that the trypsinized surface would not be in contact with the isolated epidermis. The isolated epidermis was then applied on the surface of the inverted dermis and the recombined bilayer was placed on the chorioallantoic membrane of the chick embryo, yielding the BM (Briggaman et al., 1971).

To find out whether cells from the dermis participated in the synthesis of BM, the investigators combined the epidermal layer with the dermal layer both in a viable and in a nonviable state. The latter was prepared by repeated freezing and thawing of the dermal layer, followed by a demonstration of lack of dermal cell viability (Briggaman et al., 1971). In the presence of either viable or nonviable dermis, it was observed that lamina densa was synthesized in three days, not in continuous fashion but only focally next to the intact hemidesmosomes of the epidermal basal cells. Between five and seven days after combination of the two tissue layers, lamina densa became progressively more dense and continuous at the epidermal-dermal interface. The results showed that dermal viability was not required for synthesis of lamina densa, supporting the epidermal origin of this layer in the BM. In contrast, anchoring fibrils were synthesized in the presence of viable but not nonviable dermis, suggesting the dermis as the hypothetical origin of these structures (Briggaman et al., 1971; Woodley and Briggaman, 1988). (However, evidence presented below suggested that anchoring fibrils originated in the epidermis; Carver et al., 1993b).

In two other in vitro studies, elements of the basement membrane were synthesized by culturing epidermal cell suspensions on a collagen gel (i.e., in the absence of a dermal layer) (Mann and Constable, 1977; Taniguchi and Hirone, 1983). Hemidesmosomes were synthesized along the plasma membrane of epidermal cells at the interface with collagen gel and synthesis of a continuous lamina densa was eventually observed; however, anchoring fibrils were not reported (Taniguchi and Hirone, 1983).

In vivo synthesis of a complete BM was based on use of meticulously prepared defect surfaces in skin, free of traces of BM and underlying dermis (Woodley et al., 1988a; Aihara, 1989; Carver et al., 1993b; Cooper et al., 1993). Because the BM layers are very thin, methods for detection of the main macromolecular components of BM, namely, laminin, type IV collagen, and type VII collagen, have been largely based on use of electron microscopy. These methods are destructive and the number of observations has been typically limited to a total of three to four per study with sequential observations sometimes separated by gaps as large as one to two weeks. In spite of these limitations, a useful qualitative record of BM synthesis in vivo is available.

An early demonstration that grafted KC sheets can induce synthesis of a complete basement membrane was made in the context of a clinical study (Aihara, 1989). Four patients with burn wounds were grafted with cultured KC sheets immediately after excision of the burn surface to the level of the fat or fascia (i.e., on a dermis-free defect). Just before grafting, the cultured KC sheet lacked hemidesmosomes and BM-like structures. At 9 d following grafting there were no hemidesmosomes or structures resembling the lamina densa; however, by 42 d, occasional hemidesmosomes with an associated lamina densa were observed, providing evidence of a discontinuously synthesized BM. The epidermis had become highly differentiated and cornified by 42 d. By 150 d, formation of micropapillae, structures which are normally associated with formation of rete ridges, was poor; however, the author concluded that the three characteristic layers of the BM, that is, lamina lucida, lamina densa, and the reticular layer (anchoring fibrils), had become continuous by that time (Aihara, 1989).

Somewhat different results were obtained in another clinical study in which the skin defects of four patients were prepared by excising down to fascia before grafting with the KC sheets (Woodley et al., 1988a). Observations made at 135 d showed that hemidesmosomes, a lamina lucida, and a lamina densa were present; however, anchoring fibrils and a component of the lamina densa (7-S sites of type IV collagen) were consistently absent. The lamina densa was discontinuous, absent, or reduced except under the occasional hemidesmosomes.

The role of KC sheets in synthesis of a basement membrane was described in a detailed study with dermis-free skin defects in a porcine model (Carver et al., 1993b). During preparation of these defects, the authors explicitly reported the excision of skin and fat, including all epidermal appendages, down to muscle fascia, a demonstration that the defect surface was initially free both of BM structures and of dermis. The KC sheets (Leigh et al., 1987) comprised five to six layers of flattened, undifferentiated cells, containing sparse tonofilaments and joined by desmosomes; there was no evidence of synthesis of BM structures at the completion of this in vitro stage (Carver et al., 1993b).

In contrast to these in vitro findings, progressive synthesis of a BM was observed after the KC sheets were grafted on the dermis-free defect (Carver et al., 1993b). BM was synthesized between the KC sheet graft and the muscle fascia. Newly synthesized laminin, type IV collagen, as well as type VII collagen in the BM region were all demonstrated from day 7 onward by staining with monoclonal antibodies. A discontinuous lamina lucida and lamina densa were initially observed opposite newly formed hemidesmosomes. Within 10 days, the basal lamina became continuous while the number of hemidesmosomes reached normal values. Maturation of the epidermis was considered complete at 16 d, the time when the authors first reported formation of the outermost horny layer (stratum corneum). The morphological data supported the conclusion that the newly synthesized anchoring fibrils originated with keratinocyte and not fibroblasts. During the BM maturation process, the number of hemidesmosomes in the membrane of the basal cell layer (basal plasma membrane) of the epidermis increased continuously and reached the number found in normal skin in 10 days. Although a fully stratified epidermis was formed during the period of the study, the length of individual hemidesmosomes did not reach normal size. In summary, during the 27-day period of observation, a highly developed BM was synthesized in vivo (Carver et al., 1993b). The detailed data confirming the synthesis of a BM in this model are presented in Table 5.1.

TABLE 5.1. Morphological characterization of in vivo synthesized basement membrane.[1]

Normal basement membrane	Synthesized basement membrane[2]
Keratinocytes with many tonofilaments	Keratinocytes with many tonofilaments
Hemidesmosome number per 10 μm of basal plasma membrane = 12.83 ± 0.84[3]	12.79 ± 0.98[4]
Hemidesmosome length per 10 μm of basal plasma membrane (HD length) = 3.43 ± 0.23 μm	2.45 ± 0.52 μm[4]
Subbasal dense plate length per 10 μm of basal plasma membrane (SBDP) = 1.40 ± 0.18 μm	1.30 ± 0.28 μm[4]
SBDP/HD length = 0.406 ± 0.032	0.535 ± 0.055[4]
Individual desmosome length = 0.268 ± 0.014 μm	0.191 ± 0.035 μm[4]
Monoclonal antibody (MA) staining for laminin: Yes	Yes
MA staining for type IV collagen: Yes	Yes
MA staining for type VII collagen: Yes	Yes
Anchoring fibrils: fine, plentiful	Thicker anchoring fibrils; apparently more numerous than normal
Collagen bundles beneath reticular layer: mature and well organized	Not well organized; less mature
Rete ridges: well formed	No rete ridges
Resistance of epidermis to mild abrasion: High	Very low

[1] Carver et al., 1993b.

[2] Keratinocyte autografts on muscle fascia. Swine model.

[3] Mean and 95% confidence interval reported for all numerical entries.

[4] Observed after 27 d.

Similar findings were reported in an independent study (Cooper et al., 1993). KC sheets were grafted on dermis-free defects in athymic mice, prepared by full-thickness skin excision at the lateral side, sparing the *pannicuus carnosus* muscle underneath. Electron microscopy, based on use of highly specific antibody markers, as well as light microscopy, were used to observe the formation of laminin and type IV collagen in the BM. Laminin was synthesized by 10 d; however, little or no type IV collagen could be detected at that time. Both lamina lucida and lamina densa were discontinuous by 20 d and anchoring fibrils were observed to be minimally present. At 42 d, the epidermis was mature, except at the basal cell level; it was also flat, lacking rete ridges. A continuous basal lamina was observed at that time; however, staining for type IV collagen was very light and apparently discontinuous (Cooper et al., 1993).

A much simpler pathway toward synthesis of the basement membrane was demonstrated by culturing second-passage normal human keratinocytes for 14 d in a chemically defined medium on an inert polycarbonate filter substrate at the air-liquid interface (Rosdy et al., 1993). No dermal tissue or cells (fibroblasts) were employed in this in vitro protocol. The authors prepared the primary keratinocyte cultures in serum-free conditions; keratinocytes were then subcultured in a chemically defined medium before resuspending in a simpler defined medium and inoculating onto either a cellulose filter or a polycarbonate filter. A differentiated epidermis was synthesized on the artificial substrates that was similar to living epidermis in the human adult, comprising 25 cell layers with the characteristic stratification pattern of the mature tissue. Electron microscopy showed a BM comprising a lamina lucida and a lamina densa on the surface of the polycarbonate filters. In addition, multiple hemidesmosomes with sub-basal dense plates were synthesized and numerous anchoring filaments were attached to the lamina densa. Several protein components of the BM were identified, including several non-collagenous components of anchoring filaments, heparan sulfate proteoglycan, laminin, type IV collagen, and tenascin. In contrast, type VII collagen, the essential component of anchoring fibrils, was identified inside the cytoplasm of the first layer of epidermal cells, evidence that it had been synthesized, but had not been secreted and deposited. The authors hypothesized that synthesis of anchoring filaments may require either a physically smoother substrate or the presence of dermal factors (Rosdy et al., 1993).

The combined results of the four in vivo studies (Woodley et al., 1988a; Aihara, 1989; Carver et al., 1993b; Cooper et al., 1993) lead to the conclusion that a relatively mature epidermis and a basement membrane with almost completely physiological structure can be synthesized within less than 30 days following grafting of KC sheets on dermis-free defects. There is considerable variability in the rate of the synthetic processes as well as in the morphological identification of the final structures. On the other hand, a much simpler in vitro process led to synthesis of a mature epidermis and a virtually complete basement membrane (anchoring fibrils synthesized but not expressed) (Rosdy et al., 1993).

5.2.5 Origins of Mechanical Failure of the Dermo-Epidermal Junction

In early studies of full-thickness skin defects with rodents, the dermal layer was completely excised and postage stamp–sized epidermal sheets (Thiersch grafts), free of dermal elements, were grafted on the underlying muscle. Epithelial outgrowth from the margins of the small grafts occurred through the first two weeks following grafting, eventually resulting in a single homogeneous sheet of epidermis. At this point, the epidermal sheet appeared to be adequately bonded to the defect surface and a system of rete ridges was observed histologically at the interface with the underlying defect tissue, which had become highly vascularized. By the third week, however, the epithelial grafts became progressively detached and the rete ridges eventually disappeared (Billingham and Reynolds, 1952; Billingham and Russell, 1956).

In a related experimental series, suspensions of epidermal cells, free of dermal elements, were pipetted onto the defect surface from which, as before, dermal elements had been removed. During the first two weeks the epithelial cells proliferated and covered the defect with a confluent layer that closely resembled that achieved by the use of sheets of epidermis as grafts. By the third week, however, these confluent epidermal sheets showed the same lack of attachment to the defect surface (Billingham and Reynolds, 1952; Billingham and Russell, 1956). These authors had observed the consequences of mechanical failure (avulsion) of the bond between the graft and the defect surface.

Since these early studies, methodology for culturing KC sheets has been greatly advanced but the propensity of KC sheet grafts to mechanical failure when grafted on dermis-free defects has not diminished. Frequent failure of grafted KC sheets has been observed by several independent investigators, both in animal models as well as clinically (Eldad et al., 1987; Latarjet et al., 1987; Carver et al., 1993b; Cooper et al., 1993; Kangesu et al., 1993b; Orgill et al., 1998). We will examine the possible reasons for such failure because it sheds light on the synthetic processes that are activated when KC sheets are grafted on dermis-free defects.

Any graft, whether on a skin defect or a defect in another organ, is subject to detachment by small, usually uncontrolled, mechanical forces. These are typically exogenous normal and shear forces, present during experimental or clinical handling of the grafted defect; in addition, shrinkage stresses, arising from dehydration, can cause a skin graft to become detached (Yannas and Burke, 1980). Whenever these exogenous mechanical forces become sufficiently large, or when the intrinsic strength of bond between graft and defect surface is sufficiently frail, the bond fails. Observers often describe this failure as a "spontaneous" loss of the graft or as lack of graft "take."

It has been occasionally suggested that KC sheet grafts have been avulsed after being displaced by the contracting dermal edges of the defect, especially in rodent models where contraction is a dominant mode of defect closure (Billingham and Reynolds, 1952; Banks-Schlegel and Green, 1980; Ogawa et al., 1990). Data from two studies can be used to test this suggestion. Both were carried out in the swine, a model in which contraction is a much less dominant mode of defect closure than in the rodent. In one study, the dermis-free defects were grafted with KC sheets as described above (Carver et al., 1993b); in the other, the grafts were placed on a defect that was prevented from contracting by use of a specially built rigid frame (splint) (Kangesu et al., 1993b). Extensive mechanical failure of KC sheet grafts was observed in both studies. The data showed that avulsion occurred even in the absence of contraction; the hypothesis that failure of KC sheet grafts was due to contraction was clearly not supported by the data.

In normal skin, the BM is located between the epidermis and the dermis and it is commonly assumed that it functions as an efficient adhesive layer that keeps the epidermis and dermis (the "adhints," in this analogy) bonded together. A direct demonstration of the contribution of the BM to the mechanical stability of skin was made by preparing specimens of the dermis with and without a BM, followed by incubating KC sheets in contact with these two surfaces. When the dermis lacked a BM, the KC sheet could be pulled away from its surface with negligible force; instead, the KC sheet was torn, suggesting a strong bond, when it was pulled from a dermis which had a BM (Guo and Grinnell, 1989). These observations could be used to suggest that KC sheets fail mechanically after being grafted on the dermis-free defect because no BM is synthesized. However, this hypothesis is contradicted directly by the evidence, presented in the preceding section, showing that a physiological basement membrane with nearly physiological structure is indeed synthesized under these conditions (Woodley et al., 1988a; Aihara, 1989; Carver et al., 1993b; Cooper et al., 1993).

Another hypothesis for failure can be based on the documented inability of KC sheets to synthesize the undulating BM pattern (rete ridges) that characterizes the normal epidermis (Carver et al., 1993b). The presence of an intact, extensive rete ridge pattern has been associated with resistance to shear and peel forces (Briggaman and Wheeler, 1975; Lavker, 1979). As before, the dermo-epidermal junction in skin is modeled simply as an adhesive joint, in which the BM plays the role of the adhesive and dermis/epidermis are the two adhints. Other factors remaining equal, the strength of the adhesive bond increases with the BM surface area (interfacial area for adhesion). This model predicts qualitatively that, in the absence of rete ridges, the extensive interfacial area of the BM is lowered significantly and the strength of the adhesive joint is accordingly reduced to the point where mechanical failure occurs much more readily. The readiness with which suction blisters can be raised on the skin of elderly subjects can be accounted for, according to this model, by the known absence in these subjects of a rete ridge pattern (Kiistala, 1972; Lavker, 1979). Even if correct, however, this hypothesis does not explain why rete ridges fail to form when KC sheets are grafted on dermis-free defects. It has been suggested that synthesis of rete ridges results from a specific epidermal-dermal interaction (Chapter 10); according to this hypothesis, rete ridge formation should not be expected in the absence of a dermal substrate, as is the case when KC sheets are grafted on muscle fascia.

In a clinical investigation the structural basis for the fragility of KC sheet grafts was studied by observing just where the failure occurred following formation of a standard blister both in the epidermis synthesized by grafting KC sheets and in normal skin. Blisters formed much more readily in an area grafted with a KC sheet than in intact skin. In addition, the cleavage plane of the blister at the site of KC sheet grafting was below the lamina densa of the BM while failure occurred above it in normal skin. The BM zone beneath the KC sheet grafts was found to lack a component of type IV collagen, known as 7-S sites, as well as anchoring fibrils that are present in normal skin (Woodley et al., 1988a). Results from a five-patient study showed that the tissue layer that formed in the subepidermal region contained most of the major macromolecular components of connective tissue; exceptions were the paucity of elastin fibers and poor organization of the protein linkin (microthread-like fibers). It was suggested that these structural abnormalities of skin were responsible for the observed fragility of skin that formed following grafting of KC sheets (Woodley et al., 1990).

The morphological interpretation of detachment of the epidermis was pursued in some detail in the swine model (Carver et al., 1993b). The two surfaces resulting from avulsion of grafted KC sheets were observed by electron microscopy. The cleavage plane was found to lie between the reticular layer of the BM and the uppermost part of the granulation tissue of the two-week-old defect surface. Specifically, basal keratinocytes, lamina lucida, lamina densa, and anchoring fibrils were all attached to the avulsed epidermis, while all collagen fibers remained with the fibroblasts in the granulation tissue in the defect. The authors concluded that the mechanical weakness of the dermo-epidermal junction was due to lack of integration of dermal collagen fibers with anchoring fibrils in the reticular layer of the basement membrane. In contrast, a study of normal skin controls showed that an abundance of dermal collagen fibers was intertwined with the anchoring fibrils of the basement membrane. The description of the subepidermal region at 27 d after grafting showed that collagen synthesis had taken place and that new capillaries had also formed very close, within 20 μm, to the epidermis; however, collagen fiber bundles were not well organized immediately beneath the BM (Carver et al., 1993b).

In another study, in which the KC sheets were grafted on dermis-free defects in athymic mice, one half of the keratinocyte grafts showed blistering at 20 d and 42 d (Cooper et al., 1993). Large areas of separation of the epidermis from the subepidermal region were observed over the 20-day period following grafting with the keratinocyte sheets; however, by 42 d no separation was seen at the subepidermal region. At 42 d, light microscopy revealed a persistently immature epidermis without rete ridge formation while immunohistochemical staining for type IV collagen showed discontinuous staining, consistent with disruption of the BM at the points of discontinuity. Electron microscopy showed little evidence of anchoring fibrils and a discontinuity in the basal lamina by 20 d; however, at 42 d, the basal lamina had become continuous. The morphology of the subepidermal region was not described in this study; however, blood vessels were observed underneath the keratinocyte graft at 10 d (Cooper et al., 1993).

In summary, the majority of data showed that avulsion of KC sheet grafts was caused by a critical structural flaw: the lack of a mechanically competent bond between the anchoring fibrils and collagen fibers in the subepidermal layer. Most studies discussed above showed that anchoring fibrils were synthesized underneath keratinocyte sheets that had been grafted on a dermis-free defect; in contrast, a well-vascularized, thick dermis was not synthesized. The structural defect responsible for avulsion must therefore be lack of synthesis of the dermis; put another way, the adhesive joint failed mechanically because one of the two adhints (the dermis) was either missing or, at least, was inadequately synthesized. In contrast, a sufficiently dense mass of collagen fibers, which normally becomes enmeshed with the anchoring fibrils of the BM, is present both in normal skin and in epithelialized dermal scar, thereby preventing mechanical failure in either structure. This conclusion is further supported by a study in which synthesis of a well-vascularized dermis was induced in a dermis-free defect by grafting with an active ECM analog, the dermis regeneration template; cultured KC sheets were subsequently grafted on the preformed dermal substrate. In this case, avulsion of KC sheets was not observed; in contrast, KC sheets were avulsed after being grafted on a dermis-free defect (Orgill et al., 1998).

5.2.6 Synthetic Potential and Limitations of Keratinocyte Sheet Grafts

The literature of KC sheet grafting has been strongly focused on formation of a highly differentiated epidermis and a complete basement membrane underneath the epidermis in dermis-free defects. The majority of the evidence supports the conclusion that the BM, including anchoring fibrils, derives from the epidermis (Regauer et al., 1990; Carver et al., 1993b). Photographs of histological cross sections have typically not been extended below the BM. The histological evidence demonstrates the ability of KC sheet grafts to synthesize a BM with physiological structure, including anchoring fibrils; however, there is general lack of information about the possible induction of dermis regeneration in such studies.

Although the synthesis of a dermis was not a priority in this area of research, it is worthwhile to examine the evidence in some detail for incidental references to such a synthesis. The normal dermis is a thick layer of richly vascularized, loosely assembled collagen fibers with very little preferred orientation of the average fiber axis. In an early study, a very thin layer of unidentified connective tissue, with collagen fiber axes oriented parallel to the plane of the epidermis, was evident at 108 d underneath the epidermis that formed when human cultured KC sheets were grafted in the athymic mouse (Banks-Schlegel and Green, 1980). In another study with the athymic mouse, a small, "scar-like lesion" was reported at 14 d, after the defect had contracted and the graft had been avulsed (Ogawa et al., 1990). An unidentified connective tissue was reported underneath the epidermis at 42 d in the athymic mouse (Cooper et al., 1993). In a study of the swine skin defect, very few, poorly organized collagen bundles were observed underneath the BM at 27 d (Carver et al., 1993b). In other studies of KC grafting on a dermis-free defect, the electron-microscopic (ultrastructural) finding in the subepidermal region was an immature dermis consisting of a few thin collagen fibers; the optical-microscopic (histological) finding was a connective tissue layer with collagen fibers highly oriented in the plane of the epidermis, reminiscent of scar (Eldad et al., 1987; Latarjet et al., 1987; Woodley et al., 1990; Orgill et al., 1998).

In summary, there is no evidence that a normal dermis is synthesized when KC sheets are grafted on a dermis-free defect.

5.3 Synthesis of the Dermis

Having described methods for synthesizing the epidermis and the basement membrane, we now turn to the dermis, the most important nonregenerative tissue in skin. We start with a detailed description of the tissue.

5.3.1 Structure and Function of the Dermis

The dermis is the inner layer of skin and consists of two zones. Immediately under the epidermis is the papillary dermis, comprising relatively thin collagen fibers, loosely packed, as well as the upward projections of the dermis into the epidermis (dermal papillae) with their content of vascular loops (Figure 5.2, top left). The papillary dermis also contains the fine axonal connections of unmyelinated sensory nerves that end at the epidermis. The main bulk of the dermis is the reticular layer. It comprises highly interlacing (reticular) collagen fibers that are thicker and more closely packed than those in the papillary dermis. The mechanical strength and substantial deformability of the dermis is enhanced by the presence of elastin fibers. While the collagen fibers are highly crystalline microfibrils that stretch to a modest extent, elastin fibers are much thinner, noncrystalline (amorphous), and deform extensively, almost as much as if they were the rubber bands commonly used in packaging. The combined mechanical reinforcement by these two types of fibers makes the dermis a very robust tissue (Burkitt et al., 1993).

The dermis supports the epidermis in two vital ways. First, it provides a tough base that can repeatedly absorb substantial mechanical forces of various types, including shear, tensile, and compressive forces, that would have caused an unsupported epidermis to fail. Second, it incorporates a rich vascular system that is required for the metabolic support of the avascular epidermis. The blood supply of the dermis becomes intimately available to the epidermis at the dermal papillae (Figure 5.2, top left). In addition, the dermis provides thermoregulatory control to the organism, as well as a tactile sensation. There are several skin appendages in the dermis, including hair follicles, sweat glands, and oil-secreting (sebaceous) glands, that are embryonically derived from the epidermis (Burkitt et al., 1993).

5.3.2 Sequential In Vivo Synthesis of a Dermis and an Epidermis

A small mass of dermis was synthesized when the dermis regeneration template (DRT) was grafted on a dermis-free defect in the guinea pig (DRT is a biologically active ECM analog; its structure is described in Chapter 8). A thin film of poly(dimethyl siloxane) (silicone elastomer) was bonded on top of the porous DRT in order to prevent the flow of exudate outside the defect, while also acting as bacteria filter and barrier for controlling the moisture permeability to nearly physiological levels (Yannas and Burke, 1980). A dramatic delay in onset of contraction of dermal edges, amounting to about 20 d relative to the ungrafted defect, was observed (Yannas, 1981; Yannas et al., 1981, 1982b). Following this delay, contraction started and was responsible for closure of most of the defect area; the balance, about 12% of initial defect area, closed by epithelialization. Underneath this epithelialized layer was a small mass of connective tissue that was tentatively labeled a dermis on the evidence that it was well vascularized and comprised loosely packed collagen fibers; these features stood in contrast to the avascular scar tissue, comprising tightly packed collagen fibers, that formed in ungrafted controls underneath the newly epithelialized area (Yannas, 1981; Yannas et al., 1981, 1982b).

However, the dermis was not synthesized, and scar resulted instead, when the degradation rate of the active ECM analog in the same guinea pig model either greatly exceeded a half-life of about 15 days or dropped significantly below 5 days. Inhibition of scar synthesis also required that the active ECM analog have an average pore diameter not much lower than about 20 to 40 µm (Yannas et al., 1982b). A later study confirmed that loss of regenerative activity of the ECM analog occurred when either the chemical composition, cross-link density, or average pore diameter were each displaced from a rather narrow range (Yannas et al., 1989). Early synthesis of a dermis was also observed when DRT was grafted on a dermis-free skin defect in the human; rather than waiting for the much slower epidermal migration from the edges of the defect to cover the defect, however, the neodermal layer was covered in this case with a thin, autoepidermal graft (Burke et al., 1981).

The effect of contraction on the regenerative activity of DRT was studied by comparing closure of defects in the guinea pig and the swine. As expected, a dermis-free defect in the swine spontaneously closed by contraction to a significantly lower extent than in the guinea pig. It was observed that DRT significantly delayed the onset of contraction in both models. At the end of the study, at 21 d, histological data showed a new bed

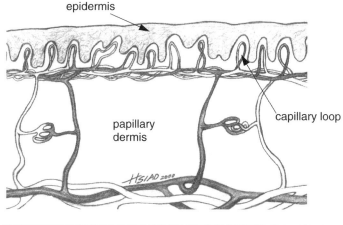

epidermis

papillary
dermis

capillary loop

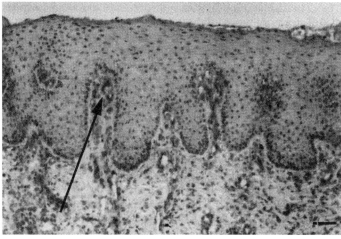

FIGURE 5.2. *Top left*: Normal skin. Diagram showing the vascular network (plexus) in the subepidermal region of normal skin (Adapted from Burkitt et al., 1993). *Bottom left*: Regenerated skin: Basement membrane zone. Regeneration was induced by grafting a dermis-free defect in the swine with dermis regeneration template seeded with autologous keratinocytes. Vascular loops in the rete ridges of the regenerated dermis (arrow) are identified by immunostaining for Factor VIII at 35 d. Notice similarity with normal plexus (top left). Bar: 75 μm. *Top right*: Regenerated skin. Anchoring fibrils in regenerated basement membrane, labeled by immunostaining for type VII collagen, are shown early during the process of synthesis (arrow) (12 d). The basal surface epithelium and the periphery of the epithelial cords are outlined by confluent linear staining, indicative of expression of these anchorage structures at the interface with the extracellular matrix by basal cells. Bar: 150 μm. *Bottom right*: Regenerated skin. The hemidesmosomal staining pattern of the epidermis in partially regenerated skin, identified by immunostaining for $\alpha_6\beta_4$ integrin, is confluent at the dermo-epidermal junction (arrow), identically to that of normal skin (35 d). Bar: 100 μm. (Photos from Compton et al., 1998.)

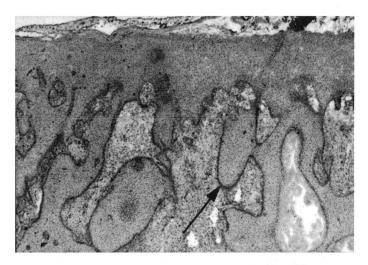

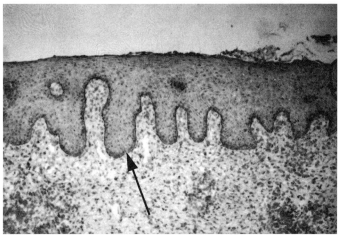

FIGURE 5.2. *Continued*

of thick collagen bundles, randomly oriented, resembling dermis rather than scar, both in the guinea pig and the swine models (Orgill et al., 1996). By 21 d, grafted defects in the guinea pig had closed largely by contraction; only 12% of the defect area was closed by an epithelialized dermis. In swine defects, contraction had virtually stopped by 21 d and defect closure was mostly completed by epithelial migration from the defect edges and over the newly synthesized dermis (Orgill et al., 1996). These results showed that the mass of dermis synthesized in the presence of DRT was strongly affected by the extent of contraction that characterized defect closure in each animal model.

In two later studies with the swine model, DRT was grafted in the cell-free state and was studied as a control of its keratinocyte-seeded version (see below). The time allocated for study of the unseeded DRT, about two weeks, was insufficient for complete re-epithelialization of the newly synthesized dermis. A well-vascularized dermis with an extensive network of capillaries had formed inside the defect (Butler et al., 1998). In a 15-day study of the unseeded DRT, the latter was degraded and replaced by a densely cellular connective tissue with a high degree of vascularity that resembled an immature dermis (Compton et al., 1998). The synthesis of basement membrane was not directly examined in these protocols; however, the available evidence suggested that, prior to eventual reepithelialization from the edges of the defect, basement membrane had not been simultaneously synthesized over the dermis in the presence of the keratinocyte-free DRT.

In clinical studies of DRT, defect closure was greatly accelerated by removing the silicone cover after about two to four weeks and grafting the newly synthesized dermis with an ultrathin autoepidermal graft, nominally about 100 μm in thickness and free of dermis (Burke et al., 1981; Heimbach et al., 1988). In these studies of massively burned patients, burns were excised down to muscle fascia prior to grafting with DRT. Detailed histological study showed that DRT fibers gradually disappeared, the newly synthesized collagen fibers became more coarse, and a distinction between papillary and reticular layers of the dermis appeared in the dermis. Scar formation was not observed either at the gross or the histological level at any time during the course of healing. No skin appendages were evident and rete ridges did not form (Stern et al., 1990). A companion immunological study showed a very small rise in immunological activity in patients' sera for the macromolecular components of DRT, bovine skin collagen and chondroitin 6-sulfate. The overall conclusion from the clinical study was that DRT presented few, if any, humoral immunological problems to patients (Michaeli and McPherson, 1990). Other clinical studies of DRT with massively burned patients have emphasized follow-up of pediatric patients over a 6-year (Burke, 1987; Tompkins et al., 1989) or 10-year period (Sheridan et al., 1994). The new integument was reported to be free of restrictions to joint function, indicative of absence of contractures; most interestingly, perhaps, from the viewpoint of organ regeneration, the new skin had the ability of growing as the child grew (Burke, 1987; Sheridan et al., 1994). The use of DRT has been described in treatment of purpura fulminans, a disorder characterized by rapidly progressing hemorrhagic necrosis of the skin (Besner and Klamar, 1998), release of contractures in massively burned patients (Spence, 1998), resurfacing of scarred areas that resulted from full-thickness burns (Lorenz et al., 1997; Pandya et al., 1998) and treatment of full-thickness wounds that had failed to close spartaneously (chronic ulcers) (Dawson, 1997).

5.3.3 Synthetic Potential and Limitations of the Cell-Free Dermis Regeneration Template

The observations described above have shown that dermis regeneration template (DRT) suppressed contraction and scar synthesis as well as induced synthesis of a dermis, a thick, richly vascularized layer of loosely arranged collagen fibers with axes that were oriented relatively randomly. In defects that closed largely by contraction (guinea pig), the synthesized dermis occupied a small area, whereas in defects that closed in greater part by epithelialization rather than contraction (swine), the dermis occupied a larger area. Clearly, the mass of dermis synthesized decreased with the intrinsic importance of contraction as a mode of defect closure in the animal model.

Contraction was poorly suppressed, and synthesis of a dermis accordingly suffered, when the chemical composition, average pore diameter, and cross-link density of DRT were modified (Yannas et al., 1989). Such modifications reflected changes in identity of cell-matrix ligands, ligand density, and duration of availability of ligands, respectively, as discussed in Chapter 10.

Clearly, the dermis synthesized using DRT was not a perfectly physiological tissue since skin adnexa (hair follicles, sweat glands, etc.) were missing. Furthermore, the cell-free DRT did not simultaneously induce synthesis of an epidermis; instead, following synthesis of the dermis, an epidermis eventually covered the neodermal substrate by spontaneous epithelial migration from the dermal edges of the defect.

5.4 Partial Synthesis of Skin

In previous sections we discussed the synthesis of the tissue components of skin. We now describe the synthesis of the organ itself. The process is described as "partial" synthesis since no skin appendages were formed. First, we describe the morphology and function of skin in greater detail in order to provide a characterization of the goal of such studies. For the convenience of the reader, part of the anatomical description of skin tissues, presented earlier, is repeated below.

5.4.1 Structure and Function of Skin

The skin forms the external surface (integument) of the body. It is the largest organ of the body, almost one-sixth of total body weight, and has four major functions. First, it prevents dehydration and invasion from microorganisms, and protects against ultraviolet light as well as mechanical, chemical, and thermal assaults. Second, it is the largest sensory organ in the body and contains receptors for touch, pressure, pain, and temperature. Third, it thermoregulates the body, insulating it against heat loss by the presence of hairs and subcutaneous fat (adipose tissue); heat loss is facilitated by evaporation of sweat from the skin surface and by increased blood flow through the rich vascular network of the dermis. Fourth, the skin supplements certain metabolic functions of the body through synthesis of vitamin D in the epidermis as well as making available triglycerides from the subcutaneous stores of adipose tissue (Burkitt et al., 1993).

The epidermis and the dermis are intimately juxtaposed via extensive indentations (rete ridges, rete pegs) in the thin basement membrane connecting them. Rete ridges can be described as the microprojections of basal cells of the epidermis into the dermis or, in a complementary fashion, as the projections of dermal capillary loops (papillae) into the epidermis. These indentations appear like undulations in a cross-sectional view of the dermo-epidermal junction and greatly increase the surface area between the two tissues. The skin of elderly subjects largely lacks rete ridges; these subjects have frequently complained of skin fragility, manifesting itself as increased susceptibility to trauma by peeling off of epidermis (Lavker, 1979). These data strongly suggest that rete ridges enhance the mechanical strength of the dermo-epidermal junction, at least by increasing the interfacial area available for binding interactions between dermis and epidermis, and possibly by other mechanisms that are not understood as well. For example, the increase in interfacial area afforded by well-formed rete ridges also increases the rate of transfer of metabolites from the dermis to the avascular epidermis. A particularly effective feature by which such proximity between the two tissues facilitates mass transfer is the presence of capillary loops, part of the vascular plexi of the dermis, that approach the epidermis closest by insinuating themselves into the dermal papillae (Figure 5.2, top left).

5.4.2 Simultaneous Synthesis of a Dermis and an Epidermis

In a series of early studies with the guinea pig model, DRT with the silicone elastomeric layer attached to it (see above) was seeded, immediately prior to grafting, with autologous, uncultured keratinocytes at a mean density of 5×10^5 ($\pm 10\%$) cells per cm^2 graft area (Yannas et al., 1981, 1982a,b, 1984, 1987b; Orgill, 1983). In this study, keratinocytes were separated from a small skin biopsy to yield a cell suspension with an estimated basal cell content of about 40% (Prunieras, 1975; Regnier et al., 1985); the balance of the cell population was not identified. The cells were driven with mild centrifugation, under conditions of carefully controlled centrifugal force and time, to the boundary of DRT with the silicone film, previously shown to be the optimum site for the seeded keratinocytes. The cell-seeded bilayer device was then grafted on dermis-free defects in the guinea pig. The entire optimized protocol for cell harvest, seeding of the DRT and grafting, required about three to four hours to implement (Orgill, 1983). These cells were not cultured for any significant period (Yannas et al., 1981, 1982a,b, 1984; Orgill, 1983).

Seeding of the DRT with uncultured keratinocytes led to a delay of 13.5 d in half-life for defect contraction relative to the ungrafted defect, significantly smaller than that observed with the cell-free DRT (about 20 d). Contraction was arrested between 35 and 50 d; at this point, the defect area was about 20% of initial area. After about 50 d, the defect area started expanding at a rate that was about twice that for skin expansion due to normal growth of the animal. This observation was consistent with an interpretation of significant synthesis of new tissue (Orgill, 1983; Yannas et al., 1989). A confluent neoepidermis formed at 12.6 ± 2 d when the density of seeded KC was 5.0×10^5 cells per cm^2 graft area. Numerous keratin cysts, present approximately after 10 d in the subepidermal region, had been extruded through the neopidermis by 25 d. After about 90 d, the defect perimeter enclosed an area of tissue over one-half that of the original defect, that grossly appeared very similar in color, texture, and touch to intact skin outside the scarred perimeter with the exception that the new skin was totally hairless (Yannas et al., 1981, 1982a,b, 1984; Orgill, 1983).

The new integument was morphologically very similar to physiological skin, both structurally and functionally, including a normal epidermis with a basement membrane, a dermo-epidermal junction with rete ridges, dermal papillae with capillaries, a well-vascularized dermis, elastin fibers, and nonmyelinated nerves in the subepidermal region. Regenerated skin was clearly different from scar (Figures 5.3 and 5.4). It was also different from normal skin; due primarily to the absence of adnexa, it could be best described as an imperfectly synthesized skin (Yannas et al., 1981, 1982a,b, 1984; Orgill, 1983). A detailed description of partially regenerated guinea pig skin is presented below as well as in Table 5.2.

Use of cultured and uncultured keratinocytes yielded a different skin in each case. In a series of studies with the swine model, a confluent epidermis was synthesized earlier when DRT was seeded with keratinocytes that had been cultured for 14 d than when it was seeded with freshly disaggregated, uncultured cells (Butler et al., 1999a). In both cases, the epidermis formed was initially hyperplastic but eventually reached near-normal thickness; it was later reorganized to form a fully differentiated, normally oriented epidermis with rete ridges. Simultaneously, a vascularized dermis with orientation of collagen fiber axes similar to that in normal dermis, and distinctly different than in scar, was formed beneath the newly formed epidermis. Many structured components of a normal dermo-epidermal junction were reconstituted, as shown by observation of confluent linear staining for anchoring fibrils (type VII collagen), a confluent

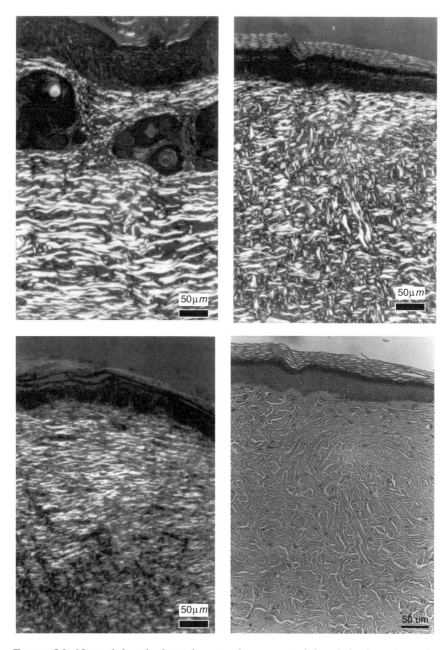

FIGURE 5.3. Normal dermis, dermal scar and regenerated dermis in the guinea pig. Comparative morphological views of connective tissue (stroma) synthesized during repair and regeneration. Observed 483 days after grafting the dermis-free defect in the guinea pig with the keratinocyte-seeded dermis regeneration template. Polarized microscopy was used to elicit differences in collagen fiber orientation in tissue sections from normal skin emphasizing hair follicles (*top left*); regenerated skin (*top right*); scar (*bottom left*). *Bottom right*: Identical field to that in top right (regenerated skin) except viewed in natural light. Bar: 50 μm. (From Orgill, 1983.)

FIGURE 5.4. The dermoepidermal region in normal skin, dermal scar and regenerated skin in the guinea pig. *Top*: Normal skin has a dermo-epidermal region characterized by complex undulations (rete ridges) and by the presence of blood vessels (v) in the subepidermal region (d). *Middle*: Dermal scar is characterized by a flat dermoepidermal junction, showing absence of rete ridges as well as absence of blood vessels in the subepidermal region (d). *Bottom*: Regenerated skin shows dermal papillae containing capillary loops that communicate with an underlying plexus of well-developed blood vessels (v) in the subepidermal region (d). Bar: 50 μm. (From Murphy et al., 1990.)

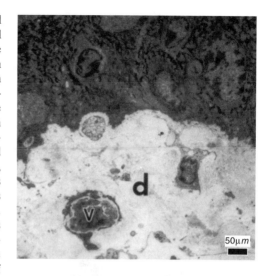

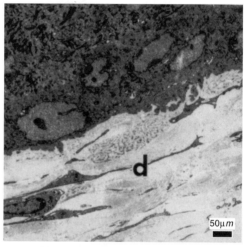

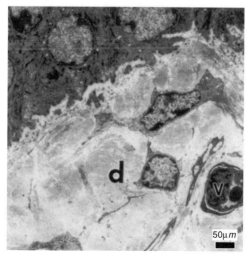

TABLE 5.2. Morphological and functional comparison of normal skin, scar, and regenerated skin (guinea pig dorsum; one year).

Normal skin[1]	Scar[1]	Regenerated skin[1]
A. Functional properties of entire skin organ		
Thickness of dermis plus epidermis: 1.325 ± 0.275 mm	Scar tissue thickness <1.2 mm	Thickness of dermis plus epidermis, 1.20 ± 0.325 mm [p(normal) < 0.6][4]
Moisture permeability: 4.5 ± 0.8 g/cm/h	NA[3]	4.7 ± 1.9 g/cm/h [p(normal) < 0.8][4]
Tensile strength: 31 ± 4 MPa	NA[3]	14 ± 4 MPa [p(normal) < 0.01][4]
Elongation at break: 90 ± 10%	NA[3]	65 ± 10%
Curvature of stress-strain curve: positive	NA[3]	Positive
Resistance of epidermis to mild abrasion: high	High	High
Neurological test (pin prick): positive	NA[3]	Positive
B. Epidermis		
Epidermal thickness: 40 μm	20–40 μm	30–40 μm (variably hyperplastic)
Keratohyaline granules	Present	Larger and more irregular than in normal
Keratinocytes joined by desmosomes	Present	Keratinocytes joined by desmosomes
Melanocytes with melanosomes	Reduced numbers of melanocytes	Melanocytes with melanosomes
Langerhans cells	NA[3]	Langerhans cells
C. Basement membrane		
Basement membrane, including hemidesmosomes, continuous lamina lucida, lamina densa and anchoring fibrils	NA[3]	Basement membrane, including hemidesmosomes, continuous lamina lucida, lamina densa and anchoring fibrils
D. Dermis		
Complex pattern of rete ridges and associated dermal papillae	No rete ridge pattern	Complex pattern of rete ridges and associated dermal papillae (less complex than normal)
Dermal papillae with subpapillary plexus, mostly venules	None	Dermal papillae with subpapillary plexus, mostly venules
Small, unmyelinated nerve fibers in subepidermal region	None	Small, unmyelinated nerve fibers in subepidermal region

TABLE 5.2. *Continued*

Normal skin[1]	Scar[1]	Regenerated skin[1]
Collagen fiber axes only slightly oriented in plane of epidermis; orientation index, $S = 0.20 \pm 0.11$[2]	Collagen fiber axes highly oriented in plane of epidermis; $S = 0.75 \pm 0.10$[2]	Moderately oriented in plane of epidermis; $S = 0.48 \pm 0.05$[2] [p(normal) < 0.001; p(scar) < 0.001][4]
Collagen fiber diameter in reticular dermis, $26 \pm 13\,\mu m$; fibers loosely packed	$11 \pm 8\,\mu m$; fibers tightly packed	$15 \pm 10\,\mu m$; fibers loosely packed [p(normal) < 0.10; p(scar) < 0.50][4]
Stellate-shaped fibroblasts	Elongated fibroblasts	Stellate-shaped fibroblasts
Elastin fibers form fine network; fibers randomly oriented in epidermal plane	Elastin fibers thinned, fragmented; highly oriented	Elastin fibers delicate, not fragmented; slightly oriented
Dermis characterized by two layers, papillary and reticular	Single layer	Single layer
E. Skin appendages		
Hair follicles and other appendages	None	None

[1] Study based on white female Hartley guinea pigs, weighing $400 \pm 50\,g$ at time of grafting. Normal guinea pig skin from the dorsum was sampled from the same pool of animals that was grafted. All defects were prepared by excising full-thickness guinea pig skin down to, but not including, the *panniculus carnosus* (dermis-free defect). Scar was synthesized by allowing healing of a full-thickness skin defect in the dorsum without grafting; ungrafted defects were bandaged (Yannas, 1981). Regenerated skin was synthesized by grafting with a keratinocyte-seeded specific analog of extracellular matrix, the dermis regeneration template (DRT). A characterization of DRT is given in Chapter 8. Data compiled from the following references: Yannas et al., 1981, 1982a,b, 1984, 1989; Orgill, 1983; Ferdman, 1987; Yannas, 1988, 1990; Murphy et al., 1990; Ferdman and Yannas, 1993. Morphological data were obtained with tissue specimens excised one year after grafting. Specimens for thickness and mechanical measurements were obtained at $280 \pm 20\,d$; for moisture permeability studies at $258 \pm 10\,d$. Data reported as mean and standard deviation.
[2] Orientation index S measured by laser light scattering. S varies from 0 (random orientation) to 1 (perfect alignment).
[3] Data not available.
[4] Probability that difference between regenerate and normal skin or scar (as indicated in parenthesis) was due to random error (calculated from t-test).

hemidesmosomal staining pattern of the epidermis ($\alpha_6\beta_4$ integrin), and a well-organized arcade of hairpin-loop capillaries (factor VIII) interdigitating with nascent epidermal rete ridges (Figure 5.2). This pattern was identical to that in normal skin. As with the guinea pig studies, skin appendages were missing (Butler et al., 1998; Compton et al., 1998; Orgill et al., 1998).

The origin of cells responsible for synthesis of the epidermis was studied with island grafts, consisting of DRT seeded with keratinocytes. In the guinea pig model it was observed that island grafts were transformed into pieces of neointegument, consisting of a normal epidermis over a dermis (no appendages). Since keratinocytes from the edges of the defect were clearly separated from the island graft and did not reach it throughout this 14-d study, the data showed that the epidermis originated exclusively with the seeded keratinocytes and not with migratory keratinocytes from the edges of the defect (Orgill and Yannas, 1998).

5.4.3 Distinction Between In Vitro and In Vivo Synthesis

In the preceding two sections, the processes described led to synthesis of skin in vivo either sequentially or simultaneously. In the sequential synthetic route, the only reactant used was DRT, a cell-free analog of ECM synthesized using an acellular reactant. In this process, synthesis of a dermis was first induced by DRT; eventually an epidermis was spontaneously synthesized over the new dermis by migratory epithelia originating at the edges of the defect. In simultaneous synthesis, the reactants included uncultured keratinocytes seeded into DRT; in this case, a new dermis and epidermis were both synthesized during the same period. A characteristic feature of these two routes was the use of reactants that either were cell-free or consisted of cells that had been manipulated in culture (in vitro) for a negligible period of time. (In a variant of this protocol, however, keratinocytes were cultured in vitro for 14 d prior to seeding in the DRT.) The resulting processes were largely, or entirely, free of cell culture methodology and will be referred to as "in vivo" synthesis.

In the next section we describe synthetic routes that made extensive use of cell culture in vitro prior to implantation in the host organism. These synthetic routes will be described as "in vitro-to-in vivo" processes. In the simplest case, only one cell type (keratinocytes) was cultured whereas, in more complex in vitro protocols, two cell types (keratinocytes and fibroblasts) were employed. In the latter approach, cells were additionally relied upon to synthesize an ECM analog in vitro rather than relying on use of a physicochemical synthetic route to prepare it.

In cases of amphibian limb regeneration, described in Chapter 1 as the basic paradigm of spontaneous regeneration, the entire synthetic activity took place in vivo. Accordingly, protocols for induced synthesis of skin in which all, or almost all, of the cell-mediated synthetic activity took place in vivo, resemble closest this basic paradigm of regeneration and are referred to as induced regeneration. Clearly, however, distinctions based on relative importance of in vitro vs. in vivo processing are somewhat arbitrary and do not justify applying the term induced regeneration to a select set of these processes. For this reason, all protocols leading to induced synthesis of a functioning organ at the correct anatomical site, irrespective of whether they make extensive or trivial use of cell culture, will be referred to below as processes of induced regeneration.

5.4.4 In Vitro to In Vivo Synthetic Routes

In this section we describe processes in which a significant part of skin was synthesized in cell culture prior to implantation at the appropriate anatomical site. The various protocols are presented in order of increasing complexity of the implant (i.e., increased extent of in vitro processing).

A slightly different protocol than one described in a preceding section also led to simultaneous synthesis of an epidermis and a dermis. Prior to grafting the dermis-free defect, the investigators seeded DRT with keratinocytes and observed synthesis of an epidermis in vitro after 11 d (Boyce and Hansbrough, 1988; Boyce et al., 1988; Cooper and Hansbrough, 1991; Cooper et al., 1993). The epidermis comprised about 10 stratified epidermal layers, the outermost among them being cornified; frequent desmosomal connections between cell layers were observed, as well as hemidesmosomes that formed between keratinocytes and the nonporous substrate (Boyce and Hansbrough, 1988). In a related study, DRT was modified prior to grafting by laminating with a layer of a nonporous version of DRT (laminated DRT) in order to localize the keratinocyte culture on one surface of the porous matrix, thereby separating keratinocytes from fibroblasts that were also cultured (Boyce et al., 1988). Laminated DRT was cultured with keratinocytes and fibroblasts in vitro to yield a "composite graft" (Cooper and Hansbrough, 1991; Cooper et al., 1993). The epidermis synthesized in vitro using the composite graft protocol comprised stratified, cohesive sheets of epithelium, approximately four to five cell layers thick (Cooper et al., 1993).

Use of the composite graft in a clinical study focused on covering defects in burn patients. The defects were prepared by excision to subcutaneous fat or fascia (dermis-free defects). Prior to placing on the defect, the composite graft consisted of a layer of cultured autologous keratinocytes on the laminated surface of the DRT sheet; autologous fibroblasts had been cultured inside the DRT pores on the opposite surface of the graft. Several days after grafting, a fully stratified epidermis with a stratum corneum had been synthesized. The components of the basement membrane, including hemidesmosomes, a continuous lamina lucida and lamina densa, and anchoring fibrils, were synthesized; rete ridges were also formed. Histological evidence for synthesis of a dermis was presented; however, skin appendages did not form (Hansbrough et al., 1989).

The athymic mouse model was also used for studies of these composite grafts. Following placement of the composite graft on the dermis-free defect, the epidermis became well keratinized with basal, spinous, and granular layers as well as a stratum corneum. Continuous and distinct staining patterns for laminin and type IV collagen, as well as anchoring fibrils and rete ridges, were observed at the dermo-epidermal junction. The available data showed that the composite graft induced simultaneous synthesis of a basement membrane and a dermis in this model (Cooper and Hansbrough, 1991; Cooper et al., 1993).

Extensive morphological data on the identity of the new tissues that had been synthesized were obtained in another clinical study of the composite graft (Boyce et al., 1993). The laminated DRT was cultured with autologous keratinocytes and fibroblasts before grafting on defects that were described as having being prepared by excising to "viable tissue (fat or deep dermis)." Although the investigators reported that grafting was done on "full-thickness" burn wounds, it was not clear whether all of the data had been obtained with dermis-free defects. At 16 d after grafting, markers of epidermal differentiation, including involucrin and filaggrin, were expressed in basal keratinocytes; lamellar bodies representing an epidermal barrier function were also present. Laminin, type IV collagen, and anchoring fibrils were observed at the dermo-epidermal junction. The dermis was characterized by collagen fibers arranged in a "basketweave" pattern characteristic of normal dermis and was described as being free of scar (Boyce et al., 1993).

In another series of studies (Cooper et al., 1991; Hansbrough et al., 1993), cells were seeded instead in a synthetic polymeric mesh consisting of a copolymer of lactic acid (10 wt.-%) and glycolic acid (90 wt.-%) (polyglactin-910 surgical mesh, PGL). The resulting graft was referred to as "living dermal replacement" (LDR). Prior to grafting, LDR consisted of a knitted mesh of PGL fibers, pore size $280 \times 400\,\mu$m and fiber thickness $100\,\mu$m, cultured with fibroblasts until all mesh openings were covered by cells that had become confluent and had synthesized several ECM components; the last step of graft preparation consisted in culturing keratinocytes to confluence on its surface. The cell content of LDR was of human origin; it was studied in the athymic mouse.

At 10 d after grafting the LDR on the dermis-free defect of the mouse, the epithelium was thin and fragile; it became cornified at 20 d. The inflammatory response to the mesh was minimal and the latter had become completely degraded at 20 d. Staining for laminin was consistent with synthesis of a continuous lamina lucida at the boundary between the graft and the surface of the defect; no evidence for other components of the basement membrane was reported. No rete ridges had formed. A large number of fibroblasts as well as vascular ingrowth were reported inside the thick layer of fibrous tissue observed underneath the epidermis; the histological evidence presented leaves an open question on the identity of this layer. When fibroblasts were omitted from the protocol for preparing the LDR, the PGL mesh separated from the defect rapidly and fibrovascular growth did not occur. The presence of keratinocytes in the LDR was required to prevent contraction of the defect (Cooper et al., 1991; Hansbrough et al., 1993).

A quite different approach was used in the preparation of the graft referred to as "living skin equivalent" (LSE). In contrast to previously described efforts, where the focus was on acellular preparation of a scaffold with one or two cell types seeded into it, the LSE protocol emphasized synthesis of as much of the structure of skin in vitro as possible, prior to grafting (Bell et al., 1979, 1981a,b, 1983). Skin fibroblasts were incorporated into a solution of collagen in tissue culture medium. The collagen solution underwent gelation at neutral pH and the resident fibroblasts contracted the gel, expressing fluid, until a coherent collagen lattice incorporating fibroblasts was formed (Bell et al., 1979). Keratinocytes were then seeded to the surface of the lattice; eventually, a multilayered, partly keratinized epidermis was synthesized in vitro, including desmosomes, tonofilaments, and keratohyalin granules (Bell et al., 1983; Hull et al., 1983b).

Following grafting of the LSE on dermis-free defects in the rat considerable remodeling of both layers of the graft took place. By 7 d, the epidermis had become fully differentiated and functional. At 14 d, the subedipermal layer of the graft (proximal layer) was vascularized and had become organized into a birefringent "basketweave" pattern, characteristic of normal dermis. The collagen fibers in this layer were much thinner and more tightly packed than in the dermis of adjacent normal skin. There were no rete ridges in the dermo-epidermal junction and no skin appendages in the dermis. The pattern of the dermis was retained at least over one year (Hull et al., 1983b).

A similar protocol was used to prepare an LSE using human cells and collagen from an animal source, followed by grafting on the athymic mouse (Bosca et al., 1988). Following grafting of the relatively immature epidermis that had been synthesized in vitro, extensive differentiation took place in vivo, with synthesis of all layers of a normal epidermis. Synthesis of a basement membrane had occurred, and hemidesmosomes, a lamina lucida, and lamina densa were clearly observed; however, anchoring fibrils were only occasionally found. The subepidermal layer contained dense collagen bundles; no other information was available on the dermis. No rete ridges or appendages were observed (Bosca et al., 1988).

In another study of the LSE with the athymic mouse, maturation of the stratum corneum of the epidermis was not observed until 30 d after grafting (Hansbrough et al., 1994). Rete ridges were not observed. Small blood vessels penetrated the neodermal layer from the underlying muscle layer. A continuous basement membrane, with hemidesmosomes, a lamina lucida, lamina densa, and large numbers of anchoring fibrils extending into the neodermal matrix, was synthesized. Hair follicles and sebaceous glands were absent. An apparently thin dermis was reported (Hansbrough et al., 1994).

A detailed study was conducted of the changes in structure of the LSE before and after grafting (Nolte et al., 1993, 1994). In vitro, the LSE had developed a well-differentiated epidermis; however, the intercorneocyte lipid lamellae in the stratum corneum did not exhibit the repeating pattern of broad and narrow electron lucent bands observed in the stratum corneum of intact skin that are largely responsible for its barrier properties. Lack of the repeat pattern in the lipids of the stratum corneum has been associated with abnormally high water permeability of skin (Cumpstone et al., 1989; Swartzendruber et al., 1989; Mak et al., 1991), the feature also observed in the LSE following in vitro culture. Although short segments of lamina densa were present at the dermo-epidermal junction, the LSE lacked a continuous basement membrane in vitro (Nolte et al., 1993, 1994).

Following grafting on the athymic mouse, the stratum corneum eventually developed a few lamellar stacks with the broad-narrow-broad configuration representing lipid bilayers; intervening monolayers were also observed in the intercorneocyte space. A continuous basement membrane, including hemidesmosomes, a lamina lucida and lamina densa, as well as an extensive network of anchoring fibrils, were also established after grafting. The dermo-epidermal junction remained flat (no rete ridges) and the dermis lacked dermal appendages. Following grafting, the collagen fibrils in the contracted gel were condensed and were eventually organized into tightly packed bundles of collagen fibrils with circular cross section. Elastic (elastin) fibrils were not detected in the collagenous matrix at any time during the 60-d study period (Nolte et al., 1994). However, nerve fibers were detected (English et al., 1992).

The deficiency in the barrier function of the LSE stratum corneum was followed up in another study (Parenteau et al., 1996). Irregularities in lipid structure were cited as probable causes for the increased permeability of LSE relative to intact human skin. The LSE was described as being deficient in fatty acids. The moisture permeability of LSE was shown to significantly decrease with the time spent at an air interface (aging) during in vitro processing, while the stratum corneum gradually formed (Parenteau et al., 1991, 1992); however, even after a lengthy 21-d exposure to the air interface, the permeability of LSE remained several times higher than that of intact skin (Parenteau et al., 1996). The length of time spent at the air interface in vitro significantly affected the structure of the LSE that developed by remodelling following grafting in the athymic mouse model (Parenteau et al., 1996). Whereas exposure of the LSE at the air interface in vitro for 4 d did not lead to development of rete ridges, lengthening of the exposure period to 10 d yielded some evidence of rete ridge formation 30 d following grafting (Parenteau et al., 1996).

In a clinical trial of the LSE, full-thickness burn wounds were grafted either with meshed (perforated) or with unmeshed LSE (Wassermann et al., 1988). By the second day, a lysis of 70 to 90% of the initial graft surface was observed when meshed grafts had been applied. With unmeshed grafts, a larger percentage of grafted area, 20 to 40%, persisted. Since lysis of the LSE appeared in all grafts a few days after application, leading to a partial graft defect, it was concluded that the LSE cannot routinely be used with burn patients (Wassermann et al., 1988). Another clinical study included patients who had a skin tumor excised and had the defect grafted with LSE; the depth of excision was not specified. A biopsy taken from a single grafted site showed evidence of scar formation. All grafted sites contracted by 10 to 15% (Eaglstein et al., 1995).

A different clinical study of the LSE focused on the treatment of chronic wounds associated with patients with venous ulcers, a chronic skin defect of variable depth (Sabolinski et al., 1996; Falanga et al., 1998). The patients were diagnosed as having venous insufficiency and had open ulcers for at least one month before treatment (median duration of ulcers in patients was about one year); however, no direct information on the depth of the wound at the time of graft application was supplied. In this study, the performance of LSE was compared with that of a multilayered compression regimen based on use of bandages. Over six months, median times to wound closure were significantly shorter in patients treated with the LSE than for those treated with standard care (Sabolinski et al., 1996; Falanga et al., 1998).

A variant of the above protocol for preparation of the living skin equivalent was developed, consisting of a collagenous graft that hypothetically simulated more closely the distribution of collagen types in normal skin (Tinois et al., 1991). The "dermal substitute" (DS) was a bilayer. It consisted of an upper (distal) layer of nonporous type IV collagen and a bottom (proximal) layer of porous type I + III collagens (average pore diameter, 50–100 µm); collagen in both layers had been cross-linked following treatment with periodic acid. The DS was cultured in keratinocytes in vitro until epidermal cell confluence was achieved. In culture, the epidermal layer was multilayered, with desmosomes and a well-organized basal cell layer with tonofilaments. A thick, horny (keratinized) layer was observed when the culture was exposed to air. The dermo-epidermal junction formed in vitro was flat (no rete ridges); it showed synthesis of hemidesmosome-like structures and an electron-dense band resembling lamina densa. Following grafting on dermis-free defects in the athymic mouse, the type IV collagen film was eventually degraded; well-differentiated hemidesmosomes, an almost continuous lamina densa, and fibrils, reminiscent of anchoring fibrils, were observed. A thick dermis was reported (Tinois et al., 1991).

5.4.5 Evidence for Synthesis of a Partly Complete Skin Organ

Skin is a complex organ and it is, therefore, futile to attempt identifying it with a single biochemical or morphological test. The analytical problem amounts to use of a large number of structural characteristics in order to differentiate between the newly synthesized organ, and two well-known standards: normal skin, preferably sampled from a location adjacent to that of the newly synthesized organ or contralateral to it; and scar, also synthesized adjacent to the newly synthesized organ.

The most complete morphological and functional comparison of normal skin, scar, and regenerated skin is available in studies where dermis-free defects in the guinea pig were grafted with the keratinocyte-seeded DRT (Yannas et al., 1981, 1982a,b, 1984, 1989; Orgill, 1983; Murphy et al., 1990). The data have been summarized in Table 5.2 and morphological comparisons of the regenerated stroma (Figure 5.3) and dermo-epidermal junction (Figure 5.4) have been presented. A detailed analysis of these data follows below. (The experimental error is given in terms of the standard deviation; the number of observations, n, is also given whenever available; the probability p that the difference between the regenerate and normal skin, or scar, was due to random error was calculated using the t-test.)

Regenerated skin was not scar in a number of significant respects. In scar, the dermo-epidermal junction was not well-formed, lacking rete ridges with the associated dermal papillae, as well as lacking capillary loops in the papillae; in contrast, regenerated guinea pig skin had all of these features ($n > 100$ fields) (Table 5.2). The subpapillary microvasculature, consisting mostly of venules, that was present in regenerated skin, was absent in scar (Figure 5.4). Unmyelinated nerves associated with the dermal papillae were present in the regenerate but missing from scar ($n > 100$ fields). Orientation of collagen fibers in the plane of the epidermis was described in terms of the orientation index S, measured by laser light scattering, that varies from 0 (random alignment of fibers) to 1 (perfect alignment). Collagen fibers in the partly regenerated dermis were significantly less oriented in the plane of the epidermis ($S = 0.48 \pm 0.05$; $n = 5$) than in scar ($S = 0.75 \pm 0.10$; $n = 7$; $p < 0.001$). However, the average diameter of collagen fibers in the regenerate ($15 \pm 10 \mu m$; $n = 5$ animals) was not significantly different than that in scar ($11 \pm 8 \mu m$; $n = 7$; $p < 0.5$). Neither regenerated skin nor scar possessed epidermal appendages (e.g., hair follicles) ($n > 100$ fields) (Yannas et al., 1981, 1982a,b, 1984, 1989; Orgill, 1983; Murphy et al., 1990).

Regenerated skin resembled normal skin in several ways. The epidermis in the regenerate was well appointed with the cell types of normal skin ($n > 100$ fields). The dermo-epidermal junction in regenerated skin was marked by a well-formed basement membrane, normal in appearance, including hemidesmosomes, a lamina lucida and a lamina densa, anchoring fibrils, and extensive rete ridge structures (Table 5.2). The dermis was endowed with the microvasculature characteristic of normal skin, including capillary loops in the papillae ($n > 100$ fields) (Figure 5.4). It was also endowed with nonmyelinated nerves in the subepidermal region ($n > 100$ fields). The thickness of regenerated skin (epidermis plus dermis; 1.20 ± 0.325 mm; $n = 3$) was not significantly different than that of normal skin

$(1.325 \pm 0.275\,\text{mm}; n = 4; p < 0.6)$. The moisture permeability of normal skin $(4.5 \pm 0.8\,\text{g/cm/h}, n = 4)$ was not significantly different from that of regenerated skin $(4.7 \pm 1.9\,\text{g/cm/h}, n = 4, p < 0.8)$. Animals were manipulated frequently during the duration of the experiment; no incidence of mechanical failure (avulsion or blistering) was, however, reported with any of the animals. Simple neurological testing (pin prick test) gave positive results in both normal and regenerated skin (Yannas et al., 1981, 1982a,b, 1984, 1989; Orgill, 1983; Murphy et al., 1990).

There were also differences between regenerated skin and normal skin (Table 5.2). The axes of collagen fibers in the regenerate were significantly less randomly oriented with respect to the plane of the epidermis $(S = 0.48 \pm 0.05; n = 5$ animals) than in normal skin $(S = 0.20 \pm 0.11; n = 21; p < 0.001; S = 1$ for ideally random orientation and zero for perfect orientation). The diameter of collagen fibers in the regenerate was smaller $(15 \pm 10\,\mu\text{m}; n = 5$ animals) than in normal skin $(26 \pm 13\,\mu\text{m}; n = 21$ animals; $p < 0.10)$. The tensile strength of regenerated dermis $(14 \pm 4\,\text{MPa}; n = 3)$ was significantly lower than that of normal skin $(31 \pm 4\,\text{MPa}; n = 4; p < 0.01)$. The rete ridge pattern in normal skin was somewhat more complex than in regenerated skin. Unlike normal skin, there were no skin appendages (e.g., hair follicles) in the regenerate $(n > 100$ fields) (Yannas et al., 1981, 1982a,b, 1984, 1989; Orgill, 1983; Murphy et al., 1990).

In summary, the morphological and functional data presented in Table 5.2, Figures 5.3 and 5.4, and analyzed above are compatible with a relatively simple conclusion: Regenerated guinea pig skin is clearly different from scar; it can be best described as an imperfectly synthesized skin.

Although less extensive, the morphological characteristics of skin synthesized in the swine model were generally similar to those reported with the guinea pig model.

5.5 Summary of Protocols

We summarize below the conditions under which each of the tissues of skin, as well as skin itself, have been synthesized. The available data make it possible to reach rather definitive conclusions about the choice of conditions that are required to induce regeneration of tissue components of skin. Nevertheless, it is essential to heed a few warnings.

First, the data summarized below have been recorded during a timescale that has been selected in a very arbitrary manner by different investigators. In certain cases, the duration of the study was probably insufficient; a lengthier study might have yielded a tissue or organ that would have been closer to normal. Second, the requirements discussed below are based on currently available data; future studies may show that some of these requirements can be relaxed. There is no absolute requirement, for example, that skin should be synthesized in vivo, even if the available evidence shows that all instances reported in which skin has been synthesized to date have been based on in vivo protocols. Third, although significantly different from the products of repair, the tissues and organ synthesized by induced regeneration are not completely physiological. For example, regenerated skin lacks appendages. Future investigators will no doubt improve on the shortcomings of today's science.

Keratinocytes cultured in vitro can form a *partly differentiated epidermis*. Previously, it had been shown that epidermal cells proliferate and are differentiated in vitro, forming an immature epidermis, in the presence of collagenous substrates (Freeman et al., 1976; Lillie et al., 1988) and in the absence of either viable fibroblasts or a fibroblast-conditioned medium (Rheinwald and Green, 1975a; Eisinger et al., 1979). In a particularly simple protocol, it sufficed to control conditions of pH, cell seeding density, and incubation temperature to synthesize a well-differentiated and partly keratinized epidermis (Eisinger et al., 1979). It has also been shown that the presence of a basement membrane is not an essential substrate for epidermal differentiation in vitro; however, epidermal adhesion on a dermal substrate appeared to be regulated by the basement membrane (Guo and Grinnell, 1989).

The data clearly show that dissociated keratinocytes can proliferate and differentiate in vitro to form an epidermis that is almost fully functional without requirement for the presence of a nonepidermal tissue component. However, the available evidence points to a requirement, a temporary one at least, for an insoluble (nondiffusible) substrate on which the proliferating keratinocytes can condense to eventually form a stratified epidermis. Furthermore, the level of epidermal differentiation appears to depend on the composition of the substrate surface (e.g., it is strongly facilitated when a connective tissue surface is used). In vivo conditions are not required in order to synthesize a partly differentiated epidermis; however, differentiation of an epidermis that has been synthesized in vitro is accelerated and appears to become more complete following grafting.

Synthesis of a *continuous basement membrane* took place when keratinocyte sheets were cultured in vitro. The membrane synthesized in vitro was complete in all respects except for the absence of secreted and deposited type VII collagen, the essential component of anchoring fibrils; however, type VII collagen was identified inside the cytoplasm of the first layer of epidermal cells (Rosdy et al., 1993). A continuous basement membrane, complete with type VII collagen deposition, was synthesized after grafting of keratinocyte sheets on the dermis-free defect surface (Aihara, 1989; Carver et al., 1993b).

A basement membrane was not synthesized when dermis regeneration template (DRT) was grafted on the dermis-free skin defect (Yannas et al., 1982a,b, 1989). It was, however, synthesized when the keratinocyte-seeded DRT (Yannas et al., 1989; Compton et al., 1998) or the fibroblast- and keratinocyte-cultured DRT (Cooper et al., 1993) were grafted on the defects. Likewise, a basement membrane was not synthesized following in vitro culture of the living skin equivalent (LSE); however, a continuous basement membrane was formed after grafting of the LSE on a dermis-free defect (Hansbrough et al., 1994; Nolte et al., 1994; Parenteau et al., 1996). A basement membrane was synthesized following grafting with the dermal substrate (Tinois et al., 1991). There is no evidence that grafting with the living dermal replacement led to formation of a basement membrane with a continuous lamina densa (Hansbrough et al., 1993). In summary, the available evidence shows that synthesis of a continuous, almost complete, BM (type VII collagen secreted but not deposited) simply requires keratinocyte culture (in vitro synthesis). An in vivo environment does not appear to be essential for synthesis of almost the entire BM structure. Neither matrix components nor fibroblasts appear to be required additives for synthesis of the basement membrane either in vitro or in vivo.

A physiological dermo-epidermal junction (DEJ), complete with *rete ridges and dermal papillae*, was not formed when cultured keratinocyte sheets were grafted on the dermis-free defect (Aihara, 1989; Carver et al., 1993b). Neither were rete ridges formed when keratinocytes were cultured in vitro on the dermal substitute, consisting of a collagenous bilayer, prior to grafting (Tinois et al., 1991). No direct synthesis of a DEJ occurred when the cell-free DRT was grafted on dermis-free defect either in the guinea pig or the swine (Yannas et al., 1982a,b; Orgill et al., 1996). Rete ridges and dermal papillae were synthesized when the keratinocyte-seeded DRT was grafted either in the guinea pig or the swine model (Yannas et al., 1989; Murphy et al., 1990; Butler et al., 1998; Compton et al., 1998; Orgill et al., 1998). However, no rete ridge formation occurred when the dermis, already synthesized after grafting with DRT, was subsequently covered with a dermis-free autoepidermal graft (Stern et al., 1990). Grafting with the fibroblast- and keratinocyte-seeded DRT led to formation of a well-defined dermo-epidermal junction (Cooper and Hansbrough, 1991; Cooper et al., 1993). Although a continuous laminin layer was reported in the presence of the keratinocyte-seeded living dermal equivalent, no data on formation of a type IV collagen layer or other structures of the DEJ were reported (Hansbrough et al., 1993). The dermo-epidermal junction following grafting with the living skin equivalent has consistently lacked rete ridges (Bell et al., 1983; Hull et al., 1983a,b; Hansbrough et al., 1994). However, synthesis of a relatively attenuated (low-frequency) pattern of rete ridges following a sufficiently lengthy exposure of the LSE to the air interface, prior to grafting, has been reported in a later study (Parenteau et al., 1996). In summary, the data are consistent with the conclusion that synthesis of rete ridges and dermal papillae occurred when either uncultured keratinocytes had been seeded into DRT or fibroblasts and keratinocytes had both been cultured with DRT. Grafting with the living skin equivalent appeared to induce synthesis of rete ridges provided that the protocol had been adjusted to allow adequate air exposure prior to grafting. Neither grafting of the cell-free DRT nor grafting with keratinocyte sheets alone yielded rete ridges and dermal papillae.

A nearly physiological *dermis without an epidermis* has been synthesized following grafting of the dermis-free defect with the cell-free DRT (Burke et al., 1981; Yannas, 1981; Stern et al., 1990; Orgill et al., 1996; Compton et al., 1998). A dermis was not synthesized when cultured keratinocyte sheets were grafted on the dermis-free defect (Eldad et al., 1987; Latarjet et al., 1987; Ogawa et al., 1990; Carver et al., 1993b; Orgill et al., 1998).

Synthesis of a *nearly physiological skin*, consisting of a well-differentiated epidermis, a continuous basement membrane, and a thick, well-vascularized dermis that was clearly not scar, was achieved in four cases: the living dermal equivalent (Bell et al., 1981b, 1983; Hull et al., 1983b; Nolte et al., 1993, 1994); the dermis regeneration template (DRT) seeded either with cultured or uncultured keratinocytes (Yannas et al., 1981, 1982a,b, 1984, 1989; Murphy et al., 1990; Butler et al., 1998; Compton et al., 1998; Orgill et al., 1998; Butler et al., 1999a); DRT seeded both with keratinocytes and fibroblasts (Cooper and Hansbrough, 1991; Cooper et al., 1993); and the dermal substitute, although the evidence reported for synthesis of a dermis was very limited (Tinois et al., 1991).

Not all of these protocols led to synthesis of physiological subepidermal structures. Rete ridges and dermal papillae, as well as elastic fibers and non-myelinated nerves in the subepidermal region were synthesized following grafting with the keratinocyte-seeded DRT (Yannas et al., 1989). All of these structures were reported to have been synthesized following grafting with the keratinocyte- and fibroblast-seeded DRT; the authors did not report on synthesis of nerves (Cooper and Hansbrough, 1991). Partial synthesis of rete ridges was observed following modification of the protocol for preparation of the living skin equivalent (Parenteau et al., 1996); although no elastic fibers were observed (Nolte et al., 1994), nerve fibers were observed in another study (English et al., 1992). Formation of subepidermal structures was not reported following grafting with the dermal substitute (Tinois et al., 1991).

It was possible to induce regeneration of skin that functioned physiologically in almost every respect (see Table 5.2); among the missing functions were absence of sweating (no sweat glands) and thermal insulation (no hair). Although very useful in the clinical context, skin regenerated so far has been an imperfect organ.

5.6 Simplest Conditions for Synthesis

We now attempt to answer questions posed at the beginning of this chapter: Which are the simplest conditions for synthesis of the tissue components of skin, and of skin itself? Which type of cell is required? Are in vivo conditions required?

An epidermis and a basement membrane were both synthesized in vitro by culturing keratinocytes, in the absence of nonepidermal components; in vivo conditions were not required. A dermis without an epidermis was directly synthesized most simply by grafting with the dermis regeneration template (DRT). Skin, including a dermis, rete ridges, a basement membrane, and an epidermis (but no appendages), was synthesized most simply by combining keratinocytes with DRT; exogenous fibroblasts did not have to be included in the graft. The final state of regenerated skin was not strikingly different whether DRT was cultured with keratinocytes prior to grafting (more extensive rete ridges formed) or was seeded with freshly disaggregated, uncultured cells. Seeding of DRT with keratinocytes was not required for synthesis of a dermis; it was required, however, for synthesis of skin.

Partial synthesis of skin (no appendages) was also accomplished by incorporating keratinocytes in a fibroblast-cultured collagen gel (living skin equivalent), or by seeding fibroblasts and keratinocytes into a modified DRT (composite graft). The last two protocols include exogenous fibroblasts and do not, therefore, make use of the simplest procedures for inducing synthesis of skin.

All successful protocols for synthesis of the dermis have required grafting on a dermis-free defect; in vitro synthesis of the dermis or of skin has not been reported.

5.7 Relative Regenerative Activity of Growth Factors, Cells, and Scaffolds

Data on the configuration of the final state following use of different reactants in the dermis-free defect are presented in Table 5.3. In many of these studies, the goal of the investigation was not tissue synthesis and, for this reason, data related to the configuration of the final state in these studies were not reported directly. In these cases, numerical data in the table were estimated by the author, based on the investigators' original data; these entries have been enclosed in parentheses. In other studies, no quantitative information was included; in these cases, excerpts from investigators' comments were quoted in this table. Only data from studies with the dermis-free defect have been included. Quantitative data have been classified using the simple defect closure rule, discussed in Chapter 4: The percent original defect area that closed by each of three closure modes (i.e., contraction (C), scar synthesis (S), and regeneration (R)) adds up to 100; or, $C + S + R = 100$.

The data in Table 5.3 show that growth factors, including platelet-derived growth factor (PDGF-BB), basic fibroblast growth factor (bFGF), and transforming growth factor-$\beta 1$ (TGF-$\beta 1$), had no effect on the configura-

TABLE 5.3. Configuration of the final state. Fraction of dermis-free defect closed by contraction (C), scar (S), and regeneration (R) in the presence of several reactants.

Animal model (day observed)	Reactant	C^1	S^1	R^1	References
A. Growth factors[2]					
Mouse (21 days)	PDGF-BB	90	10	0	Greenhalgh et al., 1990
Mouse (21 days)	bFGF	90	10	0	Greenhalgh et al., 1990
Mouse (21 days)	PDGF-BB/bFGF	90	10	0	Greenhalgh et al., 1990
Rat (7 days)	TGF-β1 in PBS	(80)	(20) scar formed	(0)	Puolakkainen et al., 1995
Rat (7 days)	TGF-β1 in poly(ethylene oxide) hydro gel	(72)	(28) scar formed	(0)	Puolakkainen et al., 1995
Rat (7 days)	TGF-β1 in DuoDERM paste	(>65)	(<35) scar formed	(0)	Puolakkainen et al., 1995
Rat (7 days)	TGF-β1 in polyoxamer gel	(>85)	(<15) scar formed	(0)	Puolakkainen et al., 1995
B. Pharmacological reactants					
Rat (12 d)	cortisone	85	15	(0)	Cuthbertson, 1959
Rat (40 d)	aspirin	96 ± 2	4 ± 2	(0)	McGrath, 1982
Rat (40 d)	prednisolone	(>83)	(<17)	(0)	McGrath, 1982
Rat (40 d)	ETA (prosta-glandin inhibitor)	96 ± 2	4 ± 2	(0)	McGrath, 1982
C. Keratinocyte (KC) sheets					
Rabbit (35 d)	Epidermal cell suspension; also, epidermal autograft	95	5	0	Billingham and Reynolds, 1952
Athymic mouse (108 d)	Cultured KC sheet	(89)	NA[3]	NA[3]	Banks-Schlegel and Green, 1980
Athymic mouse (14 d)	Cultured KC sheet	Extensive contraction	Scar-like lesion	(0)	Ogawa et al., 1990
Athymic mouse (42 d)	Cultured KC sheet	Minimal contraction; epidermal blistering	No rete ridges	NA[3]	Cooper et al., 1993
Swine	Cultured KC sheet	89	11	(0)	Carver et al., 1993a

TABLE 5.3. *Continued*

Animal model (day observed)	Reactant	C^1	S^1	R^1	References
D. Dermis regeneration template (DRT) (cell-free)					
Guinea pig (Hartley, 300 d)	DRT	88 ± 4	0	(12)	Yannas, 1981; Yannas et al., 1981, 1982a,b
Guinea pig (Hartley, 50 d)	DRT	92 ± 5	NA^3	NA^3	Yannas et al., 1989
Guinea pig (Hartley, 21 d)	DRT	(>51 ± 14)	(0)	(<49 ± 14)	Orgill et al., 1996
Guinea pig, island graft (Hartley, 14 d)	DRT	No contraction of grafted island	0	Dermis formed	Orgill and Yannas, 1998
Swine (Yorkshire pig) (21 d)	DRT	9 ± 7	0	91 ± 7	Orgill et al., 1996; Butler et al., 1998, 1999a
E. Keratinocyte-seeded DRT					
Guinea pig (Hartley, 300 d)	DRT seeded with uncultured KC	28 ± 5	0	72 ± 5	Yannas et al., 1981, 1982a,b, 1984, 1989; Orgill, 1983; Murphy et al., 1990
Athymic mouse (270 d)	DRT cultured with FB^4 and KC	77.5 ± 0.9 (42 d)	Minimal scar	Dermis formed	Cooper and Hansbrough, 1991
Athymic mouse (42 d)	DRT cultured with FB^4 and KC	Minimal contraction	NA^3	NA^3	Cooper et al., 1993
Guinea pig, island graft (Hartley, 22 d)	DRT seeded with uncultured KC	No contraction of island graft	0	Dermis formed	Orgill and Yannas, 1998
Swine (Yorkshire pig) (35 d)	DRT seeded with uncultured KC	NA^3	NA^3	Dermis formed	Compton et al., 1998
F. Synthetic polymeric mesh (PGL 910) seeded with keratinocytes and fibroblasts (living dermal replacement, LDR)					
Athymic mouse (20 d)	Polyglactin-910 mesh cultured with FB^4 (KC omitted)	Marked contraction	NA^3	NA^3	Hansbrough et al., 1993
Athymic mouse (20 d)	Polyglactin-910 mesh cultured with KC and FB^4	Minimal contraction	No rete ridges	Dermis?	Cooper et al., 1991; Hansbrough et al., 1993

TABLE 5.3. *Continued*

Animal model (day observed)	Reactant	C^1	S^1	R^1	References
G. Contracted collagen gel cultured with keratinocytes and fibroblasts (living skin equivalent, LSE)					
Rat (Sprague-Dawley) (720 d)	Contracted collagen gel cultured with KC and FB[4]	Contraction inhibited	No rete ridges	Dermis formed	Bell et al., 1981a,b; Hull et al., 1983b
Rat (Fischer)	Contracted collagen gel cultured with KC and FB[4]	Contraction inhibited	No rete ridges	Dermis formed	Bell et al., 1983; Hull et al., 1983a
Rat (Lewis) (30 d)	Contracted collagen gel cultured with KC and FB[4]	Contraction inhibited	No rete ridges	Dermis formed	Hull et al., 1983b
Rat (Lewis) (14 d)	Contracted collagen gel cultured with KC (FB[4] omitted)	No inhibition of contraction	Scar formed	No dermis formed	Hull et al., 1983b
Athymic mouse (60 d)	Contracted collagen gel cultured with KC and FB[4]	Minimal contraction	No rete ridges	Dermis formed	Hansbrough et al., 1994

[1] Numerical data entered whenever available; otherwise, investigators' comments were quoted. Values in parentheses were estimated by this author based on investigators' data.

[2] For definitions of abbreviations of growth factors used in table, see section 5.7.

[3] Data not available.

[4] Fibroblasts.

tion of the spontaneously repaired defect observed with these 20 dents (control). Use of each of these factors typically led to a configuration of the final state that was identical to that of the untreated defect (repair). Pharmacological agents, such as cortisone, prednisolone, aspirin, and prostaglandin inhibitor (ETA), did not significantly modify the final state of repair (although the kinetics of defect closure were affected occasionally). Neither did grafting with keratinocyte sheets modify the final state of repair.

In contrast to the above, insoluble substrates (scaffolds) cultured or seeded with cells were typically very effective in suppressing contraction and scar synthesis, and induced regeneration to a greater or lesser extent. In most studies, scaffolds were grafted after being cultured or seeded either with fibroblasts or keratinocytes or both. Information on the regenerative activity of most cell-free scaffolds was not available. Although cell-free DRT typically had a significant effect on the configuration of the final state, incorporation of keratinocytes significantly increased the regenerative activity of DRT and significantly reduced the extent of contraction in the final state relative to that observed with the cell-free DRT. In the guinea pig model, the cell-free DRT strongly delayed but eventually did not prevent contraction; however, seeding of DRT with keratinocytes not only delayed but eventually arrested contraction.

5.8 Summary

The dermis-free defect is suitable for experimental study of induced regeneration (synthesis) of skin and of its tissue components using a variety of reactants that are implanted in the defect.

Each of the tissue components of skin, as well as skin itself, were synthesized in a dermis-free defect using reactants comprising cell cultures and certain insoluble substrates (scaffolds) occasionally seeded with cells. Synthesis of an epidermis and a basement membrane were largely or entirely accomplished in vitro whereas synthesis of a dermis and rete ridges with dermal papillae required grafting of the reactants on the dermis-free defect (in vivo synthesis).

Synthesis of an epidermis and of a basement membrane was most simply accomplished by culturing dissociated keratinocytes in defined media. A dermis that lacked an epidermis was most simply synthesized by grafting the defect with dermis regeneration template (DRT). Regenerated skin was partially synthesized most simply using a keratinocyte-seeded DRT; it lacked appendages but comprised a physiological epidermis, basement membrane, rete ridges, and a dermis. Skin was also regenerated partially using a fibroblast- and keratinocyte-cultured DRT, as well as using a collagen gel contracted by fibroblasts and cultured with keratinocytes. Skin synthesized by each of these methods was imperfect, lacking appendages.

6
Regeneration of a Peripheral Nerve

6.1 Parameters for Study of Peripheral Nerve Regeneration

Having studied the conditions under which the tissue components of skin, and skin itself, can be induced to regenerate, we now wish to find out similar conditions for regeneration of peripheral nerves. Once more, we are interested first in establishing the experimental parameters for such a study. These parameters are the experimental space, the timescale for observation of the outcome, and the assays that define the outcome.

Unlike the majority of studies with skin defect healing in adults, in which the incidence of regeneration is typically not explicitly discussed, the literature of the peripheral nervous system (PNS) deals directly and quantitatively with regeneration. This important difference in experimental approach and style of presentation is probably associated with the relative ease with which axons can be counted in the cross section of a regenerated nerve, compared with the perceived lack of simple, well-defined and countable structures in a histological cross section of skin. As a result, the literature of PNS regeneration contains many more numerical observations. While this is encouraging, the proliferation of assays has resulted in a fragmentation of the database and a corresponding difficulty in formulating general rules that accurately summarize the data. One of the most challenging tasks in this chapter is identification of a method for measuring success in achieving nerve regeneration that can be used to evaluate the numerous, disparate data in the literature.

It is customary to find statements in the literature in which a comparison is made between the regenerative ability of the PNS and the central nervous system (CNS), often leading some authors to conclude that regeneration in the PNS is, by comparison, vigorous and extensive. Although this conclusion is apt in comparison with the CNS, it loses its value when viewed in the clinical context: Satisfactory PNS regeneration has been an elusive clinical target (Madison et al., 1992; Lundborg, 2000) and is currently a subject of very active research interest.

Following convention (Burkitt et al., 1993; Fu and Gordon, 1997), we will distinguish between neuronal (neural) tissues (i.e., neurons and their processes, the axons), and nonneuronal tissues, including Schwann cells, fibroblasts, and other cells, as well as various components of the extracellular matrix (ECM) in the nerve trunk.

As with skin, we are interested in answering fundamental questions, such as: Are in vivo conditions necessary for synthesis of nerve fibers? Can nerve trunks be synthesized in vitro? Which experimental protocols lead to in vivo synthesis of a nerve trunk?

6.1.1 Anatomically Well-Defined Defects in Peripheral Nerves

The trans-organ criteria described in a previous chapter for selection of an appropriate defect will now be applied to the PNS. As discussed in detail in Chapter 3, the criteria are satisfied with choice of a transected and tubulated nerve. A peripheral nerve usually consists of one (unifascicular) or more fascicles (multifascicular nerve trunk). Each fascicle is ensheathed in the perineurium; the entire multifascicular assembly, or the single fascicle in a unifascicular nerve, is invested in a loose collagenous tissue sheath, the epineurium (Burkitt et al., 1993). A fascicle has substantial structural and functional autonomy, being readily capable of isolation from adjacent fascicles and of separate transmission of electric signals. During unifascicular surgery the boundary of the defect can be readily established (Morris et al., 1972a; Behrman and Acland, 1981; Archibald and Fisher, 1987); the requirement for an anatomically well-bounded lesion is therefore easily satisfied by transecting a unifascicular nerve. Adjustment of gap size is a critically important experimental parameter that affects the outcome (i.e., repair vs. regeneration). Due to its importance, this parameter has been studied separately and will be discussed in detail below.

The tubular configuration as means for reconnecting cut nerves (splicing) has been extensively used both as a treatment (Weiss, 1944; Fields et al., 1989) and as an experimental configuration for containment of test substances (see review by Fu and Gordon, 1997). Tubulation profoundly affects the healing response of a transected nerve, as can be demonstrated by comparing healing in the presence and absence of tubulation (Chamberlain et al., 2000a). For this reason, the tubulated gap cannot be considered a model for study of spontaneous regeneration; instead, it properly becomes a model for study of induced regeneration.

6.1.2 Timescale of Observations: Short-Term and Long-Term Assays

One of the major differences between studies on skin and peripheral nerve regeneration is timescale of observation: It is typically reported in days with skin, in several weeks with nerves. But just how many weeks must elapse for a definitive measurement? In this section we will attempt to sort through the data in order to identify a useful timescale range for studies of PNS regeneration.

Generally, two methods have been used to monitor the kinetics of PNS regeneration. In morphological studies, a histologic tissue section is viewed by microscopy to detect and count, new structures that have been formed. Since each animal usually carries just one, or at most two, defects, this approach requires study of many animals before data with statistical significance can be obtained over any significant time period. In electrophysiological and behavioral studies, however, the same animal is monitored by these noninvasive studies through the entire experimental period, yielding a virtually continuous record of response to the experimental treatment. For this reason, it is easier to find in the literature kinetic data in the form of electrophysiological, rather than morphological, data.

During the first several weeks following surgery, axons in the regenerate are elongating across the tubulated gap and new connections in the distal stump are being made; accordingly, no electrical signal travels along the defect during this "silent" period, amounting to about eight weeks for a tubulated 10-mm gap in the rat sciatic nerve (Chang et al., 1990). The duration of the silent period depends on the gap length; obviously, morphology becomes the indispensable experimental tool during this period. The speed of axon elongation across a tubulated gap in the rat sciatic nerve has been estimated at about 1 mm/day (Williams et al., 1983), sufficient for bridging of a 10-mm gap in a fraction of the silent period; obviously, axon elongation across the gap does not alone suffice to initiate conduction of an electrophysiological signal.

Time constants of regeneration have been extensively studied with electrophysiological procedures. Typical timescales required to reach constant levels (saturation) of several functional properties were reported for electrophysiological signals following regeneration across a 10-mm gap in the rat sciatic nerve bridged with a silicone tube; they were reported to be about 12 weeks for the time necessary for stimulation of a nerve (latency) and 40 weeks for the conduction velocity (Fields and Ellisman, 1986a; Fields et al., 1989). Data from another study of a similar experimental model showed saturation of the latency by 30 weeks and of the conduction velocity by 30 weeks (Chang et al., 1990). Using long-term electrophysiological data, showing almost complete recovery to normal levels following regeneration across a 5-mm gap in the monkey median nerve, ensheathed in a collagen tube, it can be estimated that most electrophysiological parameters reached approximately constant levels by about 100 weeks (2 years) in this model (Archibald et al., 1995). Other authors, who have studied regeneration in a 4-mm and an 8-mm gap in the rat sciatic nerve, ensheathed in a silicone tube, have defined long-term recovery in terms of a 36-month period (Jenq and Coggeshall, 1985a,b).

The requirement for an approximately two-year period before the regeneration process approached normal levels was documented in a thorough kinetic study of regeneration across a 5-mm gap in the monkey median nerve (Archibald et al., 1995). The data showed clearly that recovery of electrophysiological signals resulting from regeneration across a 5-mm gap bridged with a collagen tube could be described by an S-shaped curve with a half-life of order 30 weeks; however, as many as 115 weeks were required to reach a time-independent (asymptotic) level of nearly normal recovery. Insight into the mechanism responsible for the lengthy timescales required to reach a substantial level of regeneration in the PNS was gleaned from a study of tissue remodeling in the regenerate obtained in a study of the 10-mm gap in the rat sciatic nerve that was bridged either with a collagen tube or a silicone tube (Chamberlain et al., 1998b). The total number of axons in the midline of the regenerate increased up to 30 weeks and then remained unchanged up to 60 weeks for both groups. In contrast, however, the number of a selected set of axons, characterized by a diameter larger than 6 µm and primarily responsible for the electrophysiological response (Arbuthnot et al., 1980; Strichartz and Covino, 1990), was shown to increase between 30 and 60 weeks, at which time the experiment was discontinued (Chamberlain et al., 1998b).

The long-term increase in number of large-diameter axons was significant when collagen tubes but not when silicone tubes were employed, suggesting that the hypothetical remodeling process that accounted for the increase in axon diameter was completed much earlier with silicone tubes. Since the changes were also accompanied with a significant decrease in nerve trunk diameter (as well as a corresponding increase in the fraction of trunk area occupied by myelinated axons), it was concluded that extensive synthetic processes were going on inside the nerve trunk, with the mass of non-neuronal tissue being replaced by neuronal tissue during this unexpectedly late period (Chamberlain et al., 1998b). The combined findings (Archibald et al., 1995; Chamberlain et al., 1998b) made it clear that important remodeling processes in regenerated peripheral nerves appeared to continue even beyond 60 weeks. The data showed that the kinetics of late recovery depended significantly not only on the gap length employed but on the type of tube implanted as well.

These studies also suggest that peripheral nerve regeneration is a sufficiently complex process to preclude its description by a single time constant. In practice, however, the objectives of most investigations appear to fall into one of roughly two major classes characterized by very different experimental timescales and based on use of different controls. In the first, a relatively short study is used to screen a number of experimental variables primarily for their effect on the ability of regenerated nerves to simply cross the tubulated gap and reach the distal stump safely. In this group, the early properties of the regenerates are compared with the lower limit of performance, that is, the negative control (the neuroma in a few studies; an internal tubulated control that does not lead to neuroma, in most others), in experiments that typically do not last longer than four to six weeks (Lundborg et al., 1982a,b; DaSilva et al., 1985; Williams, 1987; Williams et al., 1987; Yannas et al., 1987a; Aebischer et al., 1989; Santos et al., 1991). In a second class of investigations, a lengthy study is launched to measure the detailed extent of recovery of normal function, emphasizing comparison of properties of experimental regenerates with the highest limit of performance, the normal nerve. The experimental timescale for the latter type of investigation often extends to one year or even beyond (Fields and Ellisman et al., 1986a,b; Le Beau et al., 1988; Fields et al., 1989; Archibald et al., 1991, 1995; Tountas et al, 1993; den Dunnen et al., 1993a,b; Chamberlain et al., 1998b).

Below we discuss the selection of an assay for each of these two very different experimental timescales.

6.1.3 Short-Term Quantitative Assays (<20 wk): Frequency of Reinnervation

Unlike studies with the synthesis of skin, outcome data from in vivo studies of peripheral nerve regeneration have been mostly quantitative. Although extensive, the data cannot be used to extract direct, useful relations between reactants and tissues synthesized. The first reason, mentioned in Chapter 2, is the emphasis on axon morphology (axonocentric viewpoint) and the relative neglect of data on tissues that are not spontaneously regenerative, such as the perineurium and the endoneurium.

The second reason is the large proliferation of assays for these in vivo studies. Data on PNS regeneration have been presented in several ways, including number of unmyelinated or myelinated axons, axon diameter distribution, thickness of myelin sheath, percent of defects bridged by nerve fibers, cross section area of regenerated nerve trunk, level of vascularization, density of Schwann cells, presence of endoneurial collagen, number of axons per fascicle, density of fascicles, and so on. Data on several electrophysiological parameters, either of regenerated motor or sensory nerves, also have been reported; these have included, among others, the velocity and amplitude of the electric signal conducted through the regenerate. A large variety of neurological and behavioral tests (e.g., walking track tests, sweat gland reinnervation, pin-prick testing) has been also used to assess the extent of regeneration. The complexity increases rapidly to over 30 outcome assays or so when one considers that investigators have exercised additional degrees of freedom in planning their experiments, including choice of the gap length between the transected stumps, time of observation (1 to 150 weeks), and location of observation along the length of the regenerate (proximal stump, center of gap, distal stump), as well as variation in selection of an animal species. Although each of these outcome assays conveys valuable information about the status of the regenerated nerve, the lack of one or two standardized and widely used assays quickly defeats a reviewer's attempt to make use of the literature in order to identify the simplest protocols required to induce synthesis of specific tissues.

Fortunately, there is a widely used dimensionless measure of synthesis of a nerve trunk with myelinated axons along a gap: the frequency of reinnervation across a tubulated gap (% N), reported as percent of defects that were bridged by myelinated axons. It has been employed in numerous studies with the sciatic nerve of the rat (Lundborg et al., 1982a; Jenq and Coggeshall, 1984; Seckel et al., 1984; Williams et al., 1984, 1987; Fields and Ellisman, 1986a; Müller et al., 1987a; Williams, 1987; Chang et al., 1990; Bailey et al., 1993; den Dunnen et al., 1993b; Derby et al., 1993; Chamberlain et al., 1998b) as well as the sciatic nerve of the mouse (DaSilva et al., 1985; Aebischer et al., 1988; Santos et al., 1991; Butí et al., 1996; Navarro et al., 1996).

Values of % N can be determined using either morphological data (e.g., presence of axons at the midpoint of the gap or at the distal stump) (Lundborg et al., 1982a) or electrophysiological data (e.g., presence of an electrical signal at the target organ) (e.g., Butí et al., 1996). This metric is based on a binary outcome (i.e., either there is successful bridging of the gap by myelinated axons or there is not). Success is defined as the presence of a finite, though usually unspecified, number of axons at the midpoint of the gap or at a more distal point along the gap length, including the distal stump.

There is substantial direct evidence that a nerve trunk that has regenerated across a gap and contains myelinated axons along its length (conducting nerve trunk), thereby contributing positively to the assay for % N, also includes a regenerated perineurium (Lundborg et al., 1982a; Scaravilli, 1984; Fields et al., 1989; Azzam et al., 1991). This evidence is described in greater detail in a later section. In the absence of direct morphological evidence, the synthesis of a conducting nerve trunk across a gap will therefore be postulated to be indirect evidence for synthesis of a perineurium.

In order to use % N as a measure of differences in regenerative activity among different tubulated configurations employed by independent investigators it is necessary to account for the effect of several experimental parameters affecting its value significantly. These parameters include the time of observation, location of assay for axons either inside or outside the gap, choice of anatomical site of the defect, animal species, and gap length. The procedure for making the most significant corrections (i.e., those arising from variations in animal species and gap length) is briefly described in the next section.

6.1.4 Correction for Differences in Gap Length and Animal Species: Critical Axon Elongation

The procedure for correcting the effect of variation in gap length and animal species on the frequency of reinnervation, % N, is based on the early observation that % *N* drops sharply with a relatively small increase in the tubulated gap length (Lundborg et al., 1982a).

Data from several investigators who have used silicone tubes to bridge gaps of several lengths in the transected sciatic nerve in the rat have been used in Figure 6.1a (right curve) to construct a "characteristic curve" for the silicone tube configuration. The inflexion point of this S-shaped curve is the gap length beyond which % *N* drops below 50%; it has been referred to as the "critical axon elongation," L_c. The characteristic curve for the silicone tube has been used to define the performance of a "standard" device with $L_c = 9.7 \pm 1.8$ mm in the rat sciatic nerve. The characteristic curves of several other tubulated configurations have been systematically compared

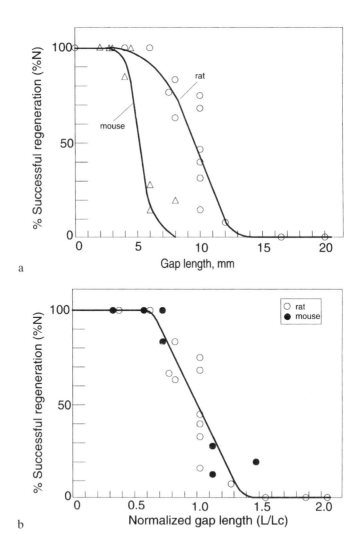

either against the internal control configuration employed by the investigators or against this standard. The difference between the values of L_c for a test configuration and either the internal control used by the investigator or the silicone standard (length shift, ΔL) has been used as a measure of the regenerative advantage or disadvantage of the tubulated configuration relative to the internal control or silicone standard. A large body of independent data from the literature has been analyzed in a self-consistent manner by hypothesizing that the characteristic curves of various devices all have the same "universal" shape and differ only with respect to the length shift, ΔL, that separates the data for the various devices along the gap length axis. The procedure used to estimate L_c and ΔL for a variety of devices is described in the appendix at the end of this text. The use of ΔL to compare a large variety of experimental configurations is described later in this chapter.

A similar analysis has led to the conclusion that mouse sciatic nerve data from several independent investigators who studied the silicone tube configuration can also be used to construct a "standard" curve for the mouse (Figure 6.1a, left curve). The mouse data are consistent with a significantly

◄────────────────────────────

FIGURE 6.1. *Top* (Figure 6.1a): Construction of the "characteristic curve" for a silicone tube used as a bridge for gaps of different lengths in the mouse (triangles) and rat (circles) sciatic nerves. Each curve summarizes data from several independent investigators (see below). Frequency of innervation of the gap, % N, is plotted against the gap length employed by the investigator. The data show a sharp drop in % N at a certain critical axon elongation, L_c, a characteristic of a given experimental configuration and animal species. L_c is defined as the gap length at which % N = 50, the length above which the chance of observing innervation is less than even. L_c for the rat sciatic nerve is estimated from the data at 9.7 ± 1.8 mm; for the mouse sciatic nerve it is 5.4 ± 1.0 mm. The S-shaped curve, comprising silicone tube data for the rat sciatic nerve, has been used as a "standard" for comparison of various tubulated configurations. *Bottom* (Figure 6.1b): Superposition of data from studies of mouse and rat sciatic nerve. Rat (open circles) and mouse (filled circles) data were superposed by plotting % N data against the reduced length, L/L_c, the ratio of the gap length at which an observation of % N was made in a rodent species divided by the critical axon elongation, L_c, for that species.

Data in Figure 6.1a for the rat sciatic nerve were reported by the following investigators who employed silicone tubes (gap lengths are shown in parentheses): Lundborg et al., 1982a (6, 10, 15, 20 mm); Williams et al., 1984 (10 mm); Jenq and Coggeshall, 1985a (0, 4, 8 mm); Fields and Ellisman, 1986a (10 mm); Williams et al., 1987 (15 mm) Yannas et al., 1987a (15 mm); Madison et al., 1988 (15 mm); Hollowell et al., 1990 (8 mm); Derby et al., 1993 (7.5, 12.5 mm); Chang et al., 1990 (10 mm; both unfilled and saline-filled tubes); Lundborg et al., 1997 (15 mm); Ansselin et al., 1997 (18 mm); Chamberlain et al., 1998a (10 mm). The mouse sciatic nerve was studied by the following investigators who also used silicone tubes: Aebischer et al., 1988 (4 mm); Santos et al., 1991 (3 mm); Butí et al., 1996 (2, 4, 6, 8 mm); Navarro et al., 1996 (6 mm); Labrador et al., 1998 (4, 6 mm).

lower value for critical axon elongation than for the rat, namely, $L_c = 5.4 \pm 1.0$ mm. Rat and mouse data were superposed simply by plotting % N data against the reduced length, L/L_c, the ratio of the gap length at which an observation of % N was made in a rodent species divided by the critical axon elongation for that species. The superposed data appear in Figure 6.1b. The ability to superpose data from two species suggests that the relation between frequency of reinnervation and gap length reflects a general phenomenon that may not be species-specific.

If sufficient data were available to construct a characteristic curve for a given device, it would be possible to estimate the value of L_c for the device; a self-consistent comparison of L_c values could then be made among different experimental configurations. In the absence of such data, one can hypothesize that the characteristic curves of all devices have the same shape and differ only by a horizontal shift along the gap length axis. On the basis of this hypothesis, L_c is estimated by use of a single experimental value of % N at a given gap length, as explained in the appendix. Furthermore, if the widely used silicone tube is accepted as a standard, values of the length shift, ΔL, the difference between the values of L_c for an arbitrarily selected configuration and the known value for the silicone tube, can be estimated. Use of the "constant shape" hypothesis has been made to construct Table 6.1.

6.1.5 Relation Between Critical Axon Elongation Data and the Defect Closure Rule

The defect closure rule describes the configuration of the final state of a healing process in an organ. Limited data showed that the critical axon elongation, L_c, for an experimental tubulated configuration in the PNS was directly related to the magnitude of the regeneration term in the defect closure rule.

The data were obtained using three widely different experimental configurations for study of the 10-mm gap in the rat sciatic nerve: the untubulated gap, the gap bridged with a silicone tube, and that bridged with a collagen tube; both tubes were filled with phosphate-buffered saline (PBS) prior to implantation. The relative frequency of reinnervation, % N, for the untubulated group (neuroma), the silicone tube group, and the collagen tube group was directly observed (Chamberlain et al., 1998b). Estimates of the critical axon elongation, L_c, for these three experimental configurations were reached using the procedure described in detail in the appendix; values of the length shift, ΔL, were also tabulated. Finally, the relative contribution of each mode of defect closure was estimated by the author based on the published histological data (Chamberlain, 1998; Chamberlain et al., 1999b, 2000a). These data are tabulated in Table 6.2.

Comparison of the data points for these three devices shows that L_c and ΔL increase regularly with percent regeneration (R) in the final state (Table 6.2). The limited data provide preliminary support to the postulate that data

TABLE 6.1. Regenerative activity of several tubulated configurations.[1]

Experimental variable X[2] (describes tubulated gap)	L_c in presence of X, mm	L_c in absence of X, mm	Shift length, ΔL, mm[2]	References
A. Effects of tubulation, insertion of distal stump, and ligation of distal tube end				
Collagen tube vs. no tubulation	≥13.4	≤6.0	>7.4	Chamberlain et al., 2000a
Distal stump inserted vs. open-ended tube	11.7	≤6.0	>5.7	Williams et al., 1984
Distal stump inserted vs. ligated distal end	11.7	≤6.0	>5.7	Williams et al., 1984
B. Tube wall composition				
Silicone tube (standard)	9.7	(9.7)[3]	0	Data and references in Figure 6.1
EVA copolymer[4] vs. silicone standard	≤11.0	(9.7)[3]	≤1.3	Aebischer et al., 1989
PLA, plasticized[5] vs. silicone standard	≥13.4	(9.7)[3]	≥3.7	Seckel et al., 1984
LA/ε-CPL[6] vs. silicone standard	≥13.4	(9.7)[3]	≥3.7	den Dunnen et al., 1993b
Collagen tube vs. silicone tube	≥13.4	8.0	≥5.4	Chamberlain et al., 1998b
C. Tube wall permeability				
Cell-permeability vs. impermeability	≥19.4	13.4	≥6.0	Jenq and Coggeshall, 1987
Cell-permeability vs. protein-permeability	≥11.4	13.4	≥3.9	Jenq et al., 1987
Protein-permeability vs. impermeability	7.5	8.9	−1.4	Jenq and Coggeshall, 1985a; Jenq et al., 1987
D. Schwann cell suspensions				
Schwann cell suspension vs. PBS	21.4	≤14.0	≥7.4	Ansselin et al., 1997
E. Tube filling: Solutions of proteins				
bFGF vs. no factor	14.3	≤11.0	>3.3	Aebischer et al., 1989
NGF vs. cyt C[7]	11.1	10.4	0.7	Hollowell et al., 1990
aFGF vs. no factor	15.5	≤11.0	≥4.5	Walter et al., 1993
F. Tube filling: Gels based on ECM components				
Fibronectin vs. cyt C[7]	19.1	18.6	0.5	Bailey et al., 1993
Laminin vs. cyt C[7]	18.6	18.6	0	Bailey et al., 1993
G. Tube filling: Insoluble substrates				
Collagen-GAG matrix vs. no matrix	16.1	≤11.0	≥5.1	Yannas et al., 1985, 1987a

TABLE 6.1. *Continued*

Experimental variable X^2 (describes tubulated gap)	L_c in presence of X, mm	L_c in absence of X, mm	Shift length, ΔL, mm^2	References
Oriented fibrin matrix across gap vs. oriented matrix only adjacent to each stump	15.5	≤11.0	≥4.5	Williams et al., 1987
Early-forming vs. late-forming fibrin matrix	15.5	12.5	3.0	Williams et al., 1987
Axially vs. randomly oriented fibrin	11.4	≤6.7	≥4.7	Williams, 1987
Rapidly degrading CG matrix (NRT[8]) vs. no CG matrix	≥13.4	8.5	≥4.9	Yannas et al., 1988; Chang et al., 1990; Chang and Yannas, 1992
Axial vs. radial orientation of pore channels in NRT[8]	≥13.4	10.0	≥3.4	Chang et al., 1990; Chang and Yannas, 1992
Laminin-coated collagen sponge vs. no laminin coating	11.7	≤6.0	>5.7	Ohbayashi et al., 1996
Polyamide filaments[9] vs. no filaments	18.4	≤11.0	≥7.4	Lundborg et al., 1997
NRT[8] in collagen tube vs. silicone tube[10] (cross-anastomosis)	>25	7.7	>17.3	Spilker, 2000

[1] Data from rat sciatic nerve. Regenerative activity of a configuration is expressed in terms of the critical axon elongation, L_c.

[2] X is a generic designation for a variety of features of the tubulated configuration. Regenerative activity increases with the shift length, ΔL, the difference between the L_c in the presence of the experimental variable X (second column) and in its absence (third column). Standard: the silicone tube, $L_c = 9.7$.

[3] Parentheses indicate use of the value for the silicone standard (used in the absence of internal control data in the investigation).

[4] EVA, ethylene-vinyl acetate copolymer (Aebischer et al., 1989).

[5] PLA, poly(lactic acid) (Seckel et al., 1984).

[6] LA/ε-CPL copolymer, copolymer of lactic acid and ε-caprolactone (den Dunnen et al., 1993a,b).

[7] Cyt C, cytochrome C.

[8] NRT, nerve regeneration template, a graft copolymer of type I collagen and chondroitin 6-sulfate, differing from dermis regeneration template by a higher degradation rate and an axial (rather than random) orientation of pore channel axes along the nerve axis.

[9] Eight polyamide filaments, each 250 μm in diameter, placed inside the silicone tube.

[10] Obtained by implanting the experimental tube in the cross-anastomosis (CA) surgical procedure (Lundborg et al., 1982a) in which both contralateral sciatic nerves of the rat are transected; the right sciatic nerve is transected proximally at the sciatic notch allowing the right distal segment to be placed near the left proximal stump inside the opposite ends of the experimental tube. The CA procedure allows study of gap lengths over 20 mm.

TABLE 6.2. Relation between length shift and defect closure by nerve regeneration.[1]

Configuration	Extent of defect closure by each closure mode			Critical axon elongation, L_c, mm	Length shift, ΔL, mm
	% Contraction	% Scar	% Regeneration		
No tube	95	5	0	≤ 6.0	≤ -2.0
Silicone tube	53	0	47	8.0	0
Collagen tube	0	0	100	≥ 13.4	≥ 5.4

[1] Data from three experimental configurations using tubes filled with PBS to bridge the 10-mm gap in the rat sciatic nerve (estimates based on 42-d data from Chamberlain et al., 2000a).

from the defect closure rule lead to the same rank ordering of tubulated configurations as do values of the critical axon elongation, L_c, and the length shift, ΔL. However, a more extensive body of data would be required to yield a definitive result.

6.1.6 Long-Term Assays (>20wk): Fidelity of Regeneration

Having described above an assay for the self-consistent evaluation of tubulated configurations from short-term data (typically <20wk), we now proceed to selection of long-term assays. These assays report the extent to which the regenerate has achieved physiological function, as shown by a comparison of functional data for the regenerate with normal values.

Long-term assays are based on the concept of "fidelity of regeneration," defined simply as the fractional value of a property Y of the regenerate relative to its normal value, as follows: Fidelity of regeneration (% *FR*) = (value of property Y in regenerate/value of property Y in normal organ). Properties Y have included those based on both morphological and functional assays and are presented in Table 6.3.

6.1.7 Summary Description of Assays

We summarize assays that can be used to describe the synthesis of various component tissues of peripheral nerves as well as the synthesis of entire nerve trunks.

In vitro synthesis of nerve fibers has been described by means of qualitative assays based on relatively standardized morphological criteria. In contrast, in vivo synthesis of PNS components has been reported in a large variety of assays; although the assays have been quantitative, their large variety makes it nearly impossible to identify the simplest conditions required to induce synthesis of specific tissues. An additional difficulty arises from the absence of assays in the literature that describe synthesis of nonregenerative tissues, such as the endoneurium.

These difficulties in comparing data from the literature have been partly overcome by introducing an assay based on corrected values of the fre-

TABLE 6.3. Long-term (>20 weeks) studies of induced regeneration of peripheral nerves in experimental animals: Electrophysiological data.[1]

Experimental parameters				Electrophysiological properties (fraction of normal value)			
Animal model (length of study, wk)	Gap length, mm	Tube	Tube filling	Latency	Conduction velocity	Amplitude	References
Sciatic, rat (43)	10	Silicone	None	(1)	0.64	0.09	Fields and Ellisman, 1986a; Fields et al., 1989
Sciatic, rat (40)	10	Silicone	NRT[2]: 5 μm 10 μm 60 μm 300 μm	1.38 1.39 1.51 1.64	0.59 0.63 0.57 0.54	0.22 0.55 0.42 0.20	Chang et al., 1990; Chang and Yannas, 1992
Sciatic, rat (60)	10	Silicone	NRT[2]: 35 μm	—	0.48	0.27	Chamberlain et al., 1998b
Sciatic, mouse (21.4)	6	Silicone	None	—	—	0.07	Navarro et al., 1996
Sciatic, mouse (21.4)	6	PTFE[3]	None	—	—	0.02	Navarro et al., 1996
Rabbit, tibial (36)	10	PGL[4]	None	—	—	(1)	Molander et al., 1983
Monkey, median (52)	<1	PGA[5]	None	—	0.94	0.32	Tountas et al., 1993
Mouse, sciatic (21.4)	6	LA/ε-CPL[6]	None	—	—	0.18	Navarro et al., 1996
Monkey, median (200)	5	Collagen	None	1.40	0.93	0.91	Archibald et al., 1995
Rat, sciatic (60)	10	Collagen	None	—	0.60	0.27	Chamberlain et al., 1998b
Rat, sciatic (60)	10	Collagen	NRT[2]: 35 μm	—	0.75	0.36	Chamberlain et al., 1998b
Mouse, sciatic (21.4)	6	Collagen	None	—	—	0.07	Navarro et al., 1996
Cat, sciatic (69)	25	PGA[5] mesh/ collagen	NGF/ bFGF laminin	1.7	<1	(ca. 1)	Kiyotani et al., 1996

[1] Expressed as fraction of normal value (fidelity of regeneration).
[2] NRT, nerve regeneration template, a graft copolymer of type I collagen and chondroitin 6-sulfate, differing from dermis regeneration template by a higher degradation rate and axial (rather than random) orientation of pore channel axes along the nerve axis. Data in the table entry are reported for NRT at four values of average pore diameter: 5, 10, 60 and 300 μm. In other table entries, the average pore diameter of NRT was 35 μm.
[3] PTFE, poly(tetrafluoroethylene).
[4] PGL, polyglactin 910.
[5] PGA, poly(glycolic acid).
[6] LA/ε-CPL, copolymer of lactic acid and ε-caprolactone.

quency of reinnervation, % N, across a tubulated gap in a peripheral nerve. The corrections applied have allowed comparison of % N data from investigators who have used different gap lengths and animal species. There is substantial direct evidence that a nerve trunk that has regenerated across a gap and contains myelinated axons along its length, thereby positively contributing to the assay for % N, also includes a regenerated perineurium. Evidence for synthesis of a conducting nerve trunk across a gap will therefore be postulated to be indirect evidence for synthesis of a perineurium.

To correct for the effect of variation in gap length and animal species in the literature data for % N, we have introduced the concept of the critical axon elongation, L_c, the gap length above which N drops below 50%. Independent data from the literature have shown that $L_c = 9.7 \pm 1.8$ mm for the rat and 5.4 ± 1.0 mm for the mouse. We have suggested that the relative regenerative activity of various tubulated configurations can be measured self-consistently by comparing L_c values for each of these configurations with the L_c value for the silicone tube; the latter has been proposed as a standard. The difference between these L_c values yields values of the length shift, ΔL, a measure of the regenerative activity of an experimental configuration relative to the standard. In data from several investigations, the L_c value for the test configuration has been compared to that of the internal control employed.

We have selected two assays to describe in vivo data, one each for the short and long term (over 20 wk). The first assay, described above, provides short-term information on whether the synthesis of a peripheral nerve trunk with myelinated nerve fibers has proceeded or not (percent reinnervation across a gap, % N). The second assay provides information about the extent of regeneration in the long term (e.g., the ability to conduct in a near-physiological fashion along the nerve trunk); it is expressed in terms of the fractional extent to which the newly synthesized nerve trunk functions normally (fidelity of regeneration, % FR).

6.2 Synthesis of Myelinated Nerve Fibers

Having concerned ourselves with problems of uniform presentation of results from assays reported by different investigators, we now turn to description of the processes that lead to synthesis of peripheral nerves and their tissue components. First we focus on the synthesis of nerve fibers, the simplest functional unit of a nerve, and the tissue immediately adjacent to them, the endoneurium.

A nerve trunk can be simply viewed as a cylinder of supporting tissue, ranging in diameter from a fraction of one mm to several mm, embedded in which are thousands of tiny cylinders, each with a diameter typically about 20 to 50 μm. The specialized function of a nerve, electrical conduction, takes place along these tiny cylinders, often referred to as nerve fibers or endoneurial tubes, each comprising a myelinated axon invested in a myelin sheath that, in turn, is ensheathed in a tubular basement membrane; the latter are surrounded by a specialized assembly of collagen fibers, the endoneurial stroma. Below we further review the structure of these elementary conducting units.

6.2.1 Structure of Myelinated and Nonmyelinated Axons and of the Endoneurium

Axons, the long processes of neuronal cells (neurons), are enveloped by Schwann cells, the specialized cells of the nervous system. Both in the intact nervous system and in a regenerating nerve, axons can be classified into those that are surrounded by a myelin sheath (myelinated) and those that are nonmyelinated. Axons comprise axoplasm that contains smooth endoplasmic reticulum and microtubules. Whether myelinated or not, axons are embedded in endoneurium, consisting of a delicate packing of loose vascular supporting tissue that includes collagen fibers. Several axons with their associated endoneurium are enclosed in a condensed layer of collagenous tissue, the perineurium, and the enclosed bundle of axons comprises a fascicle. Many peripheral nerves consist of more than one fascicle; in these nerves, fascicles are bound together by a collagenous tissue, the epineurium (Burkitt et al., 1993). Each of these three major compartments of a peripheral nerve that are bounded by endoneurium, perineurium, and epineurium, will be described below in the context of data related to their synthesis.

Myelinated axons are characterized by a diameter in the range 1 to 15 μm, and function as efficient conductors of signals that reach target organs, including muscles (motor axons) and sensory organs (sensory axons). During development, myelin is synthesized around axons whose diameter is greater than 0.7 μm, in response to a signal that includes a diffusible molecule (Garbay et al., 2000); furthermore, myelin synthesis is upregulated by contact between adjacent Schwann cell plasma membranes (Sasagasako et al., 1999). Differentiation of a Schwann cell into a myelinating cell requires simultaneous interactions with basement membrane and an axon destined for myelination (Fernandez-Valle et al., 1997).

The myelination of an individual axon is provided along its length by several Schwann cells. Each cell covers a segment along the axon length (internode); there are points located between successive Schwann cells that are not covered by myelin (nodes of Ranvier). Myelination accelerates conduction by preventing propagation of the action potential along the axon, instead forcing the potential to travel by jumping from node to node (salutatory conduction). The myelin sheath consists of the plasma membrane of the Schwann cell that is tightly wrapped around the axon perimeter at the inernode; these concentric layers are free of Schwann cell cytoplasm. Schwann cells wrapped around an individual axon are ensheathed in a tubular basement membrane that forms a continuous cover of the myelinated axon, even at the nodes. During the process of myelination, concentric layers of Schwann cell cytoplasm and plasma membrane envelop the axon; the cytoplasm is then excluded and the inner surfaces of plasma membrane fuse with each other, providing a multiplicity of membrane leaflets that comprise the mature myelin sheath.

The basement membrane surrounding a myelinated axon is very similar to that in skin but is tubular in shape rather than being primarily a flat surface with indentations (rete ridges), as in skin. Schwann cell basement membrane contains type IV collagen, laminin, type V collagen, entactin, heparan sulfate proteoglycan, and fibronectin (Bunge and Bunge, 1983; McGarvey et al., 1984; Baron-Van Evercooren et al., 1986; Olsson, 1990; Obremski and Bunge, 1995). Type IV collagen comprises the fine collagen meshwork that is exclusive to basement membranes in various organs. Laminin binds to type IV collagen via entactin; it also binds to other macromolecular constituents of the basement membrane.

Nonmyelinated axons function in the autonomic nervous system and in small pain nerves. They comprise fibers of relatively small diameter, typically less than 1 μm. These axons are also surrounded by Schwann cells. Unlike myelinated axons, however, the supporting Schwann cells have retained their cytoplasm; they ensheathe the axon but are not wrapped tightly several times around it, and myelin is also absent. Several nonmyelinating axons are frequently surrounded by a single Schwann cell (ensheathment) while the external surface of the latter is encased in a basement membrane (Burkitt et al., 1993). Below we will focus on myelinating axons.

Using standardized nomenclature, we describe a nerve fascicle as being surrounded by a perineurial sheath that forms the border between the endoneurium inside and the epineurium outside (Olsson, 1990). Both myelinated and unmyelinated axons are enclosed in the space inside the fascicle (intrafascicular space) that is bounded by the perineurial sheath (see below). Nerve fibers are closely surrounded by the endoneurial stroma (Figure 6.2, top), an extracellular matrix resembling a fiber-reinforced gel, comprising collagens, fibronectins, proteoglycans, and other macromolecular components, as well as fibroblasts, macrophages, and mast cells (Olsson, 1990). Collagen fibrils in the intrafascicular space comprise both collagens type I and III and have diameters averaging 50 nm (Thomas and Jones, 1967; Salonen et al., 1987a,b); following detailed study, a value of 56.1 ± 6.9 nm was also reported (Bradley et al., 1998). The three-dimensional architecture of collagen fibrils surrounding nerve fibers has been shown to consist of two distinct sheaths: The outer one comprises bundles of longitudinally oriented collagen fibrils whereas the inner sheath is a delicate network of interwoven collagen fibrils. Some of the collagen fibrils forming the inner network are closely attached to the basement membrane of Schwann cells. The entire architectural arrangement suggests that the two collagen sheaths serve to tether and position the nerve fibers inside the intrafascicular compartment (Ushiki and Ide, 1986).

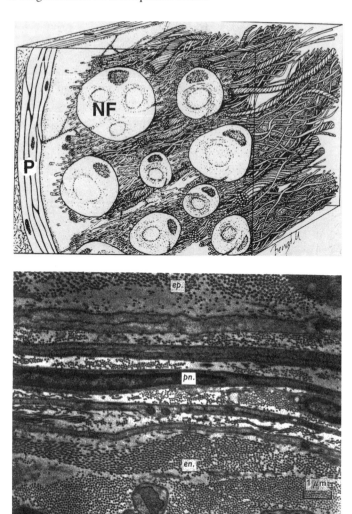

FIGURE 6.2. Structures of physiological endoneurium and perineurium. *Top* Diagram suggesting the main features of the endoneurial stroma surrounding nerve fibers. Each nerve fiber (NF) is embedded in a matrix composed of fluid, collagen fibers of the endoneurial stroma, blood vessels and cells; all these form the endoneurial microenvironment. The inner surface of the perineurium is shown on the left (P). (From Olsson, 1990.) *Bottom* Cross-sectional view of the perineurium (pn.) of rat sural nerve. Collagen fibers comprising the epineurium (ep.) and endoneurium (en.) are also shown. In this cross-sectional view, perineurial cells appear as highly elongated structures that are very intimately juxtaposed. See section 6.3.1 in text. Bar: 1 μm. (From Thomas and Jones, 1967.)

The intrafascicular space receives fluid components from the endoneurial blood vessels. The fluid comprises water, various ions and plasma proteins, as well as other soluble compounds. It is maintained under a small but finite net hydrostatic pressure; this arrangement stands in contrast to other connective tissue–rich compartments, such as subcutaneous tissue, where a net pressure does not appear to exist. Numerous vessels pierce the perineurium and join the endoneurial vascular network. The endothelial cells of endoneurial vessels are thin, contain vesicles that may be involved in transport phenomena across the endothelium, and are bound by tight junctions. Junctions between the cells contribute to a permeability barrier that protects the space immediately outside the nerve fibers from leakage of certain substances inside the endoneurial blood vessels (blood-nerve barrier, similar but much less restrictive than the blood-brain barrier). Maintenance of a constant environment around the nerve fibers provides protection from changes in ionic strength or from other substances (pathogens) that can modify the conductivity of nerve fibers or otherwise injure them (Olsson, 1990).

The nerve trunk can be viewed as comprising two separate vascularized compartments, the epineurium and the endoneurium, kept separated by the permeability barrier of the perineurium (Figure 6.2, bottom) (see below). Testing procedures, based on the selective permeability of these compartments to standard tracers, can be used to detect the presence of endoneurial blood vessels with tight junctions (Azzam et al., 1991). Soon after intravenous injection of albumin or horseradish peroxides, the epineurium shows signs of substantial leakage from blood vessels in it (extravasation), while the mass of tracer extravasated from the endoneurium is much smaller. Thus, the endoneurial environment is protected from various pathogens both by the perineurial barrier and by the barrier provided by its own endoneurial blood vessels (Olsson, 1990; Azzam et al., 1991).

6.2.2 Synthetic Pathways to Myelinated Axons and Basement Membrane

Myelinated axons with their associated basement membrane have been synthesized both in vitro and in vivo.

Explanted neurons providing an outgrowth of axons have been a basic component used in studies of synthesis of myelinated axons in vitro (Bunge and Bunge, 1978). Explants have been established in culture using various media, including human placental serum, and have been treated with antimitotic agents to eliminate nonneuronal cells (Obremski and Bunge, 1995). Axonal processes (neurites) have grown radially from the explant, serving as the source of axons for the experimental protocol. Schwann cells can be obtained from another explanted neuron, purified, dissociated, and cultured in media such as fetal calf serum or a defined medium before addition to the neuron culture under study. A neuron such as the sensory dorsal root ganglion stimulates synthesis of a myelin sheath around its neurites and is, therefore, useful for in vitro studies of myelination; in contrast, the sympathetic superior cervical ganglion supports outgrowth of axons that are predominantly nonmyelinated and provides a model for study of ensheathment, rather than myelination, of axons by Schwann cells (Obremski and Bunge, 1995).

Synthesis of a myelin sheath around axons in vitro has been reliably obtained by exposing the axons and Schwann cells in culture to a surface plated with type I collagen (Bunge and Bunge, 1978). The presence of an ECM component as a hypothetical requirement for myelination of axons by Schwann cells was supported by the data (Moya et al., 1980). In another study, a reconstructed basement membrane was added as a reactant in a neuron-Schwann cell culture that led to synthesis of a myelin sheath (Carey et al., 1986). A variety of culture media were studied in an effort to clarify the requirements for myelination and several observations were made suggesting that axons and Schwann cells suffice for myelination (Carey and Todd, 1987; Eldridge et al., 1987, 1989; Clark and Bunge, 1989). The hypothesis for an ECM requirement was further challenged in a study of the embryonic dorsal root ganglion neuron that was cultured with Schwann cells, in which use was made of a fully defined medium, rather than serum; as a result, synthesis of extracellular matrix was effectively suppressed. Myelination was nevertheless observed to occur in this study, showing that ECM synthesis, including synthesis of a basement membrane, may be linked to myelination but is not a prerequisite for synthesis of a myelin sheath in vitro (Podratz et al., 1998).

Basement membrane has been synthesized in vitro when both neurons and Schwann cells were present in culture (Bunge et al., 1980, 1982; Cornbrooks et al., 1983; Carey and Todd, 1987; Eldridge et al., 1987, 1989; Clark and Bunge, 1989). In the absence of neurons, Schwann cells have been observed to synthesize components of the basement membrane (McGarvey et al., 1984); even synthesis of a filamentous matrix resembling a basement membrane has been observed (Baron-Van Evercooren et al., 1986). The presence of neurons was, however, not required to synthesize basement membrane when fibroblasts were cultured with Schwann cells; even the presence of fibroblasts was not required when purified laminin was added to the neuron-free Schwann cell culture (Obremski et al., 1993; Obremski and Bunge, 1995).

The preceding discussion has been limited to in vitro conditions. However, in vivo synthesis of conducting nerve fibers has been described in a very large number of experimental protocols, most of which consisted of a tubulated nerve gap generated by transection. Under these conditions, not only nerve fibers but other tissue components of a peripheral nerve were also synthesized. The description of these in vivo pathways for synthesis of nerve fibers will be presented in a later section, in the context of procedures for synthesis of an entire nerve trunk.

In one noteworthy protocol conducted in vivo, however, a specialized experimental configuration was used to ensure that Schwann cells would be isolated from axons. The silicone chamber bridging a 10-mm gap in the rat sciatic nerve was prepared by tubulation of the transected nerve stumps. The chamber was exogenously filled with a collagen matrix seeded with Schwann cells; however, the tube was closed at both ends by a Millipore filter that excluded axons and allowed entry of exudate from the stumps. Even though axons were absent from this in vivo configuration, it was observed that BM was synthesized around the Schwann cells (Ikeda et al., 1989).

6.2.3 Observations Related to Synthesis of an Endoneurial Stroma

Very little attention has been focused in the literature on synthesis, either in vitro or in vivo, of an endoneurial stroma, the vascularized connective tissue immediately surrounding the nerve fibers. Although the architecture of normal endoneurial stroma has been outlined, as described above (Ushiki and Ide, 1986) (Figure 6.2, top), the morphological characterization of collagen fibrils and other endoneurial structures (e.g., endoneurial blood vessels) has been missing from studies in peripheral nerve regeneration.

There have been occasional reports of synthesis of abnormally thin collagen fibers, approximately 18 nm in diameter, outside the basement membrane of Schwann cells maintained in culture with neurons (Bunge and Bunge, 1978; Bunge et al., 1980; Moya et al., 1980); however, there is no evidence that an endoneurial stroma has been synthesized in vitro. It is not clear whether a structurally integrated endoneurium, consisting of the entire intrafascicular contents and assembled either around a nerve fiber or in its absence, can be observed in the absence of a perineurial sheath. The presence of a positive intrafascicular pressure (Olsson, 1990) indicates that a nonpermeable enclosure is required for structural stability of this tissue and suggests that an endoneurium may not be stable enough to be observed experimentally without a perineurium.

Observations made in vivo showed that, in nerve trunks that had been induced to regenerate across gaps tubulated by a silicone tube, the trunk cross section comprised minifascicles very similar in structure to those that had been observed in the absence of tubulation (i.e., under conditions of spontaneous healing) (Figure 6.3), (Cajal, 1928; Morris et al., 1972d). Morphological data describing these minifascicles are rarely reported at sufficiently high magnification to show collagen fibrils comprising the endoneurial stroma that may possibly be present. In one such study (Jenq and Coggeshall, 1984), the diameters of collagen fibrils adjacent to axons appeared to be in the range 25 to 35 nm. In another study the diameters were reported to be about 40 nm (Scaravilli, 1984). These values were close to the diameter range of endoneurial collagen fibrils reported in the proximal

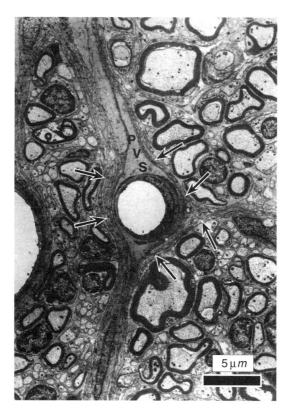

FIGURE 6.3. Regeneration of perineurial sheaths. The observation was made 26 wk after bridging a 10-mm gap in the rat sciatic nerve with a silicone tube. The perineurial sheaths of three minifascicles are indicated by the arrows. The blood vessel (hole in center) is excluded from the endoneurial space of the axons. A tracer was used to study the permeability barriers in the regenerated trunk; the blood vessel was permeable to the tracer but was retained in the perivascular space and did not enter the endoneurial space. Bar: 5 μm. (Copyright 1991. Wiley-Liss, Inc. From Azzam et al., 1991. Nerve cables formed in silicone chambers reconstitute a perineurial but not a vascular endoneurial permeability barrier. *Journal of Comparative Neurology* 314:807–819. Reprinted with permission of Wiley-Liss, Inc., a subsidiary of John Wiley & Sons, Inc.)

stump (Morris et al., 1972d) or fibrils synthesized in the distal stump (Salonen et al., 1985, 1987a) in studies of spontaneously healing transected nerves (see also Chapter 2). Although the data are very limited, the available evidence showed that the diameters of these fibrils did not match those reported in normal endoneurial stroma, observed to average 51.5 nm (Thomas and Jones, 1967) or, in another study, 56.1 ± 6.9 nm (Bradley et al., 1998).

A functional study of endoneurial stroma regeneration following tubulation in a silicone tube was based on the property of normal endoneurium to maintain a blood-nerve barrier, as described above (Azzam et al., 1991). In this study the presence of permeability barriers was determined using a tracer (horseradish peroxidase), intravenously injected and histochemically detected by light and electron microscopy. The nerve trunk had been induced to regenerate across a 10-mm gap bridged by a silicone tube. Prior to implantation, the tube was filled with dialyzed plasma, a filling previously shown to facilitate superior regeneration across the gap compared with other fillings used with silicone tubes (see Table 6.1) (Williams, 1987; Williams et al., 1987). At 26 wk, the axons and associated Schwann cells had formed minifascicles, as described above (Figure 6.3). However, blood vessels that were present in the epineurium were excluded from the immediate vicinity of the axons and there was no evidence that endoneurial blood vessels had been synthesized. Use of the tracer showed that the perineurial-like sheath was impermeable to the tracer and no tracer was detected inside the minifacicles. Detailed analysis of tracer patterns in regenerated and intact nerve led to the conclusion that the regenerate possessed a perineurial but not an endoneurial permeability barrier (Azzam et al., 1991). These data showed that bridging with a silicone tube failed to induce regeneration of physiological endoneurial vascular structures under conditions that sufficed to regenerate a functional perineurium.

Several authors have referred to the space surrounding the axons regenerated in their studies as "endoneurial space," "interstitial space," or "interaxonal space" but generally have not reported morphological data supporting the presence of a physiological endoneurial stroma.

In conclusion, there appears to be little or no direct evidence supporting the regeneration of endoneurial stroma or endoneurial vasculature in adults.

6.3 Synthesis of a Perineurium; the Epineurium

The number of publications dealing with the structure, function, or synthesis of the perineurium are a very small fraction of those focused on synthesis of nerve fibers. Nor has much attention been paid to synthesis of the epineurium. In this section we will focus on evidence related to the synthesis of these supporting tissues. Their main structural features have been briefly summarized in an earlier chapter. However, in order to establish a factual basis for the ensuing discussion of their synthesis, below we review these features and their functional correlates in greater detail.

6.3.1 Structure and Function of the Perineurium

The relation between the structural elements of the perineurium and their function is largely understood. The perineurium is a thin sheath that encases a large number of axons embedded in loose collagenous tissue (endoneurium), forming thereby a fascicle. It is a highly specialized cylindrical structure, comprising concentric layers (lamellae) of flattened polygonal cells interspersed with collagen fibrils (Figure 6.2, bottom). In cross-sectional view, perineurial cells appear as highly elongated structures that are very intimately juxtaposed, either by extensive overlapping of their contiguous margins or by interdigitation of cell processes. Occasionally, the gap separating the surface membranes of cells becomes as small as 9 nm, corresponding to "tight junctions" (*zonulae occludentes*). A feature of these cells is the presence of multiple endocytotic vesicles, considered as a possible transport system across the cells. The number of lamellae increases with the diameter of the fascicle; they number as few as 3 to 5 in the rat sural nerve (Thomas and Jones, 1967) but as many as up to 15 layers in mammalian nerve trunks (Thomas and Olsson, 1975; Olsson, 1990).

A rich content of collagen fibrils is present in the spaces that separate the cell lamellae (Figure 6.2, bottom). The diameters of fibrils are in the range 40 to 65 nm, approximately the same as in fibrils of the endoneurium but significantly smaller than those of the epineurium, where diameters average 80 nm (Thomas and Jones, 1967). The sharp gradient in diameter of collagen fibrils along the radial direction, observed to abruptly change at the outermost perineurial lamellae, has been used as the point of demarcation between the perineurium and the epineurium (Thomas and Jones, 1967). Collagen fibrils are assembled in interlamellar spaces in a lattice-like arrangement and are both longitudinally and obliquely oriented to the axis of the nerve trunk. Elastic fibers, and occasionally fibroblasts and mast cells, are also observed in the spaces between lamellae (Thomas and Olsson, 1975; Olsson, 1990).

Basement membrane (basal lamina) lines the surfaces of the cylindrical structure of the perineurium, both inside (endoneurial side) and outside (epineurial side). Unlike perineurial cells, perineurial fibroblasts are not encased in a basement membrane. Blood vessels traverse the perineurium; they connect the network of relatively large blood vessels in the epineurium with the longitudinally oriented capillary network inside the fascicles (i.e., in the endoneurium) (Thomas and Olsson, 1975; Olsson, 1990).

A major contribution of the perineurium to nerve function is maintenance of a constant chemical composition in the intrafascicular space, and therefore, of a constant level of the electrical conductivity of the nerve fibers. By forming a wall around the endoneurial space, it contributes to homeostasis at the site of conduction even when there are variations in the fluid composition outside it (e.g., during an inflammatory process). An agent with the capacity to change the electric action potential is, therefore, usually either unable to diffuse into the endoneurium or can do so only at greatly reduced rate of entry (Olsson, 1990).

The passive diffusion barrier property of the perineurium primarily depends on the close contacts between perineurial cells, described above, as well as ensheathing of these cells each in their own basement membrane. Substances moving into or out of the intrafascicular space must, therefore, always pass through at least one thickness of basement membrane. In addition, however, perineurial cells contain a wide range of phosphorylating enzymes and are considered to be well equipped to act as a metabolically active, rather than simply passive, diffusion barrier. The permeability of the perineurium has generally increased after crushing or stretching of the nerve or even after administration of a local anesthetic. Following nerve transection, or other form of trauma, blood vessels in the nerve trunk, including the perineurium, swell and become quite permeable (edema) (Olsson, 1990). Increases in vascular permeability largely account for the flow of exudate into a tubulated gap, generated by transecting the nerve trunk, a process that is repeatedly referred to below as well as in Chapter 10.

The reversible and irreversible effects of mechanical trauma on perineurial permeability have been studied. A reversible increase in permeability of a peripheral nerve was observed after stretching by 10%; however, the change became irreversible following stretching to 20% (Olsson, 1990).

6.3.2 The Epineurium

Peripheral nerves often consist of more than one fascicle. In such cases, the multifascicular bundle is surrounded by a strong cylindrical sheath, the epineurium. This outer sheath is thicker in nerves consisting of large numbers of fascicles. It comprises a layer of collagenous tissue, rather loose in the interior but much more condensed toward its periphery. It receives a rich supply of blood vessels from surrounding tissues and many of these vessels enter the perineurium (Burkitt et al., 1993).

The collagen bundles of the epineurium are predominantly oriented along the major nerve axis. As mentioned above, a significant and sharp decrease in average diameter of collagen fibers of the epineurium in the direction toward the interior of the nerve trunk has been used to distinguish the inner layers of the epineurium from the outer lamellae of the perineurium (Thomas and Jones, 1967). Fibroblasts, mast cells, and elastic fibers also have been observed in the epineurium.

There are significant structural and functional differences between the perineurium and the epineurium. Lymphatic vessels, used in tissue drainage, have been identified in the epineurium but not in the perineurium (Thomas and Olsson, 1975). Unlike the uniquely structured perineurium which acts as a permeability barrier protecting the endoneurial space, the epineurium has been described as a rather typical connective tissue, mainly useful in providing resistance to deformation, particularly in compression (Sunderland, 1990).

6.3.3 In Vitro and In Vivo Studies of Synthesis of a Perineurium

In vitro studies of synthesis of perineurial tissue appear to have been very few, and the synthesis of an epineurium in vitro appears not to have been studied. A few studies have dealt with the synthesis of the perineurium in vivo.

A perineurium was not synthesized in vitro when neurons were cultured with Schwann cells (Bunge et al., 1980). Nor was a perineurium synthesized when neurons were cultured with fibroblasts in the absence of Schwann cells (Williams et al., 1982). However, when fibroblasts were added to the culture medium that included neurons and Schwann cells, the neurons became ensheathed by Schwann cells while flattened cells with basement membrane and occasional junctions enclosed the neuron–Schwann cell units. Collagen fibrils were also synthesized (Williams et al., 1982). Although the investigators suggested that they had synthesized a fascicle complete with endoneurial space, their brief report did not provide the morphological evidence required for a detailed assessment of their conclusions.

Sensory neurons, Schwann cells, and fibroblasts were combined in a study directed toward the origin of perineurial cells; after 6 weeks in culture, perineurial cells were identified in quasi-circular arrangements, resembling fascicular sheaths, within which numerous myelinating and nonmyelinating Schwann cells were observed. The conclusion was reached that the perineurium is derived from fibroblasts and not from Schwann cells (Bunge et al., 1989). The structures presented in this study (Bunge et al., 1989) were apparently not sufficiently differentiated to make them similar to those of a mature perineurium, as these are described elsewhere (Thomas and Jones, 1967).

Significant evidence for synthesis of a perineurium in vivo was obtained in a 26-week study of the transected 10-mm gap in the rat sciatic nerve, bridged by a silicone tube (Azzam et al., 1991) (Figure 6.3). In this study, the newly synthesized nerve trunk comprised an outer circumferential layer of connective tissue and an inner core in which all myelinated and nonmyelinated axons were gathered into minifascicles surrounded by sheaths of perineurial cells. The structure that was interpreted as a perineurium consisted of a sheath surrounding bundles of axons with Schwann cells in each minifascicle. The sheath comprised 3 to 5 lamellae of flattened cells with tight junctions and endocytotic vesicles, each cell possessing basement membrane on its inner and outer surfaces. Collagen fibrils between the lamellae were not reported in this study. Strong support for the interpretation of the sheath as a physiological perineurium was obtained in the same study by observing that the sheath was a competent permeability barrier (Azzam et al., 1991). In the same study, the region of the trunk lying between the outer circumferential connective tissue layer and the inner neural core was explored in a search for the single perineurial sheath of large diameter, surrounding the entire cylindrical trunk, that might have hypothetically been regenerated in its original location. No distinct perineurium was observed at this location (Azzam et al., 1991).

A description of newly synthesized perineurial sheaths was reported in a study in which a 5-mm gap in the rat sciatic nerve was bridged by wrapping a ribbon of plastic film (not further identified) around the stumps, thereby creating a tube that contained a short segment of the severed nerve at each end. After 4 weeks, slender cell processes with all the characteristics of perineurial cells were observed surrounding bundles of nerve fibers. The cells were almost completely lined by basement membrane, their cytoplasm contained numerous endocytotic vesicles, and their thin processes were in contact with one another at their edges by means of tight junctions (*zonules occludentes*); there was also an abundance of collagen fibrils between the cell layers (Scaravilli, 1984).

Regeneration of an epineurial sheath has not been reported; however, it should be recalled that most of the studies with tubulated nerves were conducted with unifascicular nerves that lack a prominent epineurium.

In several studies, a thick sheath of tissue, with the obvious appearance of a very tight, multilayer wrapping, was reported surrounding the entire nerve trunk that was regenerated inside silicone tubes (Lundborg et al., 1982a). Authors have occasionally referred to this outer cover as a perineurial sheath. The structure of the sheath was examined and found to consist of circumferential cells that lacked, however, the encasement in basement membrane and intercellular tight junctions characteristic of mature perineurium (Williams et al., 1983). The cells comprising the multilaminated outer tissue of nerve trunk regenerated in a silicone tube were eventually identified as contractile cells (myofibroblasts), a characteristic of the early as well as chronic response of the nerve to transection (Chamberlain et al., 2000a). Further discussion of the significance of the myofibroblast capsule around the nerve trunk in the mechanism of nerve regeneration appears in Chapter 10.

In conclusion, confirmed synthesis of a perineurium inside a nerve trunk regenerated in tubulated configurations has been reported. The morphology of the perineurial sheath, as well as its permeability barrier, have both been reported to be close to normal. However, the single perineurial sheath that surrounded the original single fascicle was not regenerated; instead, the regenerated perineurium surrounded a large number of very small fascicles (minifascicles) inside the trunk.

Regeneration of an epineurium has not been reported. The outer sheath reported around a regenerated nerve trunk inside a silicone tube appears to comprise several concentric layers of contractile cells, representing a chronic response to injury rather than a regenerated perineurial or epineurial sheath.

6.4 Synthesis of a Nerve Trunk

Nerve fibers cannot survive long, much less function, in vivo without mul-
tifaceted sustenance by the supporting tissues of the nerve trunk. The evidence presented in the preceding section supports the view that a newly
synthesized nerve trunk, innervated along its entire length and capable of
conducting electrophysiological signals in a near-physiological manner,
contains not only myelinated axons but also a functional perineurium
surrounding minifascicles (Figures 6.3 and 6.4). Below we review the
conditions for synthesis of an innervated nerve trunk, an organ comprising
both nonregenerative tissues and nerve fibers.

Studies of peripheral nerve regeneration reviewed below have followed
the paradigm of tubulation of transected stumps. In this protocol, the freshly
transected stumps are inserted in a tube and the gap between the two
stumps is adjusted to a certain length that appears to provide favorable conditions for testing the experimental configuration under conditions of
regeneration across the gap. Investigators have traditionally experimented
with the contents of the gap, inserting growth factors (soluble regulators),
cell suspensions, and matrices (insoluble regulators). The chemical composition and permeability of the tube wall have also been varied in a few
instances and their effect on nerve regeneration has been noted.

Below we summarize the results of studies in which several experimental
tubulated configurations were studied. These configurations are compared
by making consistent use of the length shift, ΔL, a quantity independent of
the gap length used by the investigator. The magnitude of ΔL is a measure
of the regenerative activity of a tubulated configuration relative to the silicone tube standard (Table 6.1). Positive and negative values of ΔL signify
upregulation and downregulation, respectively, of regenerative activity over
that for the silicone tube standard.

As described above, as well as in detail in the appendix, ΔL for the
10-mm gap bridged by the silicone tube standard (filled with saline or PBS)
is, by definition, zero. Values of ΔL within ± 2 mm from zero for the rat sciatic
nerve (± 1 mm from zero for the mouse data) are considered not to be significantly different from zero. ΔL values in the range 2 to 4 mm for rat studies
and 1 to 2 mm for mouse studies will be referred to below as "significant"
(corresponding to a regeneratively "active" configuration); values above 4
mm for rat studies and 2 mm for mouse studies will be referred to as "very
significant" (regeneratively "very active" configuration). Representative
values of ΔL for several devices are presented in Table 6.1.

6.4.1 Exogenous Supply of Soluble Regulators

There is strong evidence that several soluble regulators control the growth
of nerve fibers in vitro. Nerve growth factor (NGF) (Levi-Montalcini and

FIGURE 6.4. A nerve trunk regenerated inside a silicone tube comprises several minifascicles, each surrounded by a perineurial sheath. *Top*: Minifascicles comprise several axons and associated Schwann cells (8 wk). *Bottom*: At a much later time (39 wk), the average axon diameter has increased slightly while the minifascicular structure persists. Bar: 20 μm. (Reprinted from Jenq and Coggeshall, 1985b. Long-term patterns of axon regeneration in the sciatic nerve and its tributaries. *Brain Research* 345:36, Copyright 1985, with permission from Elsevier Science.)

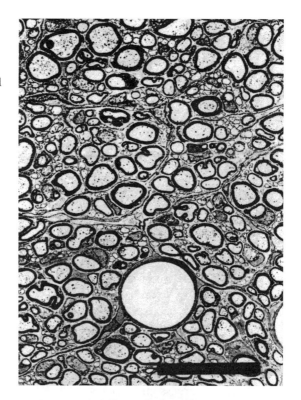

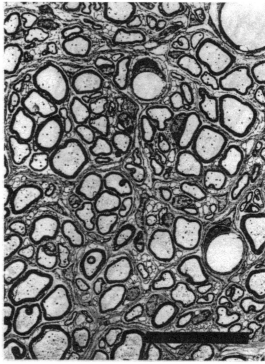

Hamburger, 1951; Cohen, 1959) has been the most frequently used model of a neuron-directed trophic agent. Several other factors also have been shown to promote survival of axotomized neurons as well as to act on non-neuronal cells that are associated with nerve regeneration. Other factors that comprise the so-called neurotrophin family include brain-derived nerve growth factor (BDNGF), neurotrophin 4/5 (NT-4/5), and neurotrophin 3 (NT-3). After axotomy, the synthesis of these neurotrophic factors, as well as of several cytokines and growth factors, is upregulated both by the axotomized neurons and by nonneuronal cells, especially Schwann cells, both in the proximal and distal nerve stumps. The list of factors produced by the two stumps resulting from complete transection is long (Lundborg et al., 1982d; Longo et al., 1983a,b). Included among these are factors that have been associated with the inflammatory response in other organs: interleukins 1, 2, and 6 (IL-1, IL-2, IL-6), ciliary neurotrophic factor (CNTF), acidic fibroblast growth factor (aFGF), transforming growth factor-β (TGF-β), platelet derived growth factor (PDGF), glial growth factor (GGF), insulin-like growth factors (IGFs), interferon-γ (IFN-γ), and others (for review see Fu and Gordon, 1997). Both acidic fibroblast growth factor (aFGF, FGF-1) and basic fibroblast growth factor (bFGF, FGF-2) have significantly upregulated proliferation and migration in vitro of fibroblasts, endothelial cells, and Schwann cells, as well as astrocytes and oligodendrocytes (Burgess and Maciag, 1989; Klagsbrun, 1989).

The tubulated gap spontaneously and completely fills with fluid within about 12 h after tubulation. The potential sources of chamber fluid have been described as bleeding, leakage of endoneurial fluid, or leakage of outside fluid through the narrow space between the inner walls of the tube edges and the outer sheath of the inserted nerve stumps (Longo et al., 1983a,b). Both stumps contribute to the spontaneous presence of soluble regulators in the tubulated gap.

Investigators have augmented or supplemented the endogenous supply of insoluble regulators by adding regulators of their own choice (exogenous supply). Methods of delivery have varied widely among investigators. As a result of such wide range of conditions, very little information has become available that relates the choice of delivery schedule on the efficacy of the regulator being delivered.

In several studies, exogenous addition of nerve growth factor (NGF) was observed to have upregulated various processes of regeneration across the tubulated gap compared with the untreated controls. These positive findings, in studies that spanned a three- to five-week period, included an increase in the diameter of the regenerated nerve trunk by a factor of two (Chen et al., 1989), a twofold (Rich et al., 1989) or a threefold increase in myelinated axons in the regenerate (Derby et al., 1993), a significant increase in regeneration of sensory neurons (DaSilva and Langone, 1989), as well as a significant increase in the rate of axonal regeneration in NGF-treated animals (Whitworth et al., 1996). However, there was evidence that the regenerative advantage conferred by such early upregulation disappeared later; after four weeks, all regenerates had similar numbers of myelinated axons (Derby et al., 1993).

The regenerative effect of an exogenous NGF supply was not confirmed in any of the following three studies: a six-week study of two methods of NGF delivery in the transected mouse sciatic nerve (Santos et al., 1991); a three-week and a five-week study of the transected buccal division of the facial nerve in the rabbit (Spector et al., 1993); and a 10-day study of Schwann cell migration as well as a 17-week study of number of myelinated axons distal to injury in the transected rat sciatic nerve (Bailey et al., 1993). Furthermore, a review of estimated values of the critical axon elongation (L_c) for NGF treatment in Table 6.1 shows no significant increase in L_c due to NGF treatment relative to the untreated control (Hollowell et al., 1990).

Exogenous addition of bFGF enhanced regeneration across gaps (Danielsen et al., 1988; Aebischer et al., 1989). Alpha-1 acid glycoprotein appeared to lag behind bFGF in regenerative activity (Aebischer et al., 1989). Values of critical axon elongation in Table 6.1 show a significant shift in critical axon elongation, $\Delta L > 3.3$, following bFGF treatment (Aebischer et al., 1989).

Acidic fibroblast growth factor (aFGF) showed significant regenerative activity in two studies (Cordeiro et al., 1989; Walter et al., 1993) and a very significant value of ΔL, ≥ 4.5, confirmed this conclusion (Table 6.1; Walter et al., 1993). Treatment with brain-derived neurotrophic factor (BDNF) was reported to have improved recovery of nerve function (Utley et al., 1996). A combination of PDGF-BB and IGF-I had no effect on PNS regeneration (Wells et al., 1997).

6.4.2 Schwann Cell Addition to the Tubulated Gap

Axons cannot regenerate in the absence of Schwann cells: axon regeneration failed when Schwann cells were completely prevented from entering a nerve repair site (Hall, 1986a,b). However, Schwann cells do not require axons in order to grow into an injured nerve (Madison and Archibald, 1994). There is evidence that Schwann cells precede axons across the gap of the nerve tubulation model (Williams et al., 1983; Kljavin and Madison, 1991; Son and Thompson, 1995; Fu and Gordon, 1997). For these reasons, several investigators have incorporated Schwann cell preparations in the tubulated model of PNS regeneration.

Seeding with Schwann cells has been shown to have had a significant regenerative effect in three independent studies. The number of myelinated axons in the regenerates inside Schwann cell-seeded tubes was clearly higher than in the unseeded controls (Guénard et al., 1992; Kim et al., 1994).

Electrophysiological recovery was significantly higher than in controls that were unseeded with Schwann cells; however, the difference did not emerge until after almost nine weeks (Kim et al., 1994). By 52 weeks, a regenerate inside a cell-seeded tube reached a conduction velocity 60% of normal, a noteworthy result considering that it had formed across a gap as long as 18 mm in the rat sciatic nerve (Ansselin et al., 1997). Furthermore, a very significant increase in critical axon elongation of Schwann cell-seeded over unseeded experimental groups, amounting to $\Delta L \geq 7.4$, was observed (Table 6.1).

In contrast to these findings, no difference was detected in degree of myelination or in electrophysiological behavior between Schwann cell-seeded and unseeded groups in a 16-week study across a 3-cm gap in the rabbit hind limb (Brown et al., 1996). In another study, seeding a tube based on a copolymer of lactic acid and ε-caprolactone with autologous Schwann cells led to recovery of mouse sciatic nerve function that was slightly lower than innervation with autograft; however, seeding with syngeneic Schwann cells did not improve regeneration over acellular grafts (Rodriguez et al., 2000).

6.4.3 Filled and Unfilled Silicone Tubes

The term *silicones* is commonly used to describe the family of polysiloxanes, inorganic polymers distinguished by having atoms of silicon in their backbone. Silicone elastomers have been extensively used in diverse demanding industrial applications, such as coatings for surfaces at high-temperature, where inertness to environmental changes is at a premium (Stevens, 1990).

The Si—O bond is resistant to enzymes or to acid-base catalyzed hydrolytic cleavage. The reputation of stability to enzymatic attack and hydrolysis, together with inertness to a variety of chemicals, has historically made silicone elastomers the first polymer family to be used in fabrication of biomaterials. As a result, the early history of research on biomaterials and artificial organs has been dominated by the use of silicone elastomers (e.g., the use of a silicone tube to drain the cerebrospinal fluid in infants with hydrocephalus) (Pudenz, 1958). The encapsulation of silicone rubber implants by scar has been studied (Ginsbach et al., 1979; Mikuz et al., 1984).

Early uses of silicone tubes in studies of peripheral nerve regeneration have focused on attempts to add primarily mechanical support (cuffing) to an injured site after the two stumps had been opposed (anastomosis) by suturing (neurorrhaphy) (Ducker and Hayes, 1967, 1968a,b). Later, it became apparent that this technique could provide unprecedented information about the soluble factors that affect the regeneration of axons in vivo and that had been previously studied only in vitro. A classical series of studies ensued that established the use of the silicone tube ("regeneration chamber") in experimental studies of axon regeneration in vivo; in addition, the presence of a critical gap length, about 10 mm, beyond which regeneration did not occur in the silicone tube, was also established (Lundborg et al., 1982a,b,c,d; Longo et al., 1983a,b; Williams et al., 1983, 1987; Jenq and Coggeshall, 1984, 1985a; Lundborg, 1987, 1988; Williams, 1987). These studies emphasized observations during the first four weeks following tubulation repair and typically did not exceed eight weeks. They led to understanding of the early cellular events following tubulation and, more importantly, provided a powerful experimental paradigm that others have since used to study the cell and molecular biology of nerve regeneration (Fu and Gordon, 1997).

Silicone tubes have been widely used as bridges for gaps in the PNS both in experimental protocols and in clinical studies. The first detailed study of the early cellular events that lead to regeneration across a gap (Williams et al., 1983) as well as the first long-term study of morphological and conductivity properties of a PNS regenerate (Fields and Ellisman, 1986a,b; Fields et al., 1989) were conducted with the aid of silicone tubes. The results of clinical studies in PNS regeneration of silicone tubes have been reported in unusual depth (Lundborg et al., 1991, 1994).

Regenerates produced across a 10-mm gap bridged by silicone tubes have typically displayed axons that were smaller in diameter and had thinner myelin sheaths compared with normal controls. After 40 weeks, values of electrical conductivity (64% normal) and amplitude (9% normal) remained significantly lower than normal controls (Fields and Ellisman, 1986a,b; Fields et al., 1989). Nerve degeneration inside silicone tubes has been observed in longer studies (Le Beau et al., 1988; Merle et al., 1989).

Below we discuss the effect of various fillings for silicone tubes, including solutions used as internal controls by investigators; gels and insoluble substrates. Extensive use is made of ΔL values from Table 6.1.

Solutions used as *internal controls* by investigators typically led to ΔL values that were not significantly different from zero. A possible exception was the observation of a very modest upregulation of regeneration, $\Delta L \geq$ 1.5, when the silicone tube was filled with PBS compared with implanting an unfilled silicone tube (Williams et al., 1987). In another study, ΔL was a low 1.2 when the activity of a silicone tube prefilled with saline was compared with an initially unfilled silicone tube (Chang et al., 1990; Chang and Yannas, 1992). Nor did twofold dilution of PBS solution, used as tube contents, affect regenerative activity; it led to a ΔL value of −0.2 (Williams et al., 1987). A cytochrome C solution led to a value of 0.7, also insignificantly different from zero (Hollowell et al., 1990).

Gels based on macromolecular substances generally displayed little, if any, regenerative activity. Values of ΔL were not significantly different from zero when silicone tubes were prefilled with gels at the following concentrations: a laminin gel at 0.5 mg/ml, a fibronectin gel at 0.5 mg/ml or a fibronectin/laminin gel at a concentration of 0.5 mg/ml for each macromolecular solute (Bailey et al., 1993); a laminin gel at 4 mg/ml (Labrador et al., 1998); a collagen gel at 1.28 mg/ml as well as at 2.56 mg/ml (Labrador et al., 1998); a collagen gel at 3 mg/ml (Itoh et al., 1999); a hyaluronate gel at 5 mg/ml in the mouse sciatic nerve (Labrador et al., 1998); and a plasma fibrin matrix, prepared by injecting $CaCl_2$ into the tube before clotting (Labrador et al., 1998). Axons did not elongate beyond 6 to 7 mm along a 15-mm gap bridged by a silicone tube filled with a collagen gel, at 2.4 mg/ml, or a laminin-containing gel, at approximately 7 mg/ml laminin (Madison et al., 1988). In contrast to the above, a solution comprising a fibronectin/laminin gel at 0.5 mg/ml for each macromolecular solute led to a significant ΔL value of 2.8 (Woolley et al., 1990). Also noteworthy was the regeneration observed using a gel, predominantly based on laminin, as filling for a nonsilicone tube, yielding a ΔL value of >5.0 (Madison et al., 1985).

At relatively high concentration levels, certain gels apparently obstructed the elongation of neuronal and nonneuronal structures. Downregulation of regeneration was observed when collagen gels at 3.0 mg/ml and 17.5 mg/ml, as well as a laminin-containing gel at 7.0 mg/ml laminin concentration, were used to fill an acrylic copolymer; physical obstruction of axon elongation by undegraded particles was implicated by the histological data (Valentini et al., 1987). The use of agarose gels, at concentration levels between 0.5 to 2 wt.-%, led to significant regenerative activity compared with the untubulated control (Labrador et al., 1995); the activity significantly decreased with an increase in agarose concentration above 1 mg/ml, presumably reflecting the rapid decrease in pore diameter of the gels along the same direction and the corresponding increase in magnitude of a physical barrier to regeneration. In another study, regeneration was moderately downregulated relative to the saline control after filling the silicone tube with a collagen gel at 2.56 mg/ml as well as after filling with a laminin gel at 4 and 12 mg/ml (Labrador et al., 1998). The combined data (Valentini et al., 1987; Labrador et al., 1998) suggested that collagen becomes a barrier to regeneration at gel concentration levels above about 1 to 2 mg/ml while laminin hypothetically became a deterrent when its gel concentration exceeded 3 to 4 mg/ml.

The presence of *insoluble substrates* with or without axially oriented structures inside a silicone tube bridging the gap was associated with significant upregulation of regenerative activity. Manipulation of the composition of the exudate that flows into the tubulated gap, to give a highly oriented macromolecular fibrous bridge as early as 24 h rather than in 7 d, led to a significant length shift, ΔL, of 3.0 (Williams et al., 1987). Early formation of a fibrin matrix with axially oriented fibrin molecules led to a very significant length shift of ≥ 4.7 relative to early formation of a fibrin matrix in which fibrin molecules were unoriented (Williams, 1987). The formation of the oriented fibrin matrix across the entire gap contributed a very significant shift of ≥ 4.4 compared with an oriented fibrin matrix that was formed only adjacent to each stump (Williams et al., 1987). A tube filling comprising a collagen sponge coated with laminin gave a very significant ΔL value of >5.8; however, the individual effect of laminin could not be separated from that contributed from the presence of the collagen sponge (Ohbayashi et al., 1996). The use of eight polyamide filaments, each 250 μm, led to a very significant shift length of ≥7.4 (Lundborg et al., 1997). Filling the silicone tube with eight collagen fibers, diameter 100 to 150 μm, also led to a very significant length shift of ≥4.6 (Itoh et al., 1999). In contrast, coating of these collagen fibers with either laminin or the YIGSR (Tyr-Ile-Gly-Ser-Arg) protein sequence, one of the cell-binding domains of laminin, did not lead to further significant increase in ΔL over that observed with the uncoated fibers (Itoh et al., 1999). The presence of a magnetically oriented type I collagen gel inside a collagen tube led to significantly improved regeneration over that obtained with the unoriented gel (Caballos et al., 1999). Although sutures have been commonly used to connect stumps that have been apposed, use of conventional sutures sufficed to lead to bridging of the stumps across a 7-mm gap in the rat sciatic nerve with a regenerated nerve trunk (Scherman et al., 2000).

The use of deliberately synthesized, insoluble ECM analogs inside gaps bridged by silicone tubes produced detailed information on the substrate preferences of regenerating nerves. A filling consisting of a highly porous, insoluble ECM analog, a graft copolymer of type I collagen and chondroitin 6-sulfate, with random orientation of pore channel axes, led to a very significant ΔL value of ≥5.1 relative to the unfilled tube (Yannas et al., 1985, 1987a). Direct comparison of two orientations of pore channel axes in the ECM analog showed that an orientation that was parallel to the nerve axis (axial) had a significant ΔL advantage of ≥3.4 compared to an orientation that was perpendicular (radial) (Chang et al., 1990; Chang and Yannas, 1992). A systematic decrease in pore diameter of the ECM analog from 300 to 5 μm for axially oriented pore channels, corresponding to a 30-fold increase in specific surface, led to a decrease in the electrophysiologically measured distal motor latency from 1.7 times normal down to 1.35 times normal, a relatively small but significant approach to normal values; an elongation shift over this range in pore diameter could, however, not be determined, probably due to the choice of a relatively short gap length of 10 mm that led to values of % N near 100 in both cases (Chang et al., 1990; Chang and Yannas, 1992). When other structural features of the ECM analogs remained constant, an increase in degradation rate was accompanied by a substantial increase in the incidence of angiogenesis in the nerve trunk (Yannas et al., 1987c) as well as by a significant decrease in the distal motor latency from 1.4 to 1.2 times normal (Yannas et al., 1988; Chang et al., 1990; Chang and Yannas, 1992); however, a shift in critical elongation could not be determined, once more probably due to the choice of a short gap length (see Appendix). A later study of the ECM analog with the axially oriented pore channels and rapid degradation rate led to a very significant ΔL value of ≥5.4 relative to the PBS-filled silicone tube (Chamberlain et al., 1998b).

6.4.4 Biodurable Tubes Other than Silicone Tubes

A few studies have been conducted on tubes that, like silicone, do not degrade following implantation. These studies were conducted using tubes based on Millipore filter material (Noback et al., 1958); polyethylene tubes filled with type I collagen gel (DaSilva and Langone, 1989); and plasticized poly(vinyl chloride) tubing filled either with a laminin-containing gel or with a type I collagen gel (Kljavin and Madison, 1991). Studies employing biodurable tubes other than silicone are very few and the data are distributed among diverse tube compositions; considering that the effect of tube wall composition is known to be significant (see below), these results do not lend themselves readily to generalizations.

6.4.5 Degradable Synthetic Polymeric Tubes

In studies with degradable tubes, the historical goal has been to improve on the silicone tube by eliminating the second surgical procedure (to remove the tube) normally required when these biodurable tubes have been implanted.

Degradable synthetic polymers intended for implantation have been commonly based on monomers, such as α-hydroxy acids, HO—CHR—COOH, that bear a similarity to amino acids. The most well-known among these are polymers derived from lactic acid ($R = CH_3$) and glycolic acid ($R = H$). Glycolic acid (GA) is not optically active and exists in only one configurational structure, while lactic acid (LA) has an optically active carbon atom and can be found in two enantiomeric forms, L- and D-lactic acid. Polymers of α-hydroxy acids are readily synthesized by ring-opening polymerization of the cyclic dimers of the corresponding α-hydroxy acids, known as lactide and glycolide cyclic diesters or simply lactide and glycolide; for this reason, poly(lactic acid) and poly(glycolic acid) are often called polylactide and polyglycolide, respectively (Stevens, 1990). Poly(glycolic acid) (PGA), poly(lactic acid) (PLA), as well as copolymers of GA and LA have been synthesized and their degradation rate in various in vitro and in vivo systems have been determined. A commonly used copolymer has the composition 90/10 glycolic acid/lactic acid (PGL; polyglactin 910). Poly(ε-caprolactone) (PCL), another polyester, is produced by ring-opening polymerization of ε-caprolactone (Stevens, 1990). Copolymers of poly(lactic acid) and ε-caprolactone have been used extensively in nerve regeneration studies.

The degradation rate of these polymers depends on the molecular weight, configurational structure, comonomer ratio, residual monomer, molding conditions, annealing, sterilization procedures, and, especially, on the fraction of crystallinity (Vert et al., 1984; Vert and Li, 1992). Poly(lactic acid) is a stiff and brittle polymer; with addition of a plasticizer such as triethyl citrate it becomes quite flexible and somewhat tougher. The most well-known uses of these polymers currently are as sutures, as orthopedic materials, and as delivery media for controlled release of drugs; however, experimental investigations of their value as implants have also been reported in practically every anatomical site.

Some information on in vivo degradation times of these polymers that have been used to tubulate transected peripheral nerves has occasionally appeared. Most of the data were obtained after long periods and represent upper bounds to the half-life of the tubes studied. A PLA tube plasticized with 10% triethyl citrate almost completely degraded by 13 weeks (Seckel et al., 1984). Rigid and meshed PGA tubes were not present one year after implantation in the monkey (Dellon and Mckinnon, 1988). A tube constructed from nonwoven PGA fabric, implanted as a nerve bridge in the monkey, was reported degraded by about 26 weeks (Tountas et al., 1993). A PGA mesh coated with collagen had degraded by 12 weeks in cats; however, small residual fragments of the tube were identified at 17 weeks (Kiyotani et al., 1996). A PGA tube was reported to have disappeared by about 26 weeks (Keeley et al., 1991; Aldini et al., 1996). Tubes constructed from PGL were also reported to have been completely degraded by about 26 weeks (Gibson et al., 1991; Aldini et al., 1996). A crystalline copolymer of lactic acid and ε-caprolactone was reduced to fragments by two years (den Dunnen et al., 1993b).

Since the hydrolytic scission of the backbone bonds in these polymers leads to production of acidic monomers, it is expected that a local inflammatory response should take place during tube degradation. The intensity of acid release from the implant and some of its consequences have been studied (Gibson et al., 1991).

Little information has been typically provided in the literature about in situ degradation rates or half-lives of these tubes following implantation in the PNS. The lack of information makes it difficult to reach definitive conclusions on the effect of tube degradability in these studies. Another complication stems from the occasional swelling or cracking of degradable tubes during the study. A third complicating factor in this group of investigations is introduced by the common lack of negative tube controls, such as silicone tubes, which makes it difficult to separate effects arising from tube degradation rate from those due to its chemical composition. Controls used in this group of studies have been mostly positive (i.e., the autograft and the normal nerve). It is recalled that the autograft can be harvested from a number of anatomic locations and is far from being a standardized treatment.

The degradation rate of the tube wall was carefully controlled at three levels and thoroughly characterized in a study of the 8-mm gap in the rat sciatic nerve (Borkenhagen et al., 1998). The total weight loss in 24 weeks was 33, 74, and 88% for the three polymers. No significant differences in fidelity of regeneration were observed after 24 weeks between the three tubes. Although in this study swelling was controlled, degradation led to development of large cracks along the length of all tubes during the first four weeks. Cracking causes loss of tubulation, an experimental configuration that is known to have a profoundly negative effect on regeneration across a gap (see Table 6.1). Accordingly, it is pertinent to question whether the regeneration data in this study should be interpreted entirely in terms of the well-documented difference in degradation rate among tubes, which appeared to have no direct effect on regenerative activity; an alternative explanation is based on the observed loss of tubulation in all three tubes resulting from a tube failure process, which may have dominated the healing process and may have hypothetically concealed possibly significant effects of the degradation rate on regenerative activity.

Tube degradability was considered as a variable in a study of the 6-mm gap in the mouse sciatic nerve in which tubes made of two biodurable polymers, silicone and poly(tetrafluorethylene), and two degradable polymers, a copolymer of lactic acid and ε-caprolactone, and collagen, were compared (Navarro et al., 1996). The results showed a superiority of the two degradable tubes in terms of frequency of reinnervation; however, tube degradability per se was not unambiguously shown to be a contributing factor in the extent of morphological or functional recovery. It is possible that the extensive data reflect an effect of chemical composition rather than of degradability of tube on the structural and functional properties of regenerated nerves.

Equivalence to an autograft control was observed in a number of studies. A tube fabricated from PGL mesh was observed after 36 weeks to lead to regenerates of similar quality with the autograft across a 10-mm gap in the rabbit tibial nerve (Molander et al., 1983). Regenerates that formed across an 8-mm gap in the rat sciatic nerve using tubes based on a copolymer of lactic acid and ε-caprolactone were found to behave equivalently to the autograft after 16 weeks (Robinson et al., 1991). Another tube, based on a copolymer of lactic acid and ε-caprolactone, but one that degraded faster than the copolymer described immediately above (Robinson et al., 1991), was found to be superior to the autograft after 11 weeks when used to bridge the 10-mm gap in the rat sciatic nerve (den Dunnen et al., 1996). The two types of tube based on the copolymer of lactic acid and ε-caprolactone differed slightly in chemical composition but significantly in porosity and in tube configuration; accordingly, it is not possible to compare their performance directly and assign it unambiguously to their differences in degradation rate. Equivalence to direct suturing was observed when a PGA tube was used to bridge the approximately 0-mm gap in the median nerve of the monkey (Tountas et al., 1993).

Using the data on critical axon elongation in Table 6.1 it is possible to reach certain useful conclusions concerning some of the degradable tubes that have been studied. Even though the investigators of degradable tubes did not employ a silicone tube as an internal control, significant improvements over the silicone tube can be deduced for several degradable tubes. This conclusion is reached on the basis of estimates of the shift in critical length, ΔL, relative to the unfilled silicone tube standard (see Table 6.1). ΔL values obtained in this manner were ≥ 3.7 for a plasticized poly(lactic acid) (Seckel et al., 1984), ≥ 3.7 for a copolymer of lactic acid and ε-caprolactone (Dunnen et al., 1993a,b), as well as ≤ 1.3 for an ethylene-vinyl acetate copolymer (Aebischer et al., 1989). The inequality signs on the first two of the length shifts reported above indicate a lower limit, suggesting that the 10-mm gap length employed in these studies with the rat sciatic nerve (Seckel et al., 1984; den Dunnen et al., 1993a,b) may have been too short to adequately evaluate the regenerative activity of these tubes.

6.4.6 Degradable Tubes Based on Natural Polymers

Components of the extracellular matrix (ECM) have been used to fabricate implants used in PNS regeneration studies. In the organism, the ECM confers stiffness, strength, and, therefore, stability of shape; it also provides strong regulatory activity to various cell types, especially during development and healing of defects. The composition and structure of ECM varies among tissues. These matrices are typically highly hydrated macromolecular networks composed of various amounts of glycoproteins such as collagen, elastin, fibronectin, laminin, and chondronectin; and proteoglycans, macromolecules that comprise a protein core with glycosaminoglycan (GAG) side chains, including chondroitin 6-sulfate, dermatan sulfate, and heparan sulfate. Macromolecular components of the ECM are synthesized in cells and are secreted in the extracellular space where further physicochemical modification takes place (e.g., crystallization and covalent crosslinking of collagen chains) (Piez and Reddi, 1984).

The major constituent of ECMs in various organs comprises the collagens, a family of fibrous proteins that account for about one-third of the total protein mass in vertebrates. Members of the collagen family show tissue-specific differences in amino acid composition and occasionally in higher levels of structural order (Miller, 1984); at least 19 unique gene products or types of collagen have been described (Van der Rest and Garrone, 1991). Almost all uses of collagen in implanted devices have been based on type I collagen, found in relative abundance in skin, tendon, and bones. An unusual amino acid composition and a characteristic wide-angle x-ray diffraction pattern, reflecting a triple helical structure, distinguish collagen from other tissue components (Piez and Reddi, 1984; Nimni, 1988). Collagen can be extracted from connective tissues and can be dispersed in aqueous acetic acid or other solvents in the form of a solution of individual triple-helical macromolecules; tissues can also be mechanically comminuted to yield a suspension of very small particles, about 50 to 200 µm, comprising naturally crosslinked aggregates of collagen macromolecules. The solid state can be recovered either by evaporation of the solvent or by precipitation by use of a nonsolvent. Reconstituted collagen prepared thereby can be fashioned into membranes (films), tubes, fibers, or tape that can be crosslinked without use of an exogenous crosslinking agent (Yannas and Tobolsky, 1967). Collagen tubes have been used in studies of PNS regeneration while ECM analogs, based on highly porous graft copolymers of type I collagen and chondroitin 6-sulfate, also have been used as filling for the tubes used in these studies (Yannas, 1990).

Among the problems associated with the use of collagen-based devices is the structural complexity of the protein component and the resulting need for multiple controls during fabrication of devices in order to avoid inadvertent loss of the native structure due to excessive changes in the environment (Yannas, 1990). Most of the collagens are poor immunogens compared with many other proteins (Timpl, 1984). The antigenicity of collagen is further decreased after processing steps, such as crosslinking, have been included in the protocol and has not been found to be clinically significant in at least one study (Michaeli and McPherson, 1990). On the other hand, autoantibodies reacting particularly against denatured collagens have been identified (Timpl, 1984); these may conceivably play a role in devices in which some of the collagen has been denatured during fabrication.

In addition to collagen, other natural polymers that have been used to fabricate tubes for the treatment of transected nerves have included fibronectin and laminin. Fibronectin is a cell-adhesion protein that is expressed at high levels during defect healing, forming a provisional matrix with fibrin (Hynes, 1990; Clark, 1996b). Laminin, also a cell-adhesion protein, is a component of the intact basement membrane (Uitto et al., 1996) as well as a participant in healing processes (Woodley, 1996; Yamada et al., 1996).

Even though collagen, fibronectin, and laminin are intrinsically degradable, the degradation rate of these natural polymers can be varied over a wide range, typically by cross-linking (as with collagen). However, the degradation rate of tubes fabricated from natural polymers rarely has been determined and, with one exception (Kline and Hayes, 1964), has not been varied in the context of a study. For this reason, although the degradability of tubes fabricated from natural polymers has clear clinical significance (no surgical procedure is needed to remove the implant), this variable appears not to have been effectively employed to maximize the regenerative activity of such tubes.

Treatment of a gap of significant length with a collagen tube was shown to be equivalent to treatment by direct suturing of near-zero gaps in a number of studies. In an early study, the nominally zero-length gap resulting from transection of the peroneal and median nerves of the chimpanzee was studied over 32 weeks; treatment both with direct suturing as well as with the collagen tube gave equivalent results (Kline and Hayes, 1964). In another study, treatment of the 4-mm gap in the rat sciatic nerve with a collagen tube was shown after 12 weeks to be substantially equivalent to treatment by direct suturing and by autografting and was equivalent to the normal control as well (Archibald et al., 1991). When the 4-mm gap in the monkey median nerve was bridged with a collagen tube, equivalence with the normal control, as well as with the autograft, was observed after 109 weeks (Archibald et al., 1991). An extensive study of collagen tubes bridging a 5-mm gap in the monkey median nerve showed that, after 200 weeks, the extent of recovery reached was the same for treatment with collagen tubes, autografting, or direct suturing; furthermore, several of the electrophysiological assays showed essential equivalence of the three surgical treatments to the normal control (Archibald et al., 1995).

A collagen tube and a synthetic degradable tube based on glycolide trimethylene carbonate performed equally well after 60 weeks, as shown in a study both of the 20-mm gap in the radial sensory nerve as well as of the 50-mm gap in the ulnar nerve of the monkey; as expected, recovery across the longer gap was of inferior quality with both types of tube (Mackinnon and Dellon, 1990). A comparison of collagen tubes with tubes based on a copolymer of lactic acid and ε-caprolactone, silicone tubes, and PTFE tubes in the mouse sciatic nerve model did not appear to lead to definitive results due to the reported low statistical significance of most functional and morphological differences between these groups (Navarro et al., 1996).

Comparison of an unfilled protein-permeable collagen tube with an unfilled silicone tube showed a very significant electrophysiological advantage and a ΔL value of ≥ 5.4 mm for the collagen tube at 60 weeks when the 10-mm gap in the rat sciatic nerve was treated with these two devices (Chamberlain et al., 1998b). Since the two tubes differed both in chemical composition and in protein permeability, it is not possible to assign the observed advantage in regenerative activity unambiguously to either property of the collagen tube. Filling the collagen tube with nerve regeneration template led to a significant increase in electrophysiological properties (conduction velocity and amplitude) of the regenerate over the PBS-filled collagen tube control after 60 weeks (Chamberlain et al., 1998b). A direct comparison of collagen tubes and silicone tubes in the mouse sciatic nerve model gave a significant advantage, corresponding to a ΔL value of 1.8 mm, in favor of the collagen tube (Navarro et al., 1996).

The effect of filling of collagen tubes with nerve regeneration template (NRT), an ECM analog with specific network structure, could not be expressed in terms of a length shift, ΔL, as both the group treated with the NRT-filled collagen tube as well as the group treated with the unfilled collagen tube were reported to lead to a frequency of reinnervation of 100%. The results suggested that the 10-mm gap length used in the study (Chamberlain et al., 1998b) was not long enough to confirm the significant advantage in electrophysiological performance of the regenerate that formed in the NRT-filled collagen tube over that which formed in the unfilled collagen tube (see above). However, morphological data clearly showed an increase in average axon diameter from 30 to 60 wk (Figure 6.5), providing

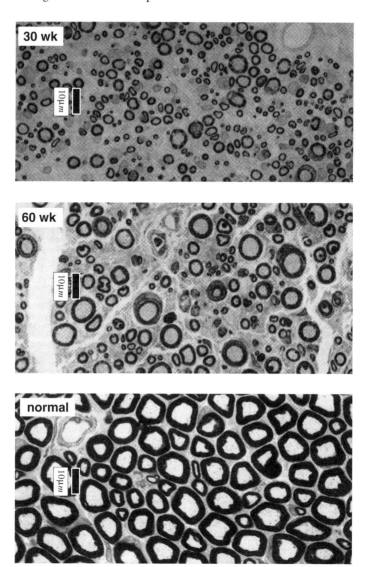

Figure 6.5. Axon diameters continued to increase significantly between 30 and 60 wk after implantation in certain experimental configurations. *Top* Regenerated after 30 wk inside a collagen tube filled with nerve regeneration template (NRT) across a 10-mm gap. *Middle* After 60 wk in the same experimental configuration, axon diameters had increased considerably but normal values were not reached; minifascicular structures persisted. *Bottom*   Cross-sectional view of normal rat sciatic nerve. Bar: 10 μm. (From Chamberlain et al., 1998b.)

evidence for continuing remodelling processes after long periods of regeneration (Chamberlain et al., 1998b).

A longer gap was provided for study of the NRT-filled collagen tube by selecting a surgical procedure that had been described earlier (Lundborg et al., 1982a). In the so-called cross-anastomosis (CA) procedure, both contralateral sciatic nerves of the rat are transected; the right sciatic nerve is transected proximally at the sciatic notch, allowing the right distal segment to be placed near the left proximal stump inside the opposite ends of the experimental tube. Unlike the more common procedure that is limited to the femoral site segment of a single sciatic nerve, the CA procedure allows study of gap lengths over 20 mm. There is some evidence that values of the critical axon elongation measured by the CA procedure lead to consistently lower values of critical axon elongation than at the commonly used femoral site, where both stumps have originated from the same nerve; for example, time-independent values of L_c for PBS-filled silicone tubes were 11.7 ± 0.5 mm for the femoral site but only 7.7 ± 0.04 mm for the CA site (Spilker, 2000). A very large value of the shift length, $\Delta L > 25$ mm, was estimated for an NRT-filled collagen tube that had been implanted by the CA procedure in the rat. The data included % $N = 100$ at 16 mm (6/6), 18 mm (5/5), 20 mm (5/5), and 22 mm (4/4), possibly the longest gap studied in the rat sciatic nerve (Spilker, 2000). The lack of sufficient independent data at the CA site makes it difficult to compare the performance of this configuration with those studied at the commonly used single-leg site.

Use of tubes fabricated from fibronectin mats gave regenerative activity equivalent to that of the nerve autograft after about nine weeks when it was used to bridge the 10-mm gap in the rat sciatic nerve (Whitworth et al., 1995). In another study, a transected rat sciatic nerve was treated by wrapping a laminin sheet around the zero-mm defect; in a control group, the stumps were connected by suturing. After about 17 weeks, it was observed that the laminin sheet was as effective as direct suturing in supporting functional recovery (Kauppila et al., 1993). The limited evidence available on tubes fabricated from fibronectin and laminin does not readily lead to generalizations.

6.4.7 Semipermeable Tubes

Acrylic copolymer tubes that allowed transfer of molecules with a molecular weight (MW) cutoff of 50 kDa did not show a significant difference in regenerative activity compared with impermeable silicone tubes (Hurtado et al., 1987; Knoops et al., 1990); however, a small increase in relative level of innervation of the same acrylic copolymer tube relative to the silicone tube was observed in another study (Aebischer et al., 1988). The comparisons were made between tubes with different chemical composition and, for this reason, they do not lead to unambiguous conclusions on the effect of protein-permeability of the tubes on regenerative activity.

Studies of silicone tubes that either were impermeable or were permeable to particles with diameter less than 1.2 µm led to the conclusion that the relative level of innervation was the same in both groups (Jenq and Coggeshall, 1985a,c; Jenq et al., 1987). In contrast, use of silicone tubes that had relatively small holes measuring 5 µm, and were confirmed to be cell-permeable, showed the same level of reinnervation as did silicone tubes that had macroscopic holes (Jenq and Coggeshall, 1985c; Jenq et al., 1987). Comparison of silicone tubes incorporating macroscopic holes with impermeable silicone tubes showed that the numbers both of myelinated and nonmyelinated axons in the distal stump were significantly higher when the tubes had holes (Jenq and Coggeshall, 1985c). In addition, tubes with macroscopic holes allowed formation of bridges of connective tissue that passed through the holes and reached all the way to the connective tissue on the surface of the regenerated trunk, suggesting the possibility that connective tissue cells, probably fibroblasts that had originated outside the nerve stumps, had facilitated the regeneration process (Jenq and Coggeshall, 1985c).

Another study in which the chemical composition of the tube was controlled while varying the permeability of the tube wall between an MW cutoff of 10^5 Da and 10^6 Da showed that regeneration across a gap could be observed even in the absence of a distal stump. Furthermore, it was shown that transfer of molecules with an MW cutoff of 10^5 Da gave superior activity compared with a cutoff of 10^6 Da, suggesting that an inhibiting factor with MW between 10^5 Da and 10^6 Da may have transferred from outside (Aebischer et al., 1989). A study of collagen tubes prepared at three levels of the permeability (macroporous, semipermeable, and nonpermeable) and conducted on a rabbit posterior tibial nerve model showed that both morphological and functional properties of the regenerated nerve trunk were significantly closer to normal when the macroporous collagen tubes were used (Kim et al., 1993).

Estimates of critical axon elongation based on rat sciatic nerve data for silicone tubes that allow particles of different sizes to transfer through the tube wall showed (Table 6.1) that the effect of cell-permeability of the tube was very significant, corresponding to $\Delta L \geq 6.0$ (Jenq and Coggeshall, 1987). The effect of cell-permeability relative to permeability for large proteins (but not to cells) was also very significant, corresponding to $\Delta L \geq 3.9$ (Jenq et al., 1987). In contrast, the effect of permeability to large proteins relative to impermeability was not significant, and was estimated at -1.4 (Jenq and Coggeshall, 1985a; Jenq et al., 1987). On the basis of mouse data (not shown in Table 6.1) with tubes that differed in chemical composition, a small but significant effect, corresponding to $\Delta L \geq 1.3$, was observed favoring an acrylic tube permeable to small proteins (cutoff at 50 kDa) relative to an impermeable silicone tube (Aebischer et al., 1988). In the same study with mice, a comparison of two acrylic tubes, both lacking a distal stump but with different permeability to small proteins, showed a very significant shift length, $\Delta L \geq 4.9$, in favor of the permeable tube (Aebischer et al., 1988).

The effect of inserting the distal stump rather than leaving the distal end open-ended can be hypothetically viewed as a study of a tube with no macroscopic hole (distal stump in) or with a hole (distal stump out). The effect of inserting the distal stump was significant to very significant, with rat data showing values of $\Delta L \geq 3.3$ (Lundborg et al., 1982a) and >5.7 (Williams et al., 1984). However, insertion of the distal stump was not equivalent to simply closing off a macroscopic hole at the distal tube end, as shown by a very significant shift length of >5.7 following insertion of the distal end compared with closing the distal end simply by tube ligation (Table 6.1, section A) (Williams et al., 1984). Mouse data (not shown in Table 6.1) also supported a very significant effect of distal stump insertion in the acrylic semipermeable tube, with a value of ΔL of ≥ 1.8 (Aebischer et al., 1988) and $\Delta L \geq 3.7$ for the silicone tube (Aebischer et al., 1988). A capped (plugged) distal tube end was significantly more supportive of regeneration than the uncapped (open-ended) tube with the acrylic semi-permeable tube, $\Delta L \geq 1.8$, while the effect of capping could not be determined using a silicone tube (Aebischer et al., 1988).

6.4.8 Long-Term Evidence for Synthesis of a Conducting Nerve Trunk

In the preceding sections we used an assay based on short-term data (i.e., data on percent reinnervation across a gap obtained within generally less than 20 weeks). This assay reports on the presence of myelinated axons along the nerve trunk; no direct information was supplied, however, on the ability of the nerve trunk to function as a conducting organ.

Data obtained after about 20 weeks, sufficient time for bridging of many tubulated gaps, frequently include electrophysiological data. An example of such data appears in Figure 6.6. Functional information of this type is useful because it strongly suggests the presence of at least one fascicle, a structural unit comprising a bundle of nerve fibers embedded in the endoneurium and encased in the perineurium. Since, however, electrophysiological data have not been confidently correlated with structural features of regenerates, they cannot replace morphological information. Other functional tests, such as permeability using protein tracers, can be used to detect the presence or absence of a physiological perineurium or endoneurium in the regenerated trunk (Azzam et al., 1991).

Electrophysiological data for several tubulated configurations are presented in Table 6.3. The data show that, in several studies, the fidelity of regeneration (fraction of property observed divided by the normal value) reached values close to or even equal to 1, corresponding to fidelity of regeneration values of 100%, indicative of normal behavior. Unfortunately,

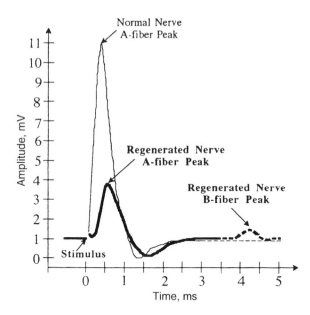

FIGURE 6.6. The conduction velocity of a regenerated nerve is typically lower than that of the normal nerve. Electrophysiological behavior of nerve trunk at 60wk, regenerated across a 10-mm gap bridged by a collagen tube filled with NRT matrix. Oscilloscope tracings of the amplitude of A-fiber and B-fiber nerve action potentials for normal rat sciatic nerve and regenerated nerve trunk. A-fiber action potential probably represents signal carried only by axons larger than about 6μm in diameter; it corresponded to conduction velocities of about 50 ± 2m/s for the regenerated nerve and 67 ± 3m/s for the normal control. B-fiber potential was observed only in regenerated trunks, corresponding to velocities of about 10 to 25 m/s. Conduction velocities were calculated from the measured distance between electrodes and from the latency, that is, the time lag between the electrical stimulus (arrow) and the peak in amplitude. (From Chamberlain et al., 1998b.)

the data cannot be compared internally because of the uncontrolled variation of basic experimental parameters (species, length of study, gap length) that are known to affect the values of electrophysiogical properties. In the majority of studies electrophysiological values were significantly lower than normal. However, the observation that the regenerated nerve conducted an electric signal shows without doubt that, in each case, nerve fibers had been synthesized along the entire length of the nerve trunk. Other data have shown that substantial numbers of large-diameter fibers (i.e., axons larger than 6μm that are responsible for values of conduction velocity) were present in the tibial and peroneal branches of the rat sciatic nerve when a 10-mm gap was bridged with a collagen tube filled with NRT (Chamberlain et al., 2000b).

6.5 Regenerative Activity for Various Tubulated Configurations

The criteria for an anatomically well-defined defect in a peripheral nerve have been satisfied by selecting transection of tissue over crushing; by extending the scale of injury beyond the scale of the nerve fiber to that of the fascicle (or the entire nerve trunk in multifasciculated nerves); avoiding generation of a hemisection and transecting instead across the entire diameter of the fascicle or nerve trunk, all the way to the perineurial tissue (single fascicle) or epineurium (multifasciculated trunk) surrounding it; and inserting the stumps in a tube in order to contain loss of exudate and invasion of extraneous tissues from neighboring organs. This tubulated configuration has been extensively used by several independent investigators.

Although a very useful experimental configuration for the study of induced regeneration, the tubulated nerve gap cannot be considered a spontaneously healing defect because it induces substantial nerve regeneration. The spontaneously healing defect is the untubulated gap, healing of which leads to synthesis of neuroma provided that the gap separating the stumps is sufficiently long.

Two assays were used in this chapter to evaluate the synthesis of nerves in vivo. The frequency of reinnervation across a tubulated gap, % N, previously used by several investigators, was the basis of a short-term assay (<20 wk) for regenerative activity of an experimental configuration. % N data from independent investigators, obtained at various levels of the gap length using two animal species (rat and mouse), were corrected for these variations in experimental protocol by use of the critical axon elongation, L_c, a measure of the maximum axon elongation across a gap. The silicone tube configuration was assigned the status of a standard and the critical axon elongation of different configurations were compared with that of the standard, yielding a parameter, the length shift, ΔL, that was used to compare a large number of configurations described in the literature on a self-consistent basis (Table 6.1). Application of the defect closure rule to the healing peripheral nerve showed that the magnitude of the regeneration term in the closure rule increased with the length shift of the configuration (Table 6.2). Electrophysiological observations, obtained in the long term (>20 wk), were used to obtain values for the fidelity of regeneration, the fraction of the normal value for a functional property that was recovered following a lengthy regeneration process (Table 6.3).

Comparison of several tubulated configurations in terms of the corresponding value of the length shift, elicited from the data in the literature, showed several significant trends in regenerative activity that are summarized below. The analysis is primarily based on data in Table 6.1.

Tubulation of nerve stumps had very significant regenerative activity relative to stumps in a nontubulated gap. Insertion of the distal stump inside the tube also had very significant regenerative activity compared with leaving the distal stump outside or to simple ligation of the distal tube end. Tubes constructed from two synthetic polymers (plasticized poly(lactic acid) and a copolymer of lactic acid and ε-caprolactone) showed significantly more regenerative activity than a tube based on an ethylene-vinyl acetate copolymer. A cell-permeable tube wall showed very significant regenerative activity compared with the impermeable tube; however, a protein-permeable tube did not show such advantage.

Tube fillings showed widely varying activity. Schwann cell suspensions had very significant regenerative activity. Incorporation of bFGF and aFGF, but not NGF, solutions showed significant to very significant regenerative activity. Solutions or gels based on ECM macromolecules such as collagen, fibronectin, and laminin did not have significant regenerative activity. Insoluble substrates that showed very significant regenerative activity were either highly oriented fibrin fibers, polyamide filaments that were axially oriented and did not fill the entire lumen, or highly porous ECM analogs with oriented pore channel axes, high specific surface, and a sufficiently rapid degradation rate.

6.6 Summary

In this section we summarize the conditions under which synthesis of tissue components of a peripheral nerve, and the entire nerve itself, was achieved.

Synthesis of a *myelin sheath* around axons elongating from neurons in culture was observed to occur when Schwann cells were present but not in their absence. The presence of ECM, including a basement membrane, was not required for the myelination process provided that Schwann cells and neurons were both present.

Encasement of myelinated axons by *basement membrane* required the presence not only of the neuron but also of laminin, one of the macromolecular components of basement membrane. Although fibroblasts synthesized basement membrane in the presence of Schwann cells, they were not required. Nor was the presence of neurons required in vivo; in other studies, the presence of laminin in the culture medium with Schwann cells sufficed to lead to synthesis of basement membrane. However, basement membrane was not synthesized when Schwann cells were present in culture in the absence both of neurons and components of the basement membrane (or of ECM).

Synthesis of a physiological *endoneurium* was not observed in vitro. However, synthesis of thin collagen fibrils, reminiscent of those comprising the endoneurium, took place in the presence of neurons and Schwann cells in culture, outside newly synthesized basement membrane, suggesting the possibility that elements of the endoneurium had been also synthesized adjacent to the myelinated fibers. Nor was a physiological endoneurium synthesized in vivo. Although endoneurial vessels were synthesized inside minifascicles of the nerve trunk that was regenerated across a gap bridged by a silicone tube, the vessels did not form tight intercellular junctions and were, therefore, deficient in their ability to provide a permeability barrier to conducting fibers of the intrafascicular space.

A mature *perineurium* was not synthesized in vitro; instead, elongated cells were observed to encircle Schwann cells and axons in culture provided that fibroblasts were also present but not in their absence. A physiological perineurium was, however, synthesized in vivo using a variety of configurations for tubulation of the transected nerve gap. The nerve trunk that was synthesized following tubulation of the transected gap in the rat sciatic nerve with a silicone tube comprised minifascicles surrounded by a mature perineurium. This newly synthesized perineurial sheath functioned as a physiological permeability barrier.

There was no evidence that a physiological *epineurium* was synthesized either in vitro or in vivo.

There was extensive evidence that a *nerve trunk*, innervated along its entire length of several mm and capable of substantial conduction of electric signals was synthesized using various kinds of tubes. In certain instances, and provided that the synthesized length generally did not exceed a few mm, the properties of the nerve trunk matched those of the normal nerve. The tubulated configurations that had the highest regenerative activity were those in which the tube wall comprised collagen rather than a synthetic polymer and had a cell-permeable rather than an impermeable wall. In addition, the following tube fillings showed very high regenerative activity: suspensions of Schwann cells; a solution either of aFGF or bFGF; crosslinked ECM networks rather than solutions or gels; polyamide filaments oriented along the tube axis; highly porous, insoluble analogs of the ECM with specific structure and controlled degradation rate.

In vitro conditions sufficed to synthesize nerve fibers encased in basement membrane. However, synthesis of more complex tissue components of a peripheral nerve, such as a perineurium with an elementary intrafascicular space, required in vivo conditions, including those found inside a tubulated gap.

7
Irreducible Processes for Synthesis of Skin and Peripheral Nerves

7.1 Reaction Diagrams

In the preceding two chapters we reviewed in great detail the conditions under which component tissues in skin and peripheral nerves, as well as the organs themselves, have been synthesized. The reactants employed, not all of them successful in yielding new tissues, have included many types of solutions of proteins, cell suspensions, synthetic polymers and natural matrices, as well as tubes. These reactants were added to media of various types and were cultured over a range of time intervals (in vitro); or they were directly implanted in an anatomically well-defined defect (in vivo) and the results were inspected after a period of time that was highly variable. Products resulting from these processes resembled the desired tissue or organ more or less in structure and function. Clearly, these processes were studied by the various investigators under conditions that were anything but standardized.

At first glance, it appears to be very difficult to generalize on these diverse data in order to answer questions such as these: Which of the reactants used were necessary to yield the desired tissue components of skin or peripheral nerves, or the organs themselves? Which was the simplest protocol that led to the desired synthesis? Are in vivo conditions (typically more complicated than in vitro) required to achieve any of these syntheses? Are the reaction conditions required for synthesis of skin similar to those for synthesis of peripheral nerves? Do any such similarities generate rules that can be hypothetically used to synthesize other organs?

A convenient way to sort through the complex information is to adopt a convention found to be very useful by chemists about two centuries ago. It consists in applying the systematics of synthetic chemistry, used to describe the preparation of chemical compounds, in order to describe the formation of a tissue or organ. The resulting symbolism is easy to use and very effective in sorting out the essential information pertinent to synthesis of tissues and organs. This approach was outlined in Chapter 1.

Proceeding along this direction we observe that all, or almost all, reactants employed can be sorted out simply as cells either of epithelial or stromal (mesodermal) origin; other reactants can be sorted out as either soluble (diffusible) or insoluble (nondiffusible) regulators of cell function. Furthermore, it is clear that certain component tissues of organs can be synthesized in vitro as well as in vivo whereas synthesis of entire organs has been reported to occur so far only in vivo. Newly synthesized tissues (reaction products) can be discussed in terms of their presence as members of the tissue triad consisting of a regenerative (epidermis in skin, myelin sheath in nerve) attached to a nonregenerative tissue (dermis in skin, perineurium in nerve) via the basement membrane. In Chapter 2, use of the tissue triad has led to interesting analogies between skin and peripheral nerves. Below we describe the simple methodology by which the complexity of protocols in the literature is reduced to a level at which useful answers can be obtained to the questions posed above.

7.1.1 Reactants and Products; Irreducible Processes

A qualitative shorthand description of a protocol for synthesizing a tissue or organ can be provided by use of a "reaction diagram", a complete listing of the insoluble reactants and insoluble products that characterize the process. An example is the reaction diagram (Dg.) shown here:

$$\text{cell type A + nondiffusible regulator B} \rightarrow \text{tissue C} \quad \text{(Dg. A)}$$

It is a report of the insoluble substances that went into the reactor (i.e., the anatomically well-defined defect) and the insoluble products that were eventually synthesized in it.

Reaction diagram A omits information about any endogenous soluble substances (e.g., cytokines and growth factors) that have regulated the function of cells involved in synthesis of the products. This omission is deliberately made to simplify the presentation of the diagram. It is justified, by postulating that the initial concentrations of soluble regulators (cytokines and growth factors) inside the defect are identical in all investigations in which the same defect was studied; it follows that information on concentration of soluble regulators can be omitted without affecting the comparison in simplicity of protocols used by different investigators who studied the same defect. This postulate is discussed in detail below. For convenience, the reaction diagram also omits reference to any soluble products that may have been synthesized during the process; such omission also does not affect a conclusion on the relative simplicity or effectiveness of a protocol.

Although most of the simplifications described above are typically followed in the formulation of chemical equations, it is important to clearly distinguish between a reaction diagram and chemical equation. Reaction diagrams do not contain stoichiometric information and should, therefore, be considered somewhat analogous to unbalanced chemical equations. The symbols employed on both sides of the arrow in a reaction diagram simply identify the addition of a reactant or the synthesis of a product inside the defect, not the relative masses of reactants or products.

A reaction diagram based on data reported in the literature usually does not describe the simplest process by which a tissue or organ can be prepared. However, comparison of several reaction diagrams can lead to the "irreducible reaction diagram," a description of the simplest known process by which the synthesis has been achieved. For example, let us hypothesize that tissue C, synthesized as shown in Dg. A above, can be synthesized by a simpler route:

$$\text{cell type A} \rightarrow \text{tissue C} \hspace{4em} \text{(Dg. B)}$$

If Dg. B is indeed the simplest route reported in the literature, the diagram representing it will be considered to be the irreducible reaction diagram for synthesis of C. In a comparison of two reaction diagrams for synthesis of the same tissue or organ, the one using fewer reactants will be considered simpler. Between two protocols that make use of the same number of reactants, that which employs fewer cell types will be considered simpler; also, in vitro conditions will be considered to be simpler than in vivo conditions.

Once identified, the irreducible diagram suggests the minimal conditions known for synthesis of the product(s). Such an identification obviously cannot be used to assert that even simpler conditions cannot or will not be discovered at a later time when investigators much more clearly understand the nature of these synthetic processes. However, the irreducible process does contain the answer to this question: Based on the data available to us today, which reactants are required to be added (necessary) in order to synthesize a given tissue or organ? Discussion of mechanism, appearing in Chapters 8 and 10 can then focus on the simplest known synthetic route.

7.1.2 Approximations Underlying the Use of Reaction Diagrams

Although reaction diagrams greatly simplify the description of complex processes involving tissues and organs, they are rough approximations of reality and must be used with caution, as discussed below.

One of these approximations is the use of a single symbol to represent a reactant or a product, suggesting the existence of a unique state for each, a convention normally used in the representation of chemical compounds. Yet, the normal morphology of a tissue may change significantly from one anatomical site to the next in the same organ, even though its name does not. Furthermore, as maturation (or remodeling) proceeds, a tissue in an organ can be present at various levels of differentiation. Assignment of a single symbol to a tissue does not take into account many of these variations in morphology or functional state with anatomical location or maturation time.

A few examples illustrate the degree of approximation involved in describing a tissue by a single name. The epidermis (E) synthesized by culturing keratinocytes in vitro with fibroblasts and a collagen gel is a product that can be prepared at various identifiable levels of differentiation, depending on timing and other reaction conditions (Parenteau et al., 1992, 1996). The same caution applies when cells are used as reactants in a process. The symbol KC is used below to represent keratinocytes in culture medium. Implicit in the use of a single symbol is the assumption that keratinocytes exist in a single state of differentiation. In a number of studies, however, keratinocytes have been isolated from a skin biopsy and have either been used to induce synthetic processes without further culture or else have been extensively cultured before being used. The uncultured keratinocytes typically comprise cells from all epidermal layers, representing various levels of differentiation, while cultured cells have typically been converted to a higher level of differentiation (Wille et al., 1984). The details of a synthetic process can be affected, often very significantly, by the precise state of differentiation of a cell that is used as a reactant. In the example of KC seeded into dermis regeneration template, a nondiffusible regulator, the skin synthesized in the process had a significantly higher number of rete ridges when the keratinocytes had been cultivated, than when the cells were freshly dissociated but not cultured, prior to seeding (Butler et al., 1999a). In a further example, a study of synthesis of basement membrane in vitro in the presence of keratinocytes, fibroblasts, and a collagen gel led to the conclusion that basement was synthesized only when keratinocytes were added to the collagen gel that had already been cultured for a period of time with fibroblasts; a basement membrane was not formed when keratinocytes were added to fibroblasts and the collagen gel without first culturing the latter two cell types together (Chamson et al., 1989).

How well differentiated need a product be in order to merit being referred to by a unique symbol? Most tissues discussed in this chapter have been synthesized in more than one distinguishable level of differentiation. In contrast to synthetic chemistry, where the term *benzene* refers to a single compound, investigators have typically not employed standard definitions of the tissues under study. Although the vast majority of investigators agree that a tissue that displays a minimum number of well-defined morphological characteristics can be uniquely identified, a formal process of standardization of tissues based on a necessary and sufficient set of morphological and functional characteristics has not yet been developed. As an example, we often find that an investigator defines the product of a reaction as the "basement membrane" of skin if it comprises at least four distinct structural characteristics of this tissue, identified immunohistochemically in terms of the major protein constituent that is uniquely associated with each layer. In this example, these constituents are the $\alpha_6\beta_4$ integrin, characteristic of hemidesmosomes; laminin, present in lamina lucida; type IV collagen, a major constituent of lamina densa; and type VII collagen, the main component of anchoring fibrils.

In addition to such evidence of tissue identification based on protein components, an investigator may provide ultrastructural evidence of normal organization of these macromolecular elements into a whole, functioning tissue. At the other extreme, another investigator may report synthesis of a "basement membrane" based on immunohistochemical identification of just two protein constituents, such as laminin and type IV collagen, without reporting on the presence of the other proteins or providing any ultrastructural data to document the organization of the tissue. In this example, both investigators have identified the product of the reaction as "basement membrane" but have employed different criteria in assaying for it. In view of this diversity in use of identifying criteria, I have arbitrarily chosen to report synthesis of a given tissue if the investigators provided clear evidence that at least one assay of widely recognized value was employed in its identification. This nominal approach clearly errs on the side of inclusion of products and probably leads to irreducible reaction diagrams that are weighted excessively toward simplicity in description of reaction conditions.

Another implicit assumption introduced by the symbolism of the reaction diagram is the synthesis of individual tissues in "out of organ context." In this hypothetical state, a tissue component of an organ is a discrete, stable entity that can be synthesized independently of the tissues to which it is connected in the complete, physiological organ. In order to discuss the level of inaccuracy introduced by use of this approximation, we will introduce the symbolism used to represent an organ in terms of its tissue components. The physical connection between two tissues in the context of an organ is represented as a dot between the symbols of adjacent tissues; use of a dot, rather than a connecting line, prevents confusion with a chemical bond. As an example, physiological skin (S) is considered below, in abbreviated fashion, to comprise only an epidermis (E), a basement membrane with hemidesmosomes, lamina lucida, lamina densa and anchoring fibrils (BM), rete ridges with dermal papillae (RR), and a thick, vascularized dermis (D) with sensory nerves and appendages (AP); the latter derive from the epidermis during development but are located in the dermis. A completely physiological dermis with nerve fibers and appendages will, accordingly, be referred to as RR·D·AP while the physiological skin organ is symbolically represented as E·BM·RR·D·AP. When only appendages are missing, the representation of skin changes to E·BM·RR·D, also referred to below as partial skin (PS). Occasionally, rete ridges in a partial organ product are missing, and the symbolic representation becomes E·BM·D.

The simplified view of an organ as a "linear assembly" of tissues is occasionally partly supported by experimental evidence. An illustration is the synthesis of an epidermis attached to a physiological basement membrane (E·BM) in a dermis-free defect (Carver et al., 1993b); even though the dermis is missing in this tissue product, the epidermis–basement membrane bilayer, E·BM, survives for days, a sufficiently long experimental period to allow the investigators to make several useful observations about its structure. Another example is the preparation of a basement membrane on a dermis in the absence of an epidermis (BM·D) (Guo and Grinnell, 1989); here, the epidermis is missing but the basement membrane-dermis bilayer persists over a period of time.

Nevertheless, there are often serious problems with this approximation. A tissue that has been synthesized in an out-of-context state eventually shows evidence of its instability. Such a tissue is typically weakly connected to the rest of the organ; it is probably unvascularized or unsupported metabolically by the organ. For example, there is strong evidence, presented in Chapter 5, that an epidermis, synthesized in vitro without a basement membrane and a dermis attached to it, fails to attach itself on the muscle surface of a dermis-free defect surface (Billingham and Reynolds, 1952; Billingham and Russell, 1956, Eldad et al., 1987; Latarjet et al., 1987; Carver et al., 1993b; Cooper et al., 1993; Kangesu et al., 1993b; Orgill et al., 1998). Furthermore, an epidermis, originally synthesized in vitro in an immature state, undergoes rapid maturation after it has been placed on a dermal substrate in vivo (Prunieras, 1975; Faure et al., 1987). The evidence clearly shows that an individual tissue can be considered as a discrete, stable entity only as a rough first approximation (e.g., in the context of an experimental protocol where the question posed is whether the tissue in question can be synthesized at all, even in a state that is only temporarily stable). We recall that chemists frequently find it very valuable to include in equations symbolic representation for free radicals, most of which are very unstable species.

Only cells, nondiffusible regulators (i.e., insoluble matrix components or matrix analogs), newly synthesized tissues, and the defect itself are explicitly included in the symbolic description of a reaction diagram. Diffusible (soluble) regulators, that is, growth factors, cytokines, clotting factors and their peptide degradation products, small ions or hormones, are omitted. At first thought, it might seem unthinkable to omit diffusible regulators that are normally expected, based on very strong evidence from in vitro studies, to be critical contributors to processes of tissue and organ synthesis in vivo. We recall, however, that our major objective in this chapter is to compare protocols employed by different investigators for synthesis of a given tissue in order to identify the simplest conditions used. In such an analysis, no advantage is gained by repetitive mention of an experimental parameter that is maintained at constant level in various investigations. Such selective omission of information has previously been practiced extensively with, for example, the temperature and the pH levels of an in vivo study; both of these parameters are widely considered, with very few exceptions, to have remained at physiological levels during each of several studies conducted using roughly the same protocol. Because they comprise a common background in different investigations, these parameters are often omitted, even from a detailed discussion of the experimental conditions.

In similar fashion, the concentration levels of diffusible regulators at the time of injury do not vary significantly among the different investigators who have studied the same type of defect (e.g., the dermis-free defect or the transected and tubulated nerve). In our review of the literature presented in Chapters 5 and 6 we were careful to include only data that were obtained in anatomically well-defined defects; the approximation discussed here appears, therefore, to be justified on face value. One may wonder whether the approximation for a given type of defect holds across several species; are diffusible regulators present at similar or widely different concentrations levels in the swine defect and the guinea pig defect? The information currently available on cytokine concentration levels in defects is so limited that the question remains unanswered.

With few exceptions for data obtained with skin defects (see Breuing et al., 1992 and Levine et al., 1993) or nerve defects (Fu and Gordon, 1997), data on concentration levels of diffusible regulators in defects have generally not been reported at all and extensive data are a rarity. Persisting with the approximation in spite of lack of such evidence we conclude that a comparison of data from different laboratories in which the anatomically well-defined defect (as defined in Chapter 3) was studied can be validly made without knowledge of the absolute concentration of soluble regulators in the defect. We will, therefore, hypothesize that concentration levels of cytokines at the time just postinjury were uniform from one laboratory to the next in the reaction diagrams discussed in this chapter that refer to a given organ. We will refer to this as the hypothesis of "uniform cytokine field." This approach appears justified when the purpose is simply to elicit information on the irreducible reaction diagram for synthesis of a tissue. Reference to cytokine concentrations will, therefore, be considered as part of the common background of all in vivo reaction diagrams that take place in a given anatomically well-defined defect and will be omitted from the reaction diagram.

The uniform cytokine field hypothesis is expected to apply only under the initial conditions for the process, that is, immediately after the injury and just before the addition of any reactant(s). The postulated uniformity is expected to fail soon after addition of a reactant to the defect. The exudate in the defect typically responds to addition of a reactant by a modification of its contents, the direction or extent of which strongly depends on the nature of the reactant.

Finally, the degree of relevance of an irreducible reaction diagram to the processes of remodeling in an adult or to developmental processes in a growing organism is unclear. The conditions in a healing defect, in which an inflammatory exudate is prominently present, should be anticipated to be significantly different from those at the equivalent anatomic site of a remodeling organ or a developing organism.

7.1.3 Tabulation of Reaction Diagrams

The collection of reaction diagrams in Tables 7.1 (skin) and 7.2 (peripheral nerves) include those in which the reactants added were well-defined and easy to reproduce in independent laboratories. Reactants that are explicitly included in the diagrams comprise dissociated (disaggregated) cells of known type, synthetic polymers of known composition, and defined components of the extracellular matrix or nondiffusible macromolecular networks synthesized from ECM components following standard synthetic methods (ECM analogs). Processes in which tissue grafts (e.g., epidermal or dermal grafts), were employed as reactants were not included in Tables 7.1 and 7.2 since, as discussed in detail in Chapters 5 and 6, their presence in the defect compromises the identification of the products. Diffusible regulators have not been included explicitly as reactants; as discussed above, since all in vivo processes in Tables 7.1 and 7.2 took place in a dermis-free defect or in a transected and tubulated nerve, they are considered to have taken place in the same (uniform) cytokine field. See the tables for the abbreviations used to construct reaction diagrams for skin synthesis (Table 7.1) and for peripheral nerve synthesis (Table 7.2).

The reaction diagrams presented in Tables 7.1 and 7.2 summarize current data in the literature. The simplest protocols for synthesizing a tissue or the organ itself have been highlighted. It should not be assumed that these irreducible conditions will not be superseded by future studies that may identify even simpler conditions for synthesis of a tissue; for example, in vivo conditions may be hypothetically shown in future studies not to be required for synthesis of a given tissue. Furthermore, the kinetics of these processes have been studied in a very sketchy manner by the various investigators; accordingly, it is not known whether the desired tissue may be synthesized if the reaction is allowed much more time to run its course in future studies.

In Tables 7.1 and 7.2, the living environment of the reaction (i.e., the dermis-free skin defect or the transected and tubulated nerve) is represented by the words "in vivo" on top of the reaction arrow; the absence of such notation implies conditions of in vitro culture. Although not explicitly shown in a reaction diagram, the defect contributes the cytokine field, that is, endogenous reactants not explicitly shown in the diagram that have been hypothesized to be present at the same initial concentrations across various investigations in which the same defect was employed. The defect also contributes cells (also classified as endogenous reactants and not explicitly reported in the reaction diagrams); most commonly (but not exclusively), these are either fibroblasts migrating from the evolving granulation tissue of the skin defect or Schwann cells and other cells migrating from the healing nerve stump. The specific contribution made by the defect to the

TABLE 7.1. Reaction diagrams for synthesis of skin.

Abbreviations. *Reactants*: KC, keratinocytes; FB, fibroblasts; COFL, cast type I collagen film; COG, type I collagen gel produced by fibroblast contraction; CBL, bilayer consisting of a type IV collagen layer and a type I + III collagen layer; DRT, dermis regeneration template, a porous graft copolymer of type I collagen and chondroitin 6-sulfate; L-DRT, dermis regeneration template laminated on one side with a nonporous type I collagen layer; PGL, polyglactin mesh; NY, nylon mesh; PL, surface of plastic dish. *Products*: E, epidermis; BM, basement membrane; RR, rete ridges with dermal papillae; D, dermis, a richly vascularized, thick tissue layer, consisting of quasi-randomly oriented collagen fibers, unlike scar; E · BM · D, partial skin consisting of an epidermis, basement membrane, and dermis but no rete ridges; E · BM · RR · D, partial skin, consisting of an epidermis, basement membrane, rete ridges, and dermis (no appendages).? next to symbol for tissue product indicates absence of confirmatory evidence for synthesis of physiological tissue; *No* indicates product not formed. *Reaction conditions*: "in vivo" over the reaction arrow indicates reaction conducted in a dermis-free defect; its absence above arrow indicates in vitro study. Bold letters indicate an irreducible reaction diagram.

No.	Reactants	Reaction conditions and structure of product	References
Response of culture medium or defect in the absence of reactants (negative controls for all reaction diagrams)			
S01	Cell-free medium (in vitro) $\xrightarrow{\text{no tissues synthesized}}$	Negative control diagram for all reactions in culture (in vitro); no tissues synthesized	—
S02	Dermis-free defect $\xrightarrow[\text{epithelialized dermal scar}]{\text{in vivo}}$	Negative control diagram for all reactions in the adult dermis-free defect (in vivo); epithelialized dermal scar synthesized	Billingham and Reynolds, 1952; Billingham and Medawar, 1955; several other authors (see Chapter 2)
A. Epidermis (E)			
S1	KC + FB → E	Lethally irradiated FB replaced with medium from FB culture; keratinizing epithelium synthesized	Rheinwald and Green, 1975a,b; Green et al., 1979; O'Connor et al., 1981; Regauer and Compton, 1990
S2	**KC → E**	KC cultured in defined medium, pH 5.6–5.8 and optimal KC density; keratinizing epithelium synthesized	Eisinger et al., 1979; Peehl and Ham, 1980; Tsao et al., 1982
S3	KC + DRT → E	KC cultured on DRT; keratinizing epithelium synthesized	Boyce and Hansbrough, 1988
S4	KC + CBL → E	KC cultured on collagenous bilayer; keratinizing epithelium synthesized	Bosca et al., 1988; Tinois et al., 1991
S5	KC + FB + L-DRT → E	Keratinocytes and fibroblasts cultured with modified (laminated) DRT; keratinizing epithelium synthesized	Cooper et al., 1991, 1993; Boyce et al., 1993
S6	KC + FB + COG → E	KC cultured with FB in collagen gel; keratinizing epithelium synthesized	Nolte et al., 1993, 1994; Hansbrough et al., 1994

B. Basement membrane (BM)

	Reaction	Description	References
S7	$KC + COG \rightarrow E \cdot BM$	KC cultured on collagen gel; typically reported evidence for synthesis of hemidesmosomes, lamina lucida and lamina densa	Mann and Constable, 1977; Hirone and Taniguchi, 1980; David et al., 1981; Cook and Van Buskirk, 1995
S8	$KC + CBL \rightarrow E \cdot BM$	KC cultured on collagenous bilayer; hemidesmosomes, lamina lucida, lamina densa, and occasionally anchoring fibrils, synthesized	Bosca et al., 1988; Tinois et al., 1991
S9	$KC \xrightarrow{\text{in vivo}} E \cdot BM$	KC formed epidermis in vitro and was grafted; lamina lucida, lamina densa and anchoring fibrils synthesized	Woodley et al., 1988a; Aihara, 1989; Carver et al., 1993b; Cooper et al., 1993; Orgill et al., 1998
S10	$KC + FB + COG \rightarrow E \cdot BM$	KC added to precultured collagen gel and fibroblasts; hemidesmosomes, lamina lucida, lamina densa, anchoring fibrils synthesized	Chamson et al., 1989; Harriger and Hull, 1992; Okamoto and Kitano, 1993; Marinkovich et al., 1993; Tsunenaga et al., 1994; Smola et al., 1998; Stark et al., 1999
S11	$KC + FB + L\text{-}DRT \xrightarrow{\text{in vivo}} E \cdot BM$	KC added to precultured fibroblasts in modified (laminated) DRT, then grafted; lamina lucida, lamina densa and anchoring fibrils synthesized	Cooper and Hansbrough, 1991; Cooper et al., 1993; Boyce et al., 1993
S12	$KC + FB + NY \rightarrow E \cdot BM$	KC added to precultured fibroblasts in nylon mesh; anchoring filaments, lamina densa, anchoring fibrils, nidogen synthesized	Contard et al., 1993; Fleischmajer et al., 1995
S13	$\mathbf{KC \rightarrow E \cdot BM}$	KC cultured in defined medium; hemidesmosomes, anchoring filaments, lamina lucida, lamina densa synthesized; collagen VII synthesized but not secreted	Rosdy et al., 1993
S14	$KC + FB + PGL \xrightarrow{\text{in vivo}} E \cdot BM(?)$	KC added to precultured fibroblasts in nylon mesh, then grafted; continuous laminin synthesized, type IV collagen not reported	Hansbrough et al., 1993
S15	$KC + FB + COG \xrightarrow{\text{in vivo}} E \cdot BM$	KC cultured on a collagen gel with FB, then grafted; hemidesmosomes, lamina lucida, lamina densa, anchoring fibrils synthesized	Hansbrough et al., 1994; Nolte et al., 1994
S16	$KC + COFL \rightarrow No\ BM$	KC cultured on collagen film; no BM synthesized	Cook and Van Buskirk, 1995

TABLE 7.1. *Continued*

No.	Reactants	Reaction conditions and structure of product	References
S17	$KC + PL \rightarrow No\ BM$	KC cultured on surface of plastic dish; no BM synthesized	Cook and Van Buskirk, 1995
S18	$KC + DRT \xrightarrow{in\ vivo} E \cdot BM$	Uncultured KC seeded into DRT, then grafted; continuous laminin, collagen VII (anchoring fibrils), $\alpha_6\beta_4$ integrin (hemidesmosomes) synthesized	Compton et al., 1998
C. Dermis (D)			
S19	$DRT \xrightarrow{in\ vivo} D$	Cell-free DRT grafted; synthesis of thick, vascularized dermis with quasi-randomly oriented collagen fibers; no BM; no dermo-epidermal junction	Yannas, 1981; Yannas et al. 1981, 1982a,b; Orgill, 1983; Orgill et al., 1996; Orgill and Yannas, 1998; Compton et al. 1998
S20	$KC + FB + COG \rightarrow No\ D$	KC cultured on a collagen gel with FB; no dermis synthesized	Bell et al., 1981a, 1983; Hull et al. 1983a
S21	$KC + FB + COG \xrightarrow{in\ vivo} E \cdot BM \cdot D$	KC cultured in vitro on collagen gel with FB, then grafted; thick dermis with basketweave pattern and vascularization was synthesized	Bell et al., 1983; Hull et al., 1983b; Hansbrough et al., 1994; Nolte et al., 1994
S22	$KC + CBL \rightarrow No\ D$	KC cultured on collagenous bilayer; no dermis synthesized	Bosca et al. 1988; Tinois et al., 1991
S23	$KC + DRT \rightarrow No\ D$	KC cultured with DRT; no dermis synthesized	Boyce et al., 1988
S24	$KC \xrightarrow{in\ vivo} No\ D$	KC cultured, then grafted; KC sheet detached from surface of defect; no dermis synthesized	Aihara, 1989; Ogawa et al. 1990; Carver et al., 1993b; Cooper et al., 1993; Orgill et al., 1998
S25	$KC + FB + L\text{-}DRT \xrightarrow{in\ vivo} E \cdot BM \cdot RR \cdot D$	FB and KC cultured on laminated DRT, then grafted; dermis with basket-weave pattern synthesized	Cooper and Hansbrough, 1991; Cooper et al., 1993; Boyce et al. 1993
S26	$KC + FB + L\text{-}DRT \rightarrow No\ D$	FB and KC cultured on laminated DRT; no dermis synthesized	Boyce et al., 1993
S27	$KC + FB + PGL \dashrightarrow No\ D$	KC cultured on polyglactin mesh with FB; no dermis synthesized	Cooper et al., 1991; Hansbrough et al., 1993

S28	$KC + FB + PGL \xrightarrow{\text{in vivo}} E \cdot BM(?) \cdot D$	KC cultured on polyglactin mesh with FB, then grafted; dermis (?) with capillaries synthesized	Cooper et al., 1991; Hansbrough et al., 1993

D. Partial skin (E · BM · RR · D; skin appendages missing)

S29	$KC + FB + COG \xrightarrow{\text{in vivo}} E \cdot BM \cdot D$	KC cultured on collagen gel with FB to synthesize epidermis, then grafted; synthesized continuous basement and thick dermis with dermal nerve fibers; no rete ridge formation (but see Parenteau et al., 1996); no elastic fibers synthesized	Bell et al., 1981b, 1983; Hull et al., 1983b; Bosca et al., 1988; English et al., 1992; Hansbrough et al., 1994; Nolte et al., 1993, 1994
S30	$KC + DRT \xrightarrow{\text{in vivo}} E \cdot BM \cdot RR \cdot D$	Uncultured (or cultured) KC seeded into DRT, then grafted; simultaneous synthesis of epidermis, basement membrane, rete ridges with dermal papillae and dermis, including elastic fibers and dermal nerve fibers	Yannas et al., 1981, 1982a,b, 1984, 1989; Orgill, 1983; Murphy et al., 1990; Compton et al., 1998; Orgill et al., 1998; Butler et al., 1998, 1999a
S31	$KC + FB + \text{L-DRT} \xrightarrow{\text{in vivo}} E \cdot BM \cdot RR \cdot D$	FB and KC cultured on modified (laminated) DRT, then grafted; simultaneous synthesis of epidermis, basement membrane, rete ridges with dermal papillae and dermis, including elastic fibers	Cooper and Hansbrough, 1991; Cooper et al., 1993
S32	$KC + CBL \xrightarrow{\text{in vivo}} E \cdot BM \cdot D$	KC cultured on collagenous bilayer to synthesize epidermis, then grafted; synthesis of BM and dermis; dermal elastic fibers not reported; no rete ridge formation	Bosca et al., 1988; Tinois et al., 1991
S33	$KC + FB + PGL \xrightarrow{\text{in vivo}} E \cdot BM(?) \cdot D$	KC cultured on polyglactin mesh with FB, then grafted; laminin stained continuously; type IV collagen synthesis not reported; dermis (?) with capillaries synthesized; dermal elastic fibers not reported; no rete ridge formation	Cooper et al., 1991; Hansbrough et al., 1993

TABLE 7.2. Reaction diagrams for synthesis of a peripheral nerve.

Abbreviations. *Reactants:* AX, axons; SC, Schwann cells; FB, fibroblasts; COFL, surface comprising type I collagen, cast from solution; COM, collagen matrix (not further described by the investigator); RBM, reconstituted basement membrane; LA, laminin; TB, tube in which nerve stumps were inserted (tubulation), consisting either of silicone, a synthetic polymer, or collagen; FI, tube filling, consisting either of cells or diffusible or nondiffusible regulators. *Tissue and organ products:* MAX, myelinated axon; BM, basement membrane encasing Schwann cells; MAX · BM, myelinated axon encased in basement membrane (endoneurial tube); COF, collagen fibrils synthesized outside basement membrane; ED, endoneurium; PN, perineurium; EN, epineurium; MAX · BM · ED · PN, a physiological nerve trunk, with fascicle(s) comprising myelinated axons, Schwann cell basement membrane, endoneurium and a perineurial sheath around each fascicle; MAX · BM · PN, nerve trunk with perineurium but lacking physiological endoneurium; ? next to symbol for tissue product indicates absence of confirmatory evidence for synthesis of physiological tissue; *No* indicates product not formed. *Reaction conditions:* "in vivo" over the reaction arrow indicates transected and tubulated nerve; its absence indicates in vitro study. Bold letters indicate an irreducible reaction diagram.

No.	Reactants	Reaction conditions and structure of product	References
Response of culture medium or defect in the absence of reactants (negative controls for all reaction diagrams)			
N01	cell-free medium → no tissues	Negative control diagram for reactions in culture (in vitro); no tissues synthesized	—
N02	transected nerve $\xrightarrow{\text{in vivo}}$ neuroma	Negative control diagram for reactions in the adult transected nerve defect (in vivo); neuroma synthesized	Weiss, 1944; Denney-Brown, 1946; Chamberlain et al., 2000a; other authors; see Chapter 2
A. Myelin sheath (MAX, myelinated axons)			
N1	AX + SC + COFL → MAX	Schwann cells cultured with neurons on collagen surface; myelin sheath synthesized	Bunge and Bunge, 1978
N2	AX → *No* MAX	No myelin sheath sythesized around axons in regions free of Schwann cells	Bunge and Bunge, 1978
N3	AX + SC + RBM → MAX	Schwann cells cultured with neurons and reconstituted BM; myelin sheath synthesized	Carey et al., 1986
N4	**AX + SC → MAX**	Schwann cells cultured with neurons; myelin sheath synthesized	Carey and Todd, 1987; Eldridge et al., 1987, 1989; Clark and Bunge, 1989; Podratz et al., 1998

N5	$AX + SC + LA \rightarrow MAX$	Schwann cells cultured with neurons and laminin; myelin sheath synthesized	Eldridge et al., 1989

B. Basement membrane encasing Schwann cells (BM)

N6	$AX \rightarrow No\ BM$	No BM synthesized in absence of Schwann cells	Bunge et al., 1980
N7	$AX + SC \rightarrow MAX \cdot BM\ (+ COF)$	Schwann cells cultured with neurons; BM synthesized; synthesis of collagen fibrils occasionally reported as well	Bunge et al., 1980, 1982; Cornbrooks et al., 1983; Carey and Todd, 1987; Eldridge et al., 1987, 1989; Clark and Bunge, 1989
N8	$SC \rightarrow No\ BM$	Schwann cells cultured without neurons; BM components, but not BM, synthesized	Bunge et al., 1982; Carey et al., 1983; McGarvey et al., 1984; Clark and Bunge, 1989; Obremski et al., 1993
N9	$AX + SC + LA \rightarrow MAX \cdot BM$	Schwann cells cultured with neurons and laminin; BM synthesized	Eldridge et al., 1989
N10	$SC + COM \xrightarrow{in\ vivo} BM$	Schwann cells with collagen matrix inside silicone tube bridging gap between transected stumps in absence of axons; BM synthesized on Schwann cell surface	Ikeda et al., 1989
N11	$SC + FB \rightarrow BM$	Schwann cells cultured with fibroblasts; BM synthesized	Obremski et al., 1993
N12	$SC + LA \rightarrow \mathbf{BM}$	Laminin added to Schwann cell culture; BM synthesized in absence of myelin sheath	Obremski et al., 1993

C. Endoneurium (ED)

N13	$AX + SC \rightarrow No\ ED$	Schwann cells cultured with neurons; no endoneurium synthesized	Bunge et al., 1980
N14	$SITB \xrightarrow{in\ vivo} MAX \cdot BM \cdot ED(?) \cdot PN$	Silicone tube bridging nerve stumps; functional perineurium synthesized; no physiological endoneurial vasculature synthesized	Azzam et al., 1991

TABLE 7.2. *Continued*

No.	Reactants	Reaction conditions and structure of product	References
D. Perineurium (PN)			
N15	AX + SC → *No* PN	Schwann cells cultured with neurons; no perineurium synthesized	Bunge et al., 1980
N16	AX + FB → *No* PN	Schwann cells cultured with fibroblasts; no perineurium synthesized	Williams et al., 1982
N17	AX + SC + FB → MAX · BM · ED(?) · PN(?)	Schwann cells cultured with neurons and fibroblasts; perineurial-like cells observed surrounding neuron-Schwann cell units	Williams et al., 1982; Bunge et al., 1989
N18	**TB** $\xrightarrow{\text{in vivo}}$ **MAX · BM · ED(?) · PN**	Filled or unfilled silicone tube bridge; functional perineurium synthesized; no physiological endoneurial vasculature synthesized	Scaravilli, 1984; Azzam et al., 1991
E. Epineurium (EN)		No confirmed synthesis reported in vitro or in vivo	see text
F. Nerve trunk (MAX · BM · ED · PN)			
N19	**TB** $\xrightarrow{\text{in vivo}}$ **MAX · BM · ED(?) · PN**	Stumps inserted into unfilled tubes; myelin sheath and supporting tissues synthesized (but not clearly identified); nerve trunk synthesized, occasionally reported conducting	Lundborg et al., 1982a,b,c,d; Uzman and Villegas, 1983; Scaravilli, 1984; Williams et al., 1984; Seckel et al., 1984; other authors (see Chapter 6)
N20	**TB + FI** $\xrightarrow{\text{in vivo}}$ **MAX · BM · ED(?) · PN**	Stumps inserted into tubes filled with exogenous reactants; myelin sheath and supporting tissues synthesized but not clearly identified; nerve trunk synthesized, occasionally reported conducting	Madison et al., 1985, 1988; Yannas et al., 1985, 1987a,c; Valentini et al., 1987; Williams et al., 1987; Aebischer et al., 1989; other authors (see Chapter 6)

synthetic process is usually not known in advance; however, it may occasionally be deduced, as discussed below.

The negative controls employed in syntheses of skin and peripheral nerves both in vitro and in vivo have been included for completeness at the top of the reaction diagram tabulations. They are designated S01, S02 (skin) and N01, N02 (peripheral nerve) and represent conditions in vitro and in vivo under which no synthesis of the desired tissues takes place in the absence of any added reactants even though the study was conducted in the identical defect.

7.2 Irreducible Reaction Diagrams for Synthesis of Skin

Although a highly simplified version of reality, the symbolic presentation of data in the form of a reaction diagram is a surprisingly effective method for summarizing the experimental evidence on synthesis of tissue components or of the organ itself. Simple inspection of the symbolic data leads to selection of the simplest (irreducible) conditions for synthesizing a particular tissue. The irreducible diagram provides information about the existence of a requirement for cells of a given type or a specific nondiffusible regulator, or both, for the desired synthesis. Furthermore, the symbolic representation rapidly informs whether a given tissue can be synthesized in vitro rather than in a more demanding in vivo protocol.

Several conclusions emerge from inspection of reaction diagrams 1 through 6 (Dgs. S1–S6) in Table 7.1. Synthesis of an epidermis did not require culturing with fibroblasts; nor did it require the presence of the following: the dermis regeneration template (DRT); a collagenous bilayer (CBL); fibroblasts cultured with a laminated modification of DRT (L-DRT); or fibroblasts cultured in a collagen gel (COG). Furthermore, synthesis of an epidermis did not require in vivo conditions; an epidermis was synthesized simply by culturing keratinocytes in vitro in a defined (serum-free) medium, as shown in Dg. S2. We conclude that Dg. S2 illustrates the irreducible conditions for synthesis of an epidermis; it is presented in bold letters in Table 7.1.

Processes for synthesis of a basement membrane are summarized in Dgs. S7–18. A basement membrane (BM), typically attached to an epidermis and comprising at least a lamina lucida as well as a lamina dense, but without rete ridges or a thick, vascularized dermis attached to it, was synthesized by grafting a construct comprising keratinocytes cultured in a fibroblast-contracted collagen gel (COG) onto the defect, as shown here:

$$KC + FB + COG \xrightarrow{\text{in vivo}} E \cdot BM \qquad \text{(Dg. S15)}$$

Subtraction of the fibroblasts and the collagen gel from the roster of reactants did not prevent synthesis of E·BM in the defect:

$$KC \xrightarrow{\text{in vivo}} E \cdot BM \qquad \text{(Dg. S9)}$$

Furthermore, conducting the process represented by Dg. S15 in vitro, rather than in the dermis-free defect, also yielded a BM:

$$KC + FB + COG \rightarrow E \cdot BM \qquad \text{(Dg. S10)}$$

Inspection of Dg. S13 shows, however, that, in order to synthesize a basement membrane (BM), there was no requirement for either fibroblasts or any of a number of nondiffusible reactants, including a type I collagen gel produced by fibroblast contraction (COG), bilayer consisting of a type IV collagen layer and a type I+III collagen layer (CBL), dermis regeneration template laminated on one side with a nonporous type I collagen layer (L-DRT), nylon mesh (NY), polyglactin mesh (PGL), cast type I collagen film (COFL), the surface of a plastic dish (PL), or dermis regeneration template (DRT). In vitro culture of keratinocytes in a defined medium, as in Dg. S13, led to synthesis of hemidesmosomes, anchoring filaments, lamina lucida, lamina densa, as well as to synthesis, but not secretion, of type VII collagen, the major protein in anchoring fibrils (Rosdy et al., 1993). We conclude that the simplest or irreducible reaction diagram for synthesis of a basement membrane is Dg. S13. As with the epidermis, in vivo conditions were not required for synthesis of a basement membrane.

A thick, well-vascularized dermis (D) was synthesized by grafting the dermis-free defect with the dermis regeneration template (DRT):

$$DRT \xrightarrow{\text{in vivo}} D \qquad \text{(Dg. S19)}$$

Use of several in vitro protocols failed to yield a dermis. A dermis was not synthesized when keratinocytes were cultured, in the absence of fibroblasts, on a collagenous bilayer (Dg. S22) or on the dermis regeneration template (Dg. S23). Nor was a dermis synthesized when keratinocytes were cultured with fibroblasts on a collagen gel (Dg. S20), on the physically modified (laminated) DRT (Dg. S26), or on a polyglactin mesh (Dg. S27). Furthermore, no dermis was synthesized when keratinocytes alone were cultured in vitro and then grafted (Dg. S24). Under in vivo conditions, a dermis (together with other tissues attached to it) was synthesized following grafting with a culture of keratinocytes and fibroblasts in a collagen gel (Dg. S21), a culture of keratinocytes and fibroblasts in the laminated DRT (Dg. S25), and a culture of keratinocytes and fibroblasts in a polyglactin mesh (Dg. S28). Diagram S19 shows that synthesis of a dermis did not require the addition of keratinocytes or fibroblasts for in vivo synthesis; however, it did require use of DRT.

The lack of a requirement for keratinocyte addition in order to synthesize the dermis in vivo needs to be examined further. Keratinocytes normally migrate from the edges of the skin defect into the center; in addition, contraction of defect edges brings these migratory epithelia closer to grafts. It might be plausibly suggested, therefore, that migrating keratinocytes may have in fact participated in the synthesis of the dermis, summarized by Dg. S19. Data from two studies can be used to reject this hypothesis. The first was conducted with the dermis-free skin defect in the swine, in which contraction was arrested early following grafting with DRT, leaving most of the initial defect area uncovered by epithelia. Meanwhile, a dermis was synthesized in the uncovered defect that was clearly free of migrating epithelia; a few days later, migratory epithelia from the edges covered the new dermis (Orgill et al., 1996). The second study was conducted with the rapidly contracting dermis-free defect in the guinea pig; in this model, DRT was applied as an island graft, allowing it to remain clear of the contracting edges by a substantial distance for at least 2 weeks, and to synthesize the dermis in the absence of migrating epithelia (Orgill and Yannas, 1998). The results of these two studies support the keratinocyte-free description of conditions for synthesis of a dermis (Dg. S19). We conclude that DRT, a nondiffusible reactant, induced synthesis of a nonregenerative tissue in vivo in the absence of exogenously added cells. Even though the reaction diagrams do not by themselves reveal the mechanism of its activity, it is highly plausible to hypothesize that DRT regulated the activity of cell type(s) that are undefined; for this reason, DRT will be referred to as a nondiffusible regulator. A hypothetical explanation for the regenerative activity of nondiffusible regulators appears in Chapters 8 and 10.

Partial synthesis of skin, with an epidermis, basement membrane, rete ridges with interdigitating dermal papillae, and a thick, well-vascularized dermis but no appendages, was accomplished by use of the following reaction diagram:

$$KC + FB + L\text{-}DRT \xrightarrow{\text{in vivo}} E\text{·}BM\text{·}RR\text{·}D \qquad \text{(Dg. S31)}$$

A simpler in vivo process, obtained by subtracting fibroblasts from the reaction conditions shown above, as well as after substitution of unmodified DRT for physically modified DRT (L-DRT), also yielded the same partial organ:

$$KC + DRT \xrightarrow{\text{in vivo}} E\text{·}BM\text{·}RR\text{·}D \qquad \text{(Dg. S30)}$$

Simplifying further by subtracting DRT from Dg. S30 led to synthesis only of E·BM (Dg. S9). Subtraction of KC from Dg. S30 yielded only D (Dg. S19). Other, less simple in vivo reaction conditions yielded a skin that not only lacked appendages but also lacked rete ridges with interdigitating dermal papillae (elastic fibers were also not reported), that is, E·BM·D. These protocols included culturing keratinocytes with fibroblasts on a collagen gel before grafting (Dg. S29); culturing keratinocytes on a bilayer fabricated from type IV and type I+III collagen layers prior to grafting (CBL) (Dg. S32); and culturing keratinocytes on a polyglactin mesh and fibroblasts before grafting (Dg. S33). There is evidence that a modification of the protocol for preparation of the keratinocyte- and fibroblast-cultured collagen gel (Dg. S29), leading to increased maturation of the epidermis prior to grafting, yielded a partial skin with some rete ridges (Parenteau et al., 1996). Also, even though rete ridges were missing for a period of 55 days after grafting with the keratinocyte culture on the collagenous bilayer (Dg. S32), a slightly undulating dermo-epidermal junction was observed by that time (Tinois et al., 1991). It is likely that the protocols described in this paragraph could be modified further in future studies to yield a partial skin with clearly defined rete ridges.

We conclude that Dg. S30 describes the simplest reaction conditions for partial synthesis of skin. Put in words, partial synthesis of skin, including an epidermis, basement membrane, rete ridges with interdigitating dermal papillae and a thick, well-vascularized dermis with elastic fibers and dermal nerve fibers, but no appendages, required grafting the defect with the keratinocyte-seeded dermis regeneration template. Neither grafting with a KC sheet alone nor with DRT alone sufficed to yield partial skin; nor was addition of fibroblasts required. In vivo conditions were clearly required. The synthesis of rete ridges and dermal elastic fibers observed when keratinocytes were grafted with DRT (Dg. 30) was not reported when other in vivo protocols were employed (Dgs. S29, S32, S33). Elastic fibers were reported when keratinocytes were grafted with fibroblasts and with the modified DRT (L-DRT) prior to grafting (Dg. S31). In conclusion, it is clear that partial synthesis of skin (no appendages) simply requires addition of keratinocytes and the appropriate nondiffusible regulator to the dermis-free defect.

Keratinocyte seeding of the dermis regeneration template (DRT) was required for the synthesis of an epidermis at the same time that a dermis was also being synthesized (simultaneous synthesis; Dg. S30). In contrast, when the KC-free template was grafted in the swine, synthesis of a dermis first proceeded as in Dg. 19 without simultaneous synthesis of an epidermis; instead, synthesis of an epidermis occurred with a several-day delay, originating with migratory epithelia from the edge of the defect (sequential synthesis) (Orgill et al., 1996; Orgill and Yannas, 1998).

Keratinocytes were not required to be uncultured in order to participate in partial synthesis of skin, as in Dg. S30. Culture of KC to subconfluence with DRT in vitro prior to grafting also led to simultaneous synthesis of a dermis and an epidermis; in this case, the number of rete ridges was significantly higher compared with the protocol in which uncultured KC were used (Butler et al., 1999a). Alternative protocols, such as those described here, lend some flexibility to the process of synthesizing an organ. The flexibility is limited: while synthesis of the noregenerative dermis preceded synthesis of an epidermis, as described above, the reverse was not observed (Dg. S9).

We conclude that all three layers that comprise the tissue triad in skin (i.e., epithelia-BM-stroma), were synthesized in sequence by first inducing synthesis of stroma and then waiting for the keratinocytes to migrate over the stroma, eventually synthesizing the epidermis and the basement membrane; or the triad was synthesized simultaneously by seeding DRT with cells from the epithelial layer.

The simplest processes for synthesizing each of the tissue components of skin, as well as partial skin itself, can now be identified, as highlighted in Table 7.1. These irreducible reaction diagrams are the following:

Epidermis:

$$KC \to E \qquad\qquad\qquad \text{(Dg. S2)}$$

Basement membrane:

$$KC \to E \cdot BM \qquad\qquad\qquad \text{(Dg. S13)}$$

Dermis:

$$DRT \xrightarrow{\text{in vivo}} D \qquad\qquad\qquad \text{(Dg. S19)}$$

Skin (no appendages): $KC + DRT \xrightarrow{\text{in vivo}} E \cdot BM \cdot RR \cdot D$ (Dg. S30)

We notice that, although in vitro conditions sufficed to synthesize an epidermis and a basement membrane, synthesis of the dermis as well as of partial skin itself required an in vivo environment. We further notice that synthesis of an epidermis and a basement membrane in vitro both required addition of keratinocytes but not fibroblasts or a nondiffusible regulator; in particular, the addition of extracellular matrix (ECM) was not required. In contrast, synthesis of a dermis and of skin in vivo required addition both of keratinocytes and of a nondiffusible regulator.

7.3 In Vitro versus In Vivo Conditions

Why was an in vivo environment required for synthesis of rete ridges or a dermis? Which indispensable reactants, apparently not available in vitro, were supplied by the dermis-free skin defect? These questions can be answered, at least in part, by considering the few irreducible reaction diagrams that were selected in the preceding section. The requirement for a distinction between in vitro and in vivo protocols (Figure 7.1) has important practical and theoretical implications.

In an effort to identify the components of a dermis-free defect that were required in the syntheses we will limit the choices by elimination. First, we look for evidence that a given reactant, exogenously supplied, participated in an irreducible reaction diagram in vivo. Such participation in the irreducible digram shows that addition of the reactant was necessary to achieve the desired synthesis; if so, it follows that the defect was not a supplier (at least, not an adequate supplier) of this required reactant. For example, keratinocytes are a reactant that had to be exogenously supplied in order to

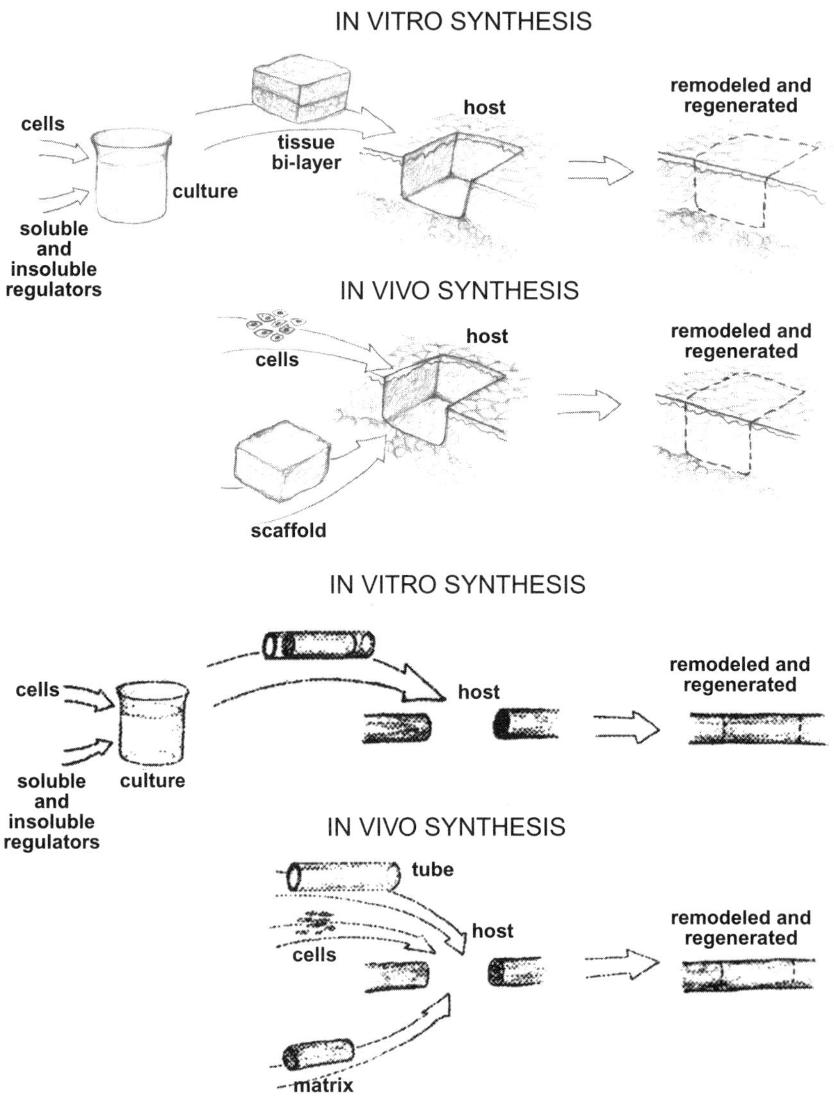

FIGURE 7.1. Experimental configurations for in vitro and in vivo synthesis of skin (top) and peripheral nerves (bottom). Reactants include cells, soluble (diffusible), and insoluble (nondiffusible) regulators. In a typical in vitro protocol, reactants are introduced in culture medium; the resulting organoid is then implanted at the anatomical site. In vivo protocols call for direct implantation at the anatomical site. In both types of protocol, remodeling and regeneration processes take place at the anatomical site before significant organ function has been resumed.

induce simultaneous synthesis of the epidermis and the dermis (Dg. S30) but not of the dermis alone (Dg. S19). Another reactant that had to be exogenously supplied to induce in vivo either synthesis of dermis (Dg. S19) or synthesis of skin (Dg. S30) is the dermis regeneration template. The data suggest, therefore, elimination of keratinocytes and the dermis regeneration template from consideration as reactants that are indispensably supplied by the defect; if these reactants had been supplied by the defect, there would have been no requirement for their addition as reactants to the irreducible digram.

Exogenous supply of fibroblasts was not required to synthesize any of the components of skin, as seen by inspection of all four irreducible reaction diagrams, S2, S13, S19, and S30. Since it is well-known that fibroblasts are critically involved in synthesis of ECM (Clark et al., 1996b; Eckes et al., 1996), it appears that the required fibroblasts were spontaneously supplied by the defect (endogenous supply). A similar argument can be made about the absence of microvascular endothelial cells from the irreducible diagrams; these cells are responsible for angiogenesis (Madri et al., 1996). Since the irreducible diagrams describe the synthesis of vascularized stroma, it follows that the defect spontaneously supplied microvascular endothelial cells; an exogenous supply was unnecessary. Of the tissue components in skin, the epidermis and the basement membrane could be synthesized by keratinocytes in vitro, in the absence of fibroblasts (Dgs. S2, S13). Synthesis of a dermis, however, required the presence of the defect (Dg. S19). Since the synthesis of tissues could not have proceeded in the absence of cells, it follows that all cells required for synthesis of a dermis (Dg. S19) must have originated in the defect (endogenous supply of cells). We arrive, therefore, at the hypothesis that synthesis of the dermis, as in Dg. S19, required in vivo conditions simply because of a requirement for an endogenous supply of fibroblasts and endothelial cells.

If this simple analysis was sufficient to explain the data, synthesis of a vascularized dermis should be possible in vitro by seeding the hypothetically required fibroblasts and endothelial cells into an appropriate non-diffusible regulator, such as DRT. One protocol that approximates these conditions in vitro is Dg. S26; however, no dermis was synthesized under these conditions. Diffusible regulators (i.e., soluble chemical messengers for cell communication) such as cytokines and growth factors are present in the exudate that flows very early into the defect; they are also secreted by degranulating platelets and are synthesized by cells migrating into the defect. The cytokine field produced in this manner comprises the time-dependent concentrations of several cytokines known to be simultaneously present in the defect during spontaneous healing; these concentrations are probably changing in response to signals from adjacent cells or tissues (paracrine signals). Several of these diffusible regulators have been identified and their individual role outlined (Clark, 1996b). However, the dynamics of the cell–cell signaling processes during spontaneous healing in the presence of multiple cytokines have not been elucidated; consequently, it is not clear just what the complex cytokine field contributes to tissue synthesis in the dermis-free defect. Clearly, however, the cytokine field is missing in studies conducted in vitro.

In conclusion, the available evidence strongly suggests that the defect is a required supplier both of fibroblasts and endothelial cells, as well as of the time-dependent cytokine field, during the synthesis of a dermis. It is well known that the two cell types are involved in cell-cell signalling (the signals being the cytokines), especially during fibroplasia and angiogenesis, the major pathways responsible for the synthesis of granulation tissue and dermal scar (McPherson and Piez, 1988; Eckes et al., 1996; Madri et al., 1996). Clearly, fibroblasts, endothelial cells and the cytokine field are intimately related and their function cannot be considered separately. We conclude that it is not the separate requirement for the cytokine field or for fibroblast or endothelial cell presence, but the specific regulation of fibroblast and endothelial cell function by the cytokine field, that must be primarily responsible for the uniqueness of the in vivo environment in the synthesis of certain skin components.

7.4 Conditions for Synthesis of Peripheral Nerves

We now examine the reaction diagrams for synthesis of tissue components of peripheral nerves, presented in Table 7.2.

Introduction of a neuron in a reaction medium will not be regarded as indicating the supply of a reactant. Certainly, axons are indispensable components of a physiologically conducting nerve fiber and axon elongation is indispensable during regeneration across a tubulated gap. Nevertheless, in the context of a chapter devoted to synthesis of tissues, the axon will be viewed simply as the substrate on the surface of which a highly specialized tissue, the myelin sheath, is synthesized. Although axons will be explicitly shown in the reaction diagrams below, their presence will be regarded as being equivalent to the presence of a constant background in the protocols.

In the symbolic language of this chapter, we will classify the silicone tube, as well as several other tube types used in tubulation of the stumps of a transected nerve, as nondiffusible regulators. Although it may appear somewhat strange to apply this term to a tube, there is strong evidence, presented in Chapter 6, that tubulation itself induces regeneration of peripheral nerves. There is also evidence that the tube suppresses the formation of a sheath of contractile cells around a healing nerve stump; such suppression is related to the extent of regeneration obtained (as described in Chapters 8 and 10) and appears also to sensitively depend on the physicochemical properties of the tube wall, including composition and perhaps also permeability (Chamberlain et al., 2000a).

The reaction diagrams in Table 7.2 provide certain clear guidelines. Considering the series Dgs. N1–N5, we notice that synthesis of a myelin sheath (myelination) around a neuron (MAX) did not require the presence of fibroblasts; nor did it require the presence of ECM in the form either of a type I collagen substrate, COFL (Dg. N1), a reconstructed basement membrane, RBM (Dg. N3), or laminin (LA) (Dg. N5). According to Dg. N2, axons did not self-myelinate in culture. An in vivo environment was not required for myelination. Synthesis of a myelin sheath was not obtained simply in the presence of Schwann cells in culture; the presence of axons was required (Dg. N4).

Synthesis of a basement membrane encasing Schwann cells was achieved in culture, in the presence of axons and Schwann cells (Dg. N7). An in vivo environment was not required for BM synthesis. The resulting nerve fiber, MAX·BM, is the elementary unit of conduction in the nerve trunk. Neither isolated axons (Dg. N6) nor isolated Schwann cells (Dg. N8) yielded a basement membrane. Although axons and Schwann cells synthesized a BM in the presence of laminin (Dg. N9), the presence of laminin was not required, as shown by Dg. N7. Interestingly, a basement membrane could be synthesized in the absence of axons (i.e., in the absence of myelination), both in vitro and in vivo. For example, BM was synthesized in culture in the presence of Schwann cells and laminin (Dg. N12) or Schwann cells and fibroblasts (Dg. N11). BM was also synthesized around Schwann cells inside a silicone chamber that bridged a 10-mm gap in the rat sciatic nerve. The chamber was filled with a collagen matrix seeded with exogenously supplied Schwann cells; however, the tube was closed at both ends by a Millipore filter that excluded axons but allowed entry of exudate from the stumps (Dg. N10). The basement membrane normally encases Schwann cells in physiological tissues, rather than existing separately from them; for this reason, we will select Dg. N7 as the irreducible reaction diagram for synthesis of a BM encasing Schwann cells that have formed a myelin sheath around axons in culture; we will also select Dg. N12 as an irreducible diagram for synthesis of a BM in culture in the absence of a myelin sheath.

A physiologically functioning endoneurium was not synthesized when neurons were cultured with Schwann cells (Dg. N13). Evidence that the vasculature of the endoneurium was not physiological was observed in a study of the transected and tubulated nerve (Dg. N14), even when synthesis of a physiological perineurium had been demonstrated in the same nerve trunk (Azzam et al., 1991).

A perineurium was not synthesized in culture in the presence of neurons and Schwann cells (Dg. N15) or in the presence of neurons and fibroblasts (Dg. N16). In the presence of all three cell types in culture (i.e., neurons, Schwann cells, and fibroblasts), perineurial-like structures were observed surrounding neuron-Schwann cells units (Dg. N17); however, these structures were only remotely suggestive of the structure of a mature perineurium, and it cannot be definitively concluded that a perineurium was synthesized in this protocol.

A structurally and functionally convincing perineurium was synthesized when the stumps of a transected nerve were bridged with a silicone tube

(Dg. N18), as clearly indicated by several investigators (Scaravilli et al., 1984, Azzam et al., 1991; see also Chapter 6). The possibility of regeneration of the endoneurium was not pursued. The presence of the tube was necessary; in its absence, each stump typically synthesized a neuroma (provided that the stumps were kept separated by a few mm), as shown in a study of the same animal model (Chamberlain et al., 2000a) as well as in other studies summarized in Chapter 6. Several other types of unfilled tube without exogenous filling, including tubes made of collagen and synthetic polymers, were probably also successful in inducing a synthesis of a perineurium; however, the morphological data are insufficient to document synthesis either of an endoneurium or of a perineurium in other types of tube.

Bridging of the nerve stumps with each of several types of tube yielded a conducting nerve trunk (Dg. N19). Furthermore, use of several tube fillings, including Schwann cells, as well as diffusible and nondiffusible regulators (Dg. N20), led to significantly closer approach of the structure of the nerve trunk to that of normal nerve, as documented in Table 6.1. The absence of morphological data on the regeneration of the endoneurium and the perineurium did not encourage us to separate these studies in additional classes according to the organ synthesized. For this reason, tubulated configurations have been lumped, simply for convenience of presentation in Table 7.2, into those in which tubes were unfilled (Dg. N19) and those in which tubes were filled (Dg. N20). Detailed data on the axon elongation length and long-term electrophysiological data of these tubulated configurations are presented in Tables 6.1 and 6.3, respectively.

Inspection of Table 7.2 leads to identification of the following irreducible reaction diagrams:

Myelin sheath (myelinated axons):

$$AX + SC \rightarrow MAX \qquad \text{(Dg. N4)}$$

Myelinated axon encased in BM (nerve fiber):

$$AX + SC \rightarrow MAX \cdot BM \qquad \text{(Dg. N7)}$$

BM around Schwann cells in absence of axons:

$$SC + LA \rightarrow BM \qquad \text{(Dg. N12)}$$

Endoneurium: no direct evidence for synthesis

Perineurium:

$$TB \xrightarrow{\text{in vivo}} MAX \cdot BM \cdot ED(?) \cdot PN \qquad \text{(Dg. N18)}$$

Epineurium: no direct evidence for synthesis

Nerve trunk (unfilled tubes):

$$TB \xrightarrow{\text{in vivo}} MAX \cdot BM \cdot ED(?) \cdot PN \qquad \text{(Dg. N19)}$$

Nerve trunk (filled tubes):

$$\text{TB} + \text{FI} \xrightarrow{\text{in vivo}} \text{MAX} \cdot \text{BM} \cdot \text{ED}(?) \cdot \text{PN} \qquad \text{(Dg. N20)}$$

We conclude that in vitro conditions were sufficient for synthesis of a myelin sheath and a basement membrane but not for synthesis of an endoneurium or a perineurium. Furthermore, neurons and Schwann cells in vitro sufficed to synthesize a nerve fiber but not an endoneurium or a perineurium. In order to synthesize a perineurium it was necessary to employ a tube in an in vivo setting.

We notice that Schwann cells were required for in vitro synthesis of a myelin sheath (Dg. N4) and of a basement membrane around a myelinated axon (Dg. N7); however, an exogenous supply of Schwann cells was not required in order to synthesize in vivo either a perineurium (Dg. N18) or a conducting nerve trunk (Dgs. N19, N20). As is well known to investigators of peripheral nerve regeneration with tubulated devices, Schwann cells are endogenously supplied (i.e., by the transected stumps) (Williams et al., 1983). It is likely, therefore, that the defect endogenously provided the hypothetically required supply of Schwann cells. Fibroblasts and endothelial cells are known to synthesize nonneuronal tissues similar to those in a nerve trunk and their presence in tubes bridging nerve defects has been amply documented (Williams et al., 1983); however, there is little direct information available on the synthetic activities of fibroblasts in tubulated nerve models. Neither fibroblasts nor endothelial cells appear as required reactants that are exogenously supplied in any of the irreducible diagrams in Table 7.2; however, in the synthesis of a perineurium and a nerve trunk, these cell types were most probably supplied by the defect.

Finally, we recall that in vitro studies were obviously conducted in the absence of a cytokine field. A similar reasoning to that employed above in the discussion of the synthesis of skin leads to the suggestion that the defect was a required supplier of fibroblasts, endothelial cells, and a cytokine field during the synthesis of a nerve trunk. As above, we suggest that the requirement does not apply independently to each of these two reactants; instead, what was probably required was the specific regulation of fibroblast and endothelial cell function by the cytokine field of the tubulated nerve gap. We conclude that Schwann cells, fibroblasts, endothelial cells, and the cytokine field should be considered as required contributions (required endogenous reactants) of the defect to the synthesis of a nerve trunk.

7.5 A Fresh Look at the Tissue Triad

In Chapter 2 we considered a threesome (triad) of tissues comprising the avascular, specialized epithelia on one side of the basement membrane and the highly vascularized, stroma (supporting tissues) on the other side. The evidence from studies of spontaneous regeneration in skin and peripheral nerves, summarized in Chapter 2, has shown that the epithelia and basement membrane are spontaneously regenerative while the stroma is not.

There is also a developmental similarity between keratinocytes in skin and Schwann cells in peripheral nerves (Bunge and Bunge, 1983) that was pointed out in Chapter 2. Like the Roman god, Janus, each cell type has two distinct sides, facing in opposite directions and engaged in totally different processes (polarized cells). On one of their two sides, keratinocytes and Schwann cells are anchored to the basement membrane that separates these cells from the extracellular matrix occupying the other surface of the basement membrane. The stroma in skin is the dermis; in the peripheral nerves, it is the endoneurium. On their other side, keratinocytes are involved in a specialized differentiation process leading to a keratinized epidermis that faces the air interface. Schwann cells are also engaged on their other side with a specialized differentiation process: they ensheathe the axon surface with the specialized myelin sheath. Neither the epidermis nor the myelin sheath contains ECM, although the cells in each tissue can, if appropriately regulated, synthesize ECM components, including the basement membrane.

The analogy between keratinocytes and Schwann cells can be further extended into the function of each cell type during the defect healing process. As was pointed out in an earlier chapter, following injury, both keratinocytes and Schwann cells abandon their stationary, anchoring connection to the basement membrane and become migratory, synthesizing a large number of cytokines and ECM components, including basement membrane. Later, each cell type recovers its stationary pose on the rebuilt basement membrane. The "go-stop" signals for the cycle have been partly identified: In the case of keratinocytes, migration begins either due to absence of neighbor cells or local release of growth factors (Clark, 1996b) and stops when laminin has been synthesized (Woodley et al., 1991). The go signal for Schwann cell migration may consist of one or more mitogens released by macrophages (Fu and Gordon, 1997) and there is evidence that, as with keratinocytes, the stop signal for Schwann cells is synthesis of laminin (Eldridge et al., 1989).

We will now review the conclusions from use of reaction diagrams in terms of the components of the tissue triad (Table 7.3). We observe that keratinocytes can synthesize an epidermis and a basement membrane without requirement for ECM presence; similarly, Schwann cells can synthesize a myelin sheath and a basement membrane without requiring ECM. Clearly no dermal elements are required for the synthesis of the epidermis with its associated basement membrane; nor are any epithelial elements required for synthesis of the dermis. Likewise, synthesis of the myelin sheath with its basement membrane can take place in the absence of endoneurial elements; however, there is insufficient evidence to decide whether an endoneurium can be synthesized in the absence of Schwann cells. Neverthe-

TABLE 7.3. Reactants required for synthesis of skin, peripheral nerves, and their tissue components.

Skin			Peripheral nerve		
Tissue	Reactant required for synthesis	Reaction conditions	Tissue	Reactant required for synthesis	Reaction conditions
Epidermis	Keratinocytes	In vitro[4]	Myelin sheath[6]	Schwann cells[6]	In vitro[4]
Basement membrane	Keratinocytes	In vitro[4]	Basement membrane	Schwann cells	In vitro[4]
Dermis[1]	DRT[3]	In vivo[5]	Endoneurium	Not observed	Not observed
Skin[2]	Keratinocytes and DRT	In vivo[5]	Nerve trunk[7]	Tube[8]	In vivo[9]

[1] Synthesized dermis had dermal papillae, elastic fibers, and dermal nerve fibers.
[2] Synthesized skin had a keratinizing epidermis, basement membrane, and dermis but no skin appendages.
[3] DRT, dermis regeneration template, a highly porous graft copolymer of type I collagen and chondroitin 6-sulfate with defined network structure.
[4] Synthesized in culture medium.
[5] Synthesized in a dermis-free defect.
[6] Neurons, with axonal processes, were also present but are considered in this context as a substrate for synthesis of myelin sheath by Schwann cells (myelination).
[7] Nerve trunk typically comprised conducting nerve fibers across entire length.
[8] Tube bridged gap between transected nerve stumps; tube wall commonly consisted of silicone, synthetic polymers, or collagen.
[9] Synthesized inside tube bridging transected nerve stumps.

less, the similarity of many synthetic processes for skin and peripheral nerve suggests that such a simple synthetic route may hypothetically exist and is worth pursuing. The tentative conclusion is that epithelial and stromal elements can be synthesized separately from each other.

Which tissue components can be synthesized in vitro? Can an entire organ be synthesized in vitro? To synthesize the epithelial-like cell layer of the tissue triad for skin or peripheral nerves (epidermis and myelin sheath, respectively) it was simply required to culture the dissociated, undifferentiated cells comprising that layer. Unassisted by cells of another type, keratinocytes and Schwann cells each eventually condensed in culture and differentiated to form its respective avascular layer as well as the associated basement membrane. In order to synthesize the stroma (dermis), however, an appropriate nondiffusible regulator as well as in vivo conditions were both required (data on endoneurium synthesis are unavailable). Both in skin and peripheral nerve, the dividing line between in vitro and in vivo protocols has been the basement membrane. Considering for a moment the regenerative character of the tissues involved, we further conclude that the regenerative tissues, the epidermis and the myelin sheath,

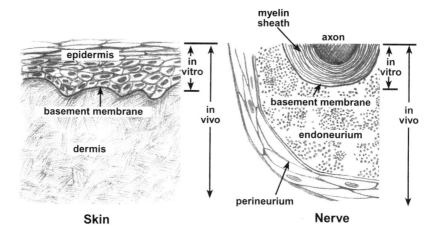

FIGURE 7.2. Current synthetic potential of in vitro and in vivo procedures in skin and peripheral nerves. Synthesis of epithelia and basement membrane in the two organs has so far been accomplished by use of in vitro as well as in vivo procedures. Synthesis of the stroma, as well as of the entire organ, has so far required use of in vivo procedures.

were synthesized in vitro while synthesis of the nonregenerative tissue (dermis) required in vivo conditions (Figure 7.2) (Yannas, 2000).

7.6 Toward Simple Protocols for Synthesis of the Entire Organ

Consideration of the tissue triad suggests similarities in protocols for synthesis of tissue components that, even though located in different organs, occupy the same relative anatomical position in the tissue triad that characterizes an organ.

Synthesis of the entire tissue triad (i.e., practically the entire organ) requires conditions that are clearly more complex than those for synthesis of tissue components (Table 7.3). For example, in order to synthesize skin, minus appendages, it is required to exogenously supply both keratinocytes and the appropriate nondiffusible regulator. Put differently, synthesis of the entire skin organ requires supply of the two reactants that must be supplied to separately synthesize each of the two major tissue components of the organ, that is, keratinocytes to synthesize the epidermis with its basement membrane and the nondiffusible regulator to synthesize the dermis. The entire skin organ, without appendages, can be synthesized using a protocol generated simply by adding the reaction diagrams for synthesis of its two major tissue components. This is a remarkably simple protocol for synthesis of an organ.

Does this simple rule also describe the protocol for synthesis of an entire peripheral nerve? Synthesis of a conducting nerve trunk requires exogenous supply of a nondiffusible regulator in the form of an appropriate tube, preferably with a filling of high regenerative activity. No other reactant need be exogenously supplied; in particular, an exogenous supply of Schwann cells, the analog of an exogenous supply of keratinocytes necessary for inducing synthesis of skin, is not required to synthesize a conducting nerve trunk comprising thousands of myelinated nerve fibers. It has been concluded above that the stumps of the defect are a supplier of Schwann cells, fibroblasts, and endothelial cells. The endogenous cell supply suffices to induce regeneration of nerve fibers; an exogenous cell supply appears, therefore, unnecessary for this task. Unlike the synthesis of skin, requiring the exogenous supply both of keratinocytes and a nondiffusible regulator, in existing protocols for synthesis of a conducting nerve trunk, the exogenous nondiffusible regulator is required but the Schwann cells are not. Do these findings suggest a fundamental dichotomy in the reactants required for these two organs?

The nerve trunks regenerated so far have resembled intact nerves closely only rarely and under narrowly defined conditions, for example, very short gaps (Table 6.3). Schwann cells have been exogenously supplied in the gap between the tubulated nerve stumps in a number of cases with very good results, as discussed in Chapter 6 (Guénard et al., 1992; Kim et al., 1994; Son and Thompson, 1995; Ansselin et al., 1997). Even in these cases, however, neither the tube type was selected to take advantage of its role as a nondiffusible regulator nor was a nondiffusible tube filling with regenerative activity employed. Each of these forms of nondiffusible regulation is separately known to profoundly affect regeneration (Chamberlain et al., 1998b, 2000a,b). Clearly, there is need for additional study to identify the tube type as well as the type of active tube filling that can lift the role of nondiffusible regulation of organ regeneration to a sufficiently higher level (Yannas, 2000). However, in these studies where an effort was made to increase the regenerative activity of the nondiffusible regulators, no use was made of an exogenous Schwann cell supply. Clearly, the success achieved with synthesis of skin suggests that an improved peripheral nerve may result from combined use of Schwann cells and nondiffusible regulators.

The ability to synthesize skin sequentially rather than simultaneously suggests yet another approach. As mentioned above, simultaneous synthesis of a dermis and an epidermis required exogenous supply of keratinocytes and an appropriate nondiffusible regulator. The same end result was reached, however, by sequential synthesis: the dermis was first induced to regenerate by use of a nondiffusible regulator; the epidermis and basement membrane were then spontaneously synthesized by the migratory keratinocytes on the existing dermal bed (see Chapter 5). In this protocol, the keratinocytes required for synthesis of the epidermis and basement membrane were endogenously supplied, in the form of migratory epithelia from the edges of the defect, and, therefore keratinocytes do not formally appear as an exogenous reactant in the symbolism of the reaction diagram for this sequential synthesis, a variant of Dg. S30:

$$DRT \xrightarrow{\text{in vivo}} E \cdot BM \cdot RR \cdot D \qquad \text{(Dg. S30a)}$$

Although this simplified protocol led to a greatly delayed synthesis of skin (Orgill et al., 1996), normally unacceptable in a clinical setting (Yannas and Burke, 1980), it is an interesting experimental alternative that can be used to improve understanding of organ synthesis.

The relative simplicity of these protocols suggests that almost the entire skin organ can be hypothetically synthesized in two spatially distinct reactor modules, each module designed to produce one of the tissue components. At a later time, the two modules could be brought together in order to synthesize the critical "transition" tissues, such as anchoring fibrils and rete ridges, thereby completing the (partial) synthesis of skin. Such a process, which I will call "modular organ synthesis," could be designed as an alternative of that in which all the reactants required to synthesize every tissue component of the organ are simultaneously fed into a single experimental volume either in vitro or in vivo. The tentative conclusion that "the whole can be synthesized as the sum of its parts" is obviously a rough approximation that does not account for synthesis of transition tissues; yet, it is an experimental approach that could shed much light into the complex processes for organ synthesis. However, transition tissue synthesis appears to require direct interaction between epithelial and meso-dermal tissues.

The synthetic approaches outlined above have been shown to be effective in the synthesis of skin and peripheral nerves. The similarity in effective synthetic protocols (Table 7.3) suggests clearly the possibility that these generic protocols could be useful in synthesis of other organs as well.

7.7 Summary

A symbolic language has been adopted to describe with economy the processes that have led to synthesis of tissues and organs in vitro and in vivo. Largely adapted from synthetic chemistry, it has been used to describe a synthetic process in terms of a reaction diagram, a shorthand report that includes the exogenously supplied insoluble reactants, the reaction conditions, and the insoluble product(s). Reactants have been classified simply as cells, diffusible (soluble) and nondiffusible (insoluble) regulators. Reaction conditions were specified as being conducted either in vitro (i.e., in a culture medium), or in vivo (as in an anatomically well-defined defect (Figure 7.1)). It was recognized that the concentrations of endogenous cytokines at the time, following injury, when (exogenous) reactants are being supplied to the defect (initial cytokine field) depend only on the nature of the defect. Provided, therefore, that different investigators have used the same defect, the initial cytokine field becomes a constant background in studies conducted in vivo and can be omitted from the reaction diagrams.

The shorthand notation has been used to conveniently identify the simplest conditions, or the irreducible reaction diagram, for synthesizing a desired tissue or organ. These diagrams summarize empirical, not theoretical, rules; they describe what has been observed, not what may be observed in future studies that may be conducted under different conditions.

Inspection of irreducible reaction diagrams for skin, peripheral nerves, and their tissue components leads to simple empirical rules that may be hypothetically applicable to the synthesis of other tissue and organs. The rules are presented in terms of the tissue triad that characterizes each organ. The tissue triad for skin and peripheral nerve, respectively, includes the basement membrane in the center, together with the epithelia-like, avascular tissue on one side (epidermis or myelin sheath), and the vascularized stroma on the other (dermis or endoneurium).

In both organs, the epithelia and the basement membrane of the triad were synthesized by culturing, in their undifferentiated state, only the cells that constitute the epithelia (i.e., keratinocytes and Schwann cells, respectively) for skin and peripheral nerve. There was no requirement for a cell of another type or for presence of extracellular matrix (nondiffusible regulator). The stroma in skin was synthesized in vivo by the exogenous addition of a nondiffusible regulator possessing regenerative activity. Synthesis of endoneurial stroma in peripheral nerves was not directly observed. Synthesis of the perineurium also required a nondiffusible regulator in vivo, in the form of a tube connecting the nerve stumps. No dermal elements were required for the synthesis of the epidermis with its associated basement membrane; nor were any epithelial elements required for synthesis of the dermis. Likewise, synthesis of the myelin sheath with its basement membrane took place in the absence of endoneurial or perineurial elements; however, since Schwann cells were endogenously supplied in all protocols by the nerve stumps, the available data cannot be used to test the hypothesis that a perineurium can be synthesized in the absence of Schwann cells. The epithelia (i.e., the epidermis or myelin sheath) were synthesized in vitro as well as in vivo; however, synthesis of the stroma (i.e., the dermis or the perineurium) required in vivo conditions (Figure 7.2).

Synthesis of the entire skin organ appeared to require simply a combination of the two reactants that were necessary for synthesis of the individual tissues of skin (i.e., keratinocytes and the appropriate nondiffusible regulator). The entire organ could be hypothetically synthesized by two distinct processes (modular organ synthesis) in which the individual synthetic reactions for the two tissue components take place in separate modules (reactors); in a later step, the two tissues are hypothetically brought together to synthesize transition tissues, such as anchoring fibrils and rete ridges. Alternatively, as with skin, the tissue components comprising the entire organ can be conceivably synthesized sequentially in the same reactor (i.e., the stroma is first synthesized by induction, followed by spontaneous regeneration of the epithelia and basement membrane on the presynthesized stroma); such a synthetic route may require fewer exogenous reactants.

These conclusions suggest challenging synthetic routes for organs other than skin and peripheral nerves. In one of these routes, for example, the anatomically well-defined defect in an organ such as the kidney or lung is supplied simply with cells of the type that comprise the epithelia of the organ and with a nondiffusible regulator that has the appropriate regenerative activity (the activity of nondiffusible regulators is discussed in Chapter 8). The findings made in this chapter with skin and peripheral nerves are similar enough to suggest that these reactants suffice to synthesize the epithelia, basement membrane, and stroma of other organs at the correct anatomical site.

8
The Antagonistic Relation Between Contraction and Regeneration

8.1 Contraction and Scar Formation Versus Induced Regeneration

Irreversible injury leads to contraction and scar formation. These two indispensable processes provide spontaneous closure of a severe defect in the adult organ; the result is repair. Any successful effort to bypass repair must inevitably include a strategy for dealing effectively with these two fundamental processes for defect closure.

In the preceding chapter we identified several protocols, some simpler than others, that can be used to reverse repair and induce regeneration instead. We now need to study these protocols, in order to find out just how such a reversal took place. In the remainder of this volume we will try to identify the pathways through which regeneration was induced. In this chapter we will focus primarily on the configuration of the final state in an effort to identify a general pattern that suggests the direction we should take in a study of the mechanistic steps. In subsequent chapters we will study the elementary steps that comprise the mechanism of induced regeneration.

Using the simple symbolism of the defect closure rule (Chapter 4), in which C, S, and R represent percentages of initial defect area that closed by contraction, scar, and regeneration, respectively, we represent healing of irreversible defects in the adult ($R = 0$) by Equation 2:

$$C + S = 100$$

Equation 2 embodies the obvious rule that, in the absence of regeneration, an increase in extent of contraction must be accompanied by a decrease in extent of scar formation, and vice versa. The defect closure rule is not unlike a description of a zero-sum game, in which the gains of one party must necessarily be compensated by the losses of another. The rule is illustrated by data of C and S values for spontaneously healing skin defects in various species, presented in Table 4.3.

Although it is obvious that any successful effort to induce regeneration must be done at the expense of the two terms, C and S, the defect closure rule gives no clue as to which of these closure modes need be expended. Most theories of failure to regenerate in adults, reviewed in Chapter 1, clearly favor scar formation as the closure process that needs to be suppressed in order to achieve regeneration. In this chapter we look for clues in the data that suggest that either one or the other of these processes of closure contribute most to the irreversibility of injury; or that perhaps each process contributes independently.

8.1.1 Reduction in Extent of Contraction in the Final State Coincided with Induced Regeneration

Although scar formation has been commonly considered the barrier to regeneration in adults, the quantitative evidence shows clearly that contraction is the more extensive mode of spontaneous closure in skin and peripheral nerve defects (Table 4.3). Accordingly, we will start our analysis by focusing on studies in which observations of induced regeneration in a given defect were accompanied with reports of changes in the extent of contraction that is observed spontaneously in that defect.

A collection of reports of induced regeneration in animal models together with the observed incidence of a change in extent of contraction is presented in Table 8.1. Two types of table entries have been made. The first consists of eight sets of quantitative data from studies with skin, peripheral nerves and the conjunctiva, presented in the format of the defect closure rule. Two of these entries are illustrated in Figure 8.1. The second set of entries in Table 8.1 comprises qualitative reports by the investigators on the incidence of a change in contraction compared to the spontaneously healing control defect. Several studies were not included in Table 8.1; these are studies of animal models in which regeneration was induced but no information was supplied by the authors on the pattern of contraction. Studies that were not referred to in Table 8.1 due to lack of information on contraction include studies on skin regeneration that have been described in detail in Chapter 5 (Bosca et al., 1988; Tinois et al., 1991) and the vast majority of studies in peripheral nerve regeneration in which the transected nerve was tubulated (see Table 6.1 for detailed references to these studies). Also not included from Table 8.1, due to lack of specific evidence on changes in contraction patterns, are data with humans.

With the exception of data on the conjunctival stroma, all other data in Table 8.1 were conducted with the anatomically well-defined defects described in Chapter 3 for skin and peripheral nerves. In the conjunctiva study (Figure 8.2), the investigators prepared an anatomically well-defined defect by removing the conjunctiva and the underlying stroma, together

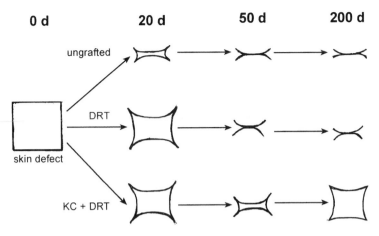

FIGURE 8.1. Schematic representation of skin regeneration in the adult guinea pig. The dermis-free defect was either ungrafted, grafted with dermis regeneration template (DRT) or grafted with keratinocyte(KC)-seeded DRT. Changes in the initial area of the defect are shown at 0 d, 20 d, and 200 d after injury and grafting. *Top*: Ungrafted defect eventually closed rapidly mostly by contraction and formation of a characteristic "stellate" scar. *Middle*: Grafting with the cell-free DRT led to strong delay in contraction and synthesis of a small mass of dermis, followed by synthesis of an epidermis over it. The resulting scar was more rounded than the stellate scar in the ungrafted defect. *Bottom*: Grafting with the keratinocyte-seeded DRT led to a significant delay in contraction, followed by arrest of contraction at 35–40 d and prolonged expansion of the defect perimeter. Simultaneous synthesis of a new skin organ, consisting of a physiological dermis and an epidermis with a basement membrane (but lacking appendages), covering an area about 2/3 of initial defect area, was observed. (Based on data from Yannas, 1981; Yannas, et al., 1989.)

with Tenon's capsule, down to the bare sclera. In this study, the shortening of the fornix adjacent to the stroma-free defect was reported in grafted and ungrafted groups as a measure of contraction of the defect (Hsu et al., 2000).

The quantitative set of data in Table 8.1 (eight sets of numbers in brackets) provides all the information necessary to deduce the presence or absence of a significant relationship between induction of regeneration and change in extent of contraction in these eight studies. The evidence clearly shows that in four of the five studies in which regeneration was induced ($\Delta R > 0$), the extent of contraction was very significantly reduced ($\Delta C < 0$). In the fifth study (Yannas, 1981), the reported small decrease in contraction is probably not significant. In contrast, in the three studies that failed to show induction of regeneration ($\Delta R = 0$), there was no change in the extent of contraction ($\Delta C = 0$).

TABLE 8.1. Induced regeneration and extent of contraction in animal models.

Species	Reactant (added to defect)	Configuration of final state, [C, S, R][1]		References
		Untreated defect	Treated defect	
A. SKIN (dermis-free)				
mouse	PDGF-BB[2]	[90, 10, 0]	[90, 10, 0]	Greenhalgh et al., 1990
mouse	bFGF[3]	[90, 10, 0]	[90, 10, 0]	Greenhalgh et al., 1990
swine	cultured KC[4] sheets	[89, 11, 0]	[89, 11, 0]	Carver et al., 1993a
rat, mouse	cultured KC on FB[5]-contracted collagen gel	not reported[8]	skin synthesis[11]; minimal contraction	Bell et al., 1981a,b, 1983; Hull et al., 1983b; Hansbrough et al., 1994b
guinea pig	DRT[6]	[91, 9, 0]	[89, 0, 11]	Yannas, 1981; Yannas et al., 1981, 1982a,b
guinea pig	DRT[6] seeded with KC[4]	[92, 8, 0]	[28, 0, 72]	Yannas et al., 1982a,b, 1989; Ogill, 1983; Murphy et al., 1990
mouse	FB[5] and KC[4] cultured on modified (laminated) DRT[6]	not reported[8]	skin synthesis[11]; minimal contraction	Cooper and Hansbrough, 1991; Cooper et al., 1993
mouse	KC[4] cultured on polyglactin mesh with FB[5]	not reported[8]	skin synthesis[11]; minimal contraction	Cooper et al., 1991; Hansbrough et al., 1993
swine	DRT[6] seeded with KC[4]	(reported in Orgill et al., 1996)	skin synthesis[11]; reduced contraction[12]	Compton et al., 1998; Orgill et al., 1998; Butler et al., 1998, 1999a

B. PERIPHERAL NERVE (transected and tubulated)

rat	silicone tube filled with NRT[7]	[95, 5, 0][9]	[53, 0, 47][9]	Chamberlain et al., 2000a,b
rat	collagen tube filled with NRT[7]	[95, 5, 0][9]	[0, 0, 100][9]	Chamberlain et al., 2000a,b

C. CONJUNCTIVA (stroma-free)

rabbit	DRT[6]	[45, 55, 0][10]	[13, 0, 87][10]	Hsu et al., 2000

[1] Configuration of the final state of defect healing is represented by the percentage of initial defect area closed by contraction (C), scar formation (S) and regeneration (R). See Chapter 4 for detailed discussion of defect closure rule and for data on untreated defects (Table 4.3). See Chapter 5 for detailed data on configuration of final state of treated defects (skin) and Chapter 6 for data on treated defects in the peripheral nerve.

[2] PDGF-BB, platelet-derived growth factor.

[3] bFGF, basic fibroblast growth factor.

[4] KC, keratinocytes.

[5] FB, fibroblasts.

[6] DRT, dermis regeneration template.

[7] NRT, nerve regeneration template.

[8] Untreated dermis-free defects in various rodents, in the swine and the human close spontaneuously by extensive contraction and scar synthesis; see Table 4.3.

[9] Author's estimate obtained from literature data, as discussed in Chapter 4.

[10] Reported as shortening of the fornix adjacent to the stroma-free defect.

[11] The level of completeness of skin synthesis varied among different protocols. See Tables 5.3 and 7.1, as well as Chapter 5 for details.

[12] Although contraction data were not reported in these studies with KC-seeded DRT in the swine, other data from the same laboratory showed that contraction was reduced following grafting of the same animal model with cell-free DRT (see Orgill et al., 1996).

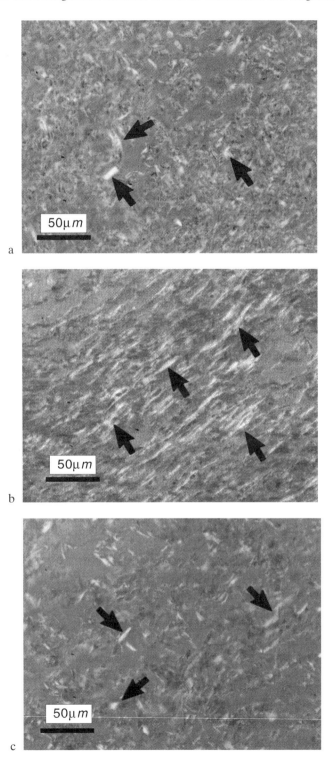

The second set of data in Table 8.1 consists of qualitative reports of the investigators on the extent to which contraction was affected in studies of induced skin regeneration. In all four studies, contraction was reported to be minimal or reduced relative to the untreated control.

In conclusion, in eight of the nine studies in which regeneration was induced, a significant reduction in contraction was also documented. In one study, the small reduction in contraction reported was not significant. In contrast, in the three studies in which no regeneration was induced, contraction was not affected. We conclude that eleven of the twelve sets of data reported in Table 8.1 are clearly consistent with the conclusion that a reduction in contraction was observed when regeneration was induced but was absent when regeneration did not take place. The available final state data suggest a hypothetical relation between suppression of contraction and induction of regeneration.

8.1.2 Delay in Closure by Contraction in Regenerating and Nonregenerating Defects

The observation, made above, that a reduction in the extent of contraction coincided with regeneration in several studies suggests that we take a closer look at other evidence of interference with contraction, such as changes in contraction rate. Much of the available evidence is in the form of quantitative data (e.g., delay in half-life) or qualitative observations related to contraction rate. These data have been included in Table 8.2.

Data in Table 8.2 were obtained in studies of anatomically well-defined defects in the skin. Investigators either reported the complete kinetics of contraction, from which the delay in half-life relative to the ungrafted control was estimated, or else reported qualitatively a change (or absence of change) in contraction rate. Some of the kinetic data on suppression of contraction were reported in studies for which final state data were presented in Table 8.1. The histological observations reported in Table 8.2 have been discussed in Chapters 5 and 6. The delay in half-life of the

◄───

FIGURE 8.2. Regeneration of conjunctival stroma in the adult rabbit. Polarized light micrographs illustrate differences in collagen fiber organization in the stroma at 28 d after excision of the conjunctival epithelium, substantia propria, and Tenon's capsule down to the level of bare sclera, taking care to avoid damage to the underlying sclera. Arrows point at parallel bands of birefringence, indicative of collagen fiber orientation. *Top* (Figure 8.2a): Normal conjunctival stroma, showing a quasi-random assembly of collagen fibers. *Middle* (Figure 8.2b): Ungrafted defect, showing highly oriented collagen fiber structure. *Bottom* (Figure 8.2c): Grafted with cell-free dermis regeneration template, showing a quasi-randomly organized arrangement of collagen fibers. Bar: 50 µm. (From Hsu et al., 2000.)

TABLE 8.2. Relation between delay in contraction and induced regeneration in skin defects.

Species (duration of study)	Reactant[1] (added to defect)	Contraction delay[2], Δt, d	Histological identification of product	References
rabbit (>25 d)	cortisone acetate	9.5	granulation tissue by 25 d	Billingham and Russell, 1956
mouse (21 d)	PDGF-BB	0	scar synthesized	Greenhalgh et al., 1990
mouse (21 d)	bFGF	0	scar synthesized	Greenhalgh et al., 1990
rat (10 d)	aFGF	0	granulation tissue; histology shows scar	Mellin et al., 1992
mouse (7 d)	TGF-b1	0	granulation tissue	Ksander et al., 1990
mouse (7 d)	TGF-b2	0	granulation tissue	Ksander et al., 1990
swine (24 d)	cultured KC sheets	0	granulation tissue	Carver et al., 1993a,b
guinea pig (120 d)	DRT	17.5 ± 3	small mass of dermis synthesized	Yannas, 1981; Yannas et al., 1981, 1982b
guinea pig (420 d)	DRT seeded with KC	13.5 ± 1.5; contraction arrested at 35–40 d	epidermis and dermis simultaneously synthesized	Yannas et al., 1982a,b, 1989

[1] Abbreviations used in this table have been defind in Table 8.1 (footnotes).
[2] Contraction delay, Δt, is the difference between contraction half-life of treated and untreated skin defects. In many studies, direct measurements of contraction were not made; instead, the investigators' verbal report was noted.

contraction process, Δt, of the treated compared with the untreated defect has been used as a standard measure of the change in rate at which a defect is closed by contraction (Billingham and Russell, 1956). Δt typically takes values over 5 d when the onset of contraction was significantly delayed by the treatment.

The data in Table 8.1 show that a significant delay in contraction coincided with induced regeneration. There was one exception to this conclusion; treatment with cortisone acetate led to granulation tissue formation (absence of regeneration). This case is discussed below in detail. In one case contraction was not only delayed but also arrested while, regeneration was being induced. Regeneration was not induced when a delay in contraction kinetics was not observed. With the exception of data on treatment with the steroid, the data on the kinetics of the contraction process are consistent with a hypothetical relation between suppression of contraction and regeneration.

8.1.3 Spontaneously Healing Defects: Relation Between Contraction and Regeneration

The data presented in the preceding two sections (also in Tables 8.1 and 8.2) were obtained in models of induced regeneration. How are contraction and regeneration related in models of spontaneously healing wounds? We will now review evidence from quantitative studies of spontaneous healing of skin defects in the frog larva (tadpole) and the rabbit ear.

The relative importance of the three modes of defect closure during development was studied with the North American bullfrog (Table 4.4). Changes in the relative percentage of contraction, scar synthesis, and regeneration in the configuration of the final state were measured before (tadpole) and after metamorphosis (frog). Contraction and regeneration alone accounted for defect closure at each of four developmental stages of the tadpoles that were studied; scar synthesis was not observed in the tadpoles. At each of four successive stages of tadpole development, the configuration of the final state changed as follows (development proceeds from left to right):

$$[41, 0, 59] \rightarrow [62, 0, 38] \rightarrow [66, 0, 34] \rightarrow [90, 0, 10]$$

With increasing development, contraction gradually became the dominant process for defect closure while regeneration correspondingly declined (Figure 8.3).

In the rabbit, a sharp difference in healing outcome of dermis-free defects has been observed in two anatomical sites: the dorsal region and the ear. While the defect in the dorsal region closed by vigorous contraction and synthesis of scar, the defect in the ear almost failed to contract at all and, instead, regenerated completely, including the synthesis of hair follicles and sebaceous glands; scar was not observed (Joseph and Dyson, 1966; Goss

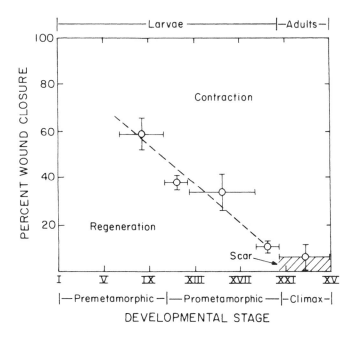

FIGURE 8.3. Contraction dominated regeneration increasingly as a mode of defect closure in the developing tadpole (larva). Time-independent values of each defect closure mode from Table 4.4 were used to construct the diagram. The broken line connecting the data divides the defect closure diagram into three regions, each corresponding to a mode of closure. Regeneration and contraction, without scar formation, combined to close dermis-free defects in the larvae of Rana catesbeiana at four stages of development. The percentage of each closure mode is indicated by the length of the ordinate inside the region corresponding to the mode. Following the developmental stage where metamorphosis occurred, indicated along the x-axis at the top of diagram as the transition from larvae to adults, regeneration was completely inhibited; instead, defects closed by contraction and scar formation in adults (cross-hatched region). (From Yannas et al., 1996.)

and Grimes, 1972, 1975) (Figure 8.4). Based on data that have been presented in Table 4.3, the configuration of the final state in these two anatomical sites is shown below:

(rabbit dorsal region)   vs.   (rabbit ear)
[96, 4, 0]   vs.   [3, 0, 97]

The striking lack of contraction in the rabbit ear defect has been attributed to particularly tight binding of the skin to the underlying cartilage (Joseph and Dyson, 1966; Mustoe et al., 1991). In contrast to the rabbit and other lagomorphs, dermis-free defects in the vast majority of mammals close by repair rather than by regeneration (Goss and Grimes, 1972; Goss, 1992). In conclusion, a comparison of closure modes of defects in these two anatomical sites of the rabbit, showed that spontaneous regeneration of skin occurred in the absence of contraction.

The two sets of data on spontaneously healing skin defects are consistent with the conclusion that regeneration was observed ($\Delta R > 0$) when contraction was suppressed ($\Delta C < 0$).

8.1.4 Scar Synthesis Was Abolished When Contraction Was Inhibited

A rather surprising conclusion emerges when attention is focused on the percentage of scar synthesis observed in quantitative studies of induced regeneration (Table 8.1).

Inspection of the data (numbers in brackets in Table 8.1) shows that, in all five instances in which regeneration was induced as a result of a given treatment, the extent of scar synthesis was reduced to an apparent level of zero. What is especially striking is that it was not necessary to entirely block contraction; scar synthesis was totally suppressed even when contraction was reduced to a relatively moderate extent (in one case, contraction appears to have remain unchanged). Although the histological data in Table 8.1 were based on detailed observation, the lack of precise quantitative data on scar content leaves open the possibility that traces of scar were synthesized but remained undetected in some of these studies in which regeneration was induced. However, the data allow no ambiguity to the conclusion that scar synthesis was essentially abolished in all cases when contraction was suppressed, even partly, while regeneration was induced. These data suggest that the extent of scar formation, S, was highly dependent on the extent of contraction, C, and that scar was a by-product of the contraction process.

8.1.5 Suppression of Contraction Did Not Suffice to Induce Regeneration

The preceding discussion brings up the obvious question: If, hypothetically, inhibition of contraction is required for regeneration, is it also sufficient?

Treatment of defects with agents that are known to suppress the inflammatory response in full-thickness skin defects, including steroids, has been studied extensively. While the rate of contraction was often strongly inhibited, regeneration was not induced. This conclusion is supported by data on delay of contraction (Table 8.2) as well as several independent data on the configuration of the final state (Table 5.3). In an early study of the effect of steroids, cortisone acetate was supplied daily to the dermis-free defect in

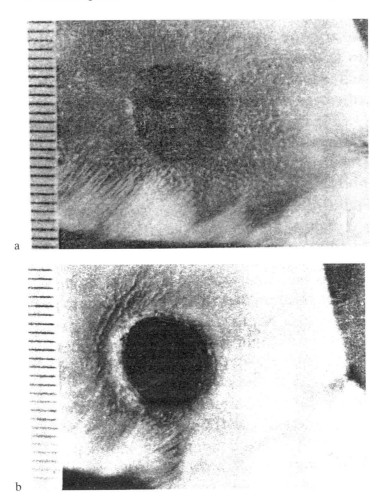

FIGURE 8.4. Regeneration, rather than closure by contraction is observed following cutting a full-thickness hole, 1 cm in diameter, in the rabbit ear. *Top left* (Figure 8.4a): 1 d. *Bottom left* (Figure 8.4b): 2 wk. *Top right* (Figure 8.4c): 4 wk. *Bottom right* (Figure 8.4d): 6 wk. (From Goss, 1980.)

a rabbit model and a significant delay in contraction was noted relative to the untreated control ($\Delta t = 9.5$ d); however, the investigators reported that granulation tissue eventually filled the defect by 25 d (Billingham and Russell, 1956). Administration of cortisone in a rat model led to a small delay in contraction; however, no regeneration was induced (Cuthbertson, 1959). In another study with the rat model, significant delays in contraction were observed following treatment with prednisolone, ETA (prostaglandin inhibitor) and aspirin; however, no regeneration was reported (McGrath,

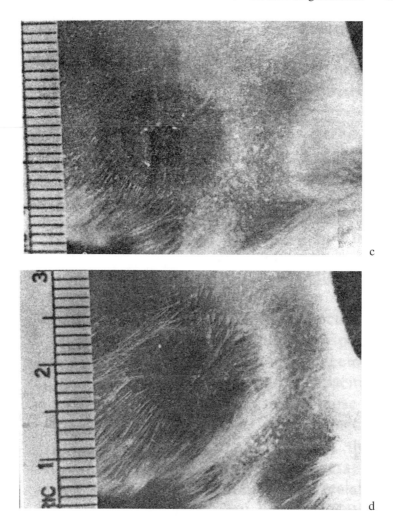

c

d

FIGURE 8.4 *Continued*

1982). In conclusion, the available data do not support a regenerative activity for any of the pharmacological agents used in these studies even though contraction was significantly inhibited.

Impaired healing due to a genetic disorder or bacterial contamination typically involves suppression of contraction. Its description is of some interest in a search of a relation between inhibition of contraction and regeneration. Dermis-free defects in the genetically diabetic mouse have been shown to close by contraction with substantial delay (delay in half-life for contraction, $\Delta t = 10 \pm 2\,d$) compared with defects in nondiabetic mice (Klingbeil et al., 1991); however, in a study of normal and diabetic mice from the same source as in the preceding study, it was observed that the configuration of the final state of healing was [90, 10, 0] in normal and [40, 60, 0] in diabetic healing, consistent with suppression of contraction without incidence of regeneration in either group of animals (Greenhalgh et al., 1990). Studies with genetically obese mice showed that contraction was delayed by about 9 d in these animals that exhibited impaired healing; however, no regeneration was observed (Klingbeil et al., 1991). In studies of defects contaminated with E. coli, delays in contraction half-life of 7 d (Fiddes et al., 1991) and 4 d (Hayward et al., 1992) due to the contamination were observed without incidence of regeneration. The combined data show that, in spite of a significant delay in contraction of impaired wounds, no regeneration was observed. In particular, in one study of diabetic animals in which relatively detailed histological data on the final state were reported (Greenhalgh et al., 1990), the deficit in defect closure due to impaired contraction was replaced by scar synthesis rather than regeneration.

Mechanical splinting has often been used to control contraction of skin defects. In a well-documented study, a modest delay in contraction of dermis-free defects in rats was reported as a result of particularly effective splinting; however, the defects eventually closed almost completely by contraction to the same extent as in the unsplinted control (Kennedy and Cliff, 1979). Modest delays in contraction were reported to result from mechanical splinting in other studies of dermis-free defects as well; however, contraction resumed after the splint was removed and played a dominant role in closure, as with unsplinted defects (Lindquist, 1946; Abercrombie et al., 1960; Zahir, 1964; Stone and Madden, 1975). In conclusion, there appears to be no evidence that inhibition of contraction by mechanical splinting induced regeneration of the dermis.

Full-thickness skin grafts have a well-documented, powerfully inhibitory effect on contraction; the latter is arrested (Billingham and Russell, 1956; Sawhney and Monga, 1970; Rudolph, 1975; Peacock and Van Winkle, 1976; Orgill, 1983). As extensively discussed in Chapter 3, grafting of a full-thickness skin wound with an autograft complicates greatly the effort to understand whether regeneration of the dermis has occurred; these data will not be discussed further in this context.

The effect of anti-inflammatory agents on wound contraction has not been studied in models of peripheral nerve regeneration. Studies of mechanical splinting have also been absent in this area.

The data discussed above show that suppression of contraction of skin defects by treatment with pharmacological agents (steroids, a prostaglandin inhibitor, aspirin), as well as in cases where contraction was impaired due to diabetes, obesity, or infection, or were retarded due to mechanical splinting, did not induce regeneration. We conclude that inhibition of contraction alone did not suffice to induce regeneration.

8.1.6 Summary of Data; a Theory Relating Inhibition of Contraction and Induction of Regeneration

In this section we will review the quantitative evidence relating contraction, scar formation, and regeneration and propose a theoretical interpretation.

Contraction or scar synthesis, or both, must be controlled in order to induce regeneration in an adult. Independent data from studies of induced regeneration in skin, peripheral nerves, and the conjunctival stroma showed that a significant reduction in the extent of contraction (Table 8.1), as well as delay in contraction (Table 8.2), coincided with induced regeneration. There were also studies in which contraction was not affected by the treatment (exogenous growth factors, keratinocyte sheet grafting); nor was regeneration induced in these studies. Two sets of data from studies of spontaneous regeneration were also reviewed. A progressive reduction in extent of spontaneous regeneration, observed with advancing ontogenetic development in an amphibian model, was accompanied by corresponding gradual increases in extent of contraction.

A rare anatomical site in an adult mammalian model (rabbit ear skin) in which spontaneous regeneration has been reported was also one in which contraction of a dermis-free defect did not occur; in contrast, vigorous contraction was observed, while regeneration was not induced, in dermis-free defects in other anatomical sites in the same species. In studies of induced regeneration in adults, even a modest reduction in extent of contraction coincided with apparently total abolition of scar synthesis. However, regeneration was not induced when contraction was delayed by treatment of dermis-free defects with anti-inflammatory agents; nor was regeneration induced in cases of impaired healing that are accompanied by strongly delayed contraction, such as in defects that were infected, or mechanically splinted, or defects in genetically diabetic or obese animals.

The available evidence supports the general theory that inhibition of contraction is necessary but not sufficient to induce synthesis of nonregenerative tissues in skin and peripheral nerves. The theory further predicts that scar is synthesized as a byproduct of the contraction process; and that even modest suppression of contraction suffices to abolish scar formation. Finally, the theory specifically predicts that regeneration is induced only when contraction is selectively suppressed and not when contraction is being abolished in the context of a general debilitation of the healing process.

The theory can be summarized by the following general condition for induction of regeneration in adult defects in skin and peripheral nerves:

$$\Delta R > 0 \text{ and } S \to 0 \text{ if } \Delta C < 0$$

where "if" denotes a necessary but not sufficient condition.

The evidence supporting the theory stated above has so far been almost entirely empirical consisting of data that simply identify those reactants that lead to a final state of regeneration rather than repair. No mechanistic data have been used. The mechanistic steps that lead to regeneration will be discussed in the remainder of this volume. In particular, examples of selective suppression of contraction are discussed in detail in Chapter 10.

8.2 Nondiffusible Regulators as Probes of Contraction

In the preceding section we summarized certain protocols that led to regeneration of skin, peripheral nerves, and the conjunctiva (Table 8.1). The data presented above as well as additional data presented in Tables 7.1 and 7.2 showed that a nondiffusible regulator was required in every case that led to synthesis of a nonregenerative tissue, including the dermis, a peripheral nerve trunk over a 10-mm gap or longer, and the conjunctival stroma. In this section we answer questions such as these: What are nondiffusible regulators? How can we use them to learn more about the mechanism of induced regeneration? Do they selectively suppress contraction and, if so, how?

8.2.1 Diffusible and Nondiffusible Regulators

Diffusible (soluble) regulators are widely known, in the form of growth factors, cytokines, and other molecules, as the indispensable actors in what has been called "crosstalk" between cells (Clark, 1996b). In sharp contrast, nondiffusible (insoluble) regulators are much less well known as regulators of cell function. Although soluble macromolecular regulators, such as fibronectin, have been long known to possess binding domains (ligands) that specifically link with cell receptors (Hynes, 1990), the specificity of action of insoluble regulators has not been as extensively described.

It is very likely that the wide difference in familiarity with soluble and insoluble regulators is due, at least in major part, to differences in familiarity with methodology for the study of each class. Chromatographic, electrophoretic, and other well-known methods for isolating and characterizing macromolecules in dilute solution are extensively described in any biochemistry text. Insoluble macromolecular networks can be characterized by the average molecular weight between crosslinks, classical methodology that is commonly included in most textbooks of polymer chemistry (Flory, 1953; Tobolsky, 1960); or by emerging techniques such as ligand identification by antibody titration. Yet these methods for analysis of nondiffusible regulators have not yet been widely used by scientists engaged in study of cell-matrix interactions.

8.2.2 Nondiffusible Regulators Are Insoluble Macromolecular Solids

The critical importance of nondiffusible regulators in processes of induced regeneration becomes immediately evident on inspection of relevant data

(Tables 5.3, 6.1, 7.1, 7.2, 8.1 and 8.2). The data show that several non-diffusible regulators induced partial synthesis of skin, peripheral nerves, and the conjunctival stroma.

A collection of nondiffusible regulators in this volume appears in Tables 7.1 and 7.2, the reaction diagrams for partial synthesis of skin and peripheral nerves, respectively. Among the examples included in Table 7.1, in protocols for synthesis of skin, are a collagen gel contracted by fibroblasts (Bell et al., 1981a,b, 1983; Hull et al., 1983b); an extracellular matrix (ECM) analog synthesized as a highly porous graft copolymer of type I collagen and chondroitin 6-sulfate (Yannas et al., 1981, 1982a,b, 1984, 1989); a laminated version of the preceding ECM analog allowing seeding of cells of different types in separated compartments (Cooper and Hansbrough, 1991; Cooper et al., 1993); a bilayer consisting of a type IV collagen layer and a type I + III collagen layer (Bosca et al., 1988; Tinois et al., 1991); and a mesh comprising fibers of polyglactin 910 (Cooper et al., 1991; Hansbrough et al., 1993).

The tabulation of reaction diagrams for synthesis of a peripheral nerve, Table 7.2, includes various tubes as well as tube fillings based on several insoluble substrates and filaments. Included among the latter, and discussed in Chapter 6, are the following: cables comprising oriented fibrin fibers (Williams et al., 1987; Williams, 1987); extruded fibers consisting either of a polyamide (Lundborg et al., 1997) or type I collagen (Itoh et al., 1999); an oriented collagen gel (Caballos et al., 1999); and a highly porous graft copolymer of type I collagen and chondroitin 6-sulfate with oriented pore channel axes (Chang et al., 1990; Chamberlain et al., 1998b; Spilker, 2000).

This is a large and somewhat bewildering collection. Represented in it are various synthetic polymers and ECM components in a variety of states. What do these materials have in common other than their insolubility and their polymeric nature?

8.2.3 Homologous Series of ECM Analogs as Probes of Induced Regeneration

Considerable information about the mechanism of induced regeneration has become available from studies with series (referred to below as homologous series) of highly porous ECM analogs. Each series comprises well-defined members that differ from each other in only one structural characteristic, for example, variation in identity of ligands for cell surface receptors; increases in average pore diameter that reduce ligand density; changes in average orientation of pore channel axes; and increases in density of covalent crosslinks between macromolecular chains that affect the degradation rate in vivo and, therefore, the period of time (duration) during which the regulator persists in a nondiffusible state.

Use of these homologous series has led to recognition of certain quantitative requirements of a mechanistic pathway that leads to induced regeneration, such as a minimum in ligand density and an optimal level of its duration in the nondiffusible state. Provided that the density of ligands available on the extensive pore surface (specific surface) of an ECM analog exceeds a certain level, a minimum number of cell receptors can be bound on the insoluble scaffold; such binding implies the transient "capture" on the scaffold of a large number of cells present inside the defect. Cell capture can lead to a phenotypic change such as a change in migration pattern or in expression of a protein that is associated with contractility; in this manner, the nondiffusible regulator can be used to control cell function.

An example of such modification in cell behavior appears to lead to cancellation of the contractile forces that lead to closure of a defect. One pathway for such a modification has involved deliberate changes in the specific surface of the ECM analog, without other changes in its structure, that can be brought about simply by modifying the average pore diameter. In an example that is discussed in detail in Chapter 10, when the average pore diameter of the ECM analog has been reduced to a relatively low level, the specific surface, and with it the ligand density, increases; accordingly, the number of contractile cells that are immobilized ("captured") on the surface increases as well, perhaps to two-thirds of the total cell population inside the defect. A further decrease in average pore diameter, with a resulting increase in ligand density, is required to immobilize almost all contractile cells inside the defect; the result is arrest of contraction (Yannas, 1997).

The length of time during which capture of contractile cells on the insoluble scaffold is effective depends on the rate at which the macromolecular chains of the scaffold are degraded, eventually becoming readily diffusible. A deliberate increase in the chemical composition of the ECM, such as an increase in the glycosaminoglycan (GAG) content or the density of covalent cross links that bind the macromolecular chains, lengthens the period of time (duration) during which the scaffold retains its insoluble character and its function as an effective cell captor. When the duration is much shorter than this limit, the scaffold very rapidly degrades and the capture of the contractile cell population does not last as long as the contraction process going on inside the defect; the result is inadequate control of contraction (Yannas, 1997).

Understanding of other structural requirements for an ECM analog with high regenerative activity, such as the precise limitation on the identity of ligands, and the requirement for pore channel orientation in peripheral nerve regeneration, are still being pursued.

8.2.4 Biological Activity of Certain ECM Analogs

The surprisingly strong and specific effect of certain nondiffusible regulators was discovered following synthesis of simple, well-defined models of the extracellular matrix (ECM analogs), initially based on type I collagen and later on type I collagen together with a glycosaminoglycan (GAG) (Yannas, 1972a,b; Huang, 1974; Wang, 1975; Yannas et al., 1975a). In a typical case, glycosaminoglycan (GAG) chains, especially chondroitin 6-sulfate, have been chemically "grafted" onto chains of type I collagen. Stabilized by covalent bonds, these analogs, known as graft copolymers, are intrinsically insoluble at physiological pH. In thermodynamic equilibrium with a good solvent, these three-dimensional network structures swell highly but do not dissolve to their component macromolecules. Biologically significant parameters of such a well-defined macromolecular network that have been controlled include collagen/GAG ratio, density of covalent cross-links, pore volume fraction, average pore diameter, and orientation of pore channel axes. Detailed methodology for synthesizing ECM analogs has been published (Yannas et al., 1980; Yannas, 1989; Chamberlain and Yannas, 1998) and detailed methods of solid-state characterization based on optical rotation, infrared spectroscopy and viscoelastic measurements have been also described (Yannas et al., 1972; Yannas and Huang, 1972; Gordon et al., 1974).

Preliminary evidence of unexpected biological activity was detected during studies in which ECM analogs were brought in contact with tissues in standardized assays. For example, whereas a network based on GAG-free type I collagen aggregated human platelets vigorously in vitro, platelet aggregation was almost totally suppressed in contact with certain collagen-GAG copolymers (Yannas and Silver, 1975; Silver et al., 1978, 1979). Since platelet aggregation and the resulting release of growth factors and inflammatory cytokines are early events in the processes of spontaneous defect healing that lead to repair, these results suggested the possibility of suppression of normal inflammatory activity by use of these copolymers.

Another early unexpected finding was observed in studies of ECM analogs that were subcutaneously implanted in the guinea pig. Whereas GAG-free collagen specimens were degraded relatively rapidly and apparently without inducing synthesis of tissue, collagen-GAG copolymers of approximately the same cross-link density resisted degradation over significantly longer periods at the same anatomical site; these copolymers also induced synthesis of connective tissue that attached the implant firmly to the subcutaneous tissues of the host (Yannas et al., 1975a,b). Synthesis of new tissue occurred when the degradation rate of the ECM analog reached an intermediate level, estimated to be of the same order of magnitude as the rate of synthesis of new tissue during the healing process at that anatomical site (Yannas et al., 1979; Yannas and Burke, 1980; Yannas, 1981). Also, while the nonporous version of a collagen-GAG copolymer, subcutaneously implanted, was eventually surrounded by a scar capsule, the identical copolymer with its pore structure intact was not surrounded by scar but instead induced synthesis of a tissue that appeared to be identical to the adjacent dermis and to have become continuous with it (Yannas, 1981; Yannas et al., 1981, 1982a,b).

In later studies it was eventually recognized that certain ECM analogs were inducing synthesis of physiological, or nearly physiological, tissues (regeneration). When seeded with keratinocytes, one of the ECM analogs arrested contraction and induced simultaneous regeneration of a dermis and an epidermis over about two-thirds of the initial defect area (Yannas et al., 1981, 1982a,b, 1984). Another ECM analog induced regeneration of a peripheral nerve across an unusually large gap between two tubulated nerve stumps (Yannas et al., 1985, 1987a; Chang et al., 1990; Chang and Yannas, 1992; Chamberlain et al., 1998b). A cell-free ECM, identical to that used in skin regeneration, analog has been used to regenerate the conjunctival stroma (Hsu et al., 2000).

Implants based on type I collagen had been studied much earlier than the ECM analogs described above. In a study of various forms of collagen, it had become clear that the level of cross-link density controlled the degradation rate of implanted collagen sutures (Grillo and Gross, 1962; Kline and Hayes, 1964). In addition, the immune response to reconstituted collagen had been found to be minimal (Grillo and Gross, 1962). In another study it had been shown that the average pore diameter of collagen implants controlled the migration of cells into collagen implants (Chvapil and Holusa, 1968; Chvapil et al., 1969). However, the studies with ECM analogs described above marked the first time that a complex biological activity, such as the ability to induce tissue regeneration, could be incorporated in a collagen-based macromolecular network (Yannas et al., 1981, 1982a,b, 1984, 1989).

In early studies, the cell-free ECM analog that induced dermis regeneration was referred to as "synthetic skin" (Yannas et al., 1977), "artificial skin" (Yannas et al., 1979, 1980; Dagalakis et al., 1980; Yannas and Burke, 1980), and "artificial dermis" (Burke et al., 1981). Its unprecedented biological activity eventually led to use of the term *dermis regeneration template* (DRT) as a means of distinguishing the specific ECM analog from the large number of other analogs that have been synthesized. DRT was recognized as a singular macromolecular network after it was observed that its ability to suppress contraction, a hypothetically required precursor of induced regeneration, rapidly dropped when the network structure significantly deviated from one characterized by an apparently critical chemical composition, average pore diameter, and cross-link density (Yannas et al., 1989). DRT was first described as "a biodegradable template for synthesis of neodermal tissue" (Yannas and Burke, 1980) and was the first "molecular scaffold" with biological activity reported in the patent (Yannas et al., 1977), the abstract (Yannas et al., 1975a, 1979) or the journal literature (Yannas et al., 1981, 1982a,b). Several innovative methods for synthesizing scaffolds based on synthetic polymers and intended for various applications in tissue engineering have been reported (Langer and Vacanti, 1993; Freed et al., 1994; Griffith Cima, 1994; Peppas and Langer, 1994; Griffith, 2000; Saltzman, 2000; Thomson et al., 2000). Model scaffolds for the study of ligands involved in cell-ECM interactions have been synthe-sized (Hubbell, 2000).

8.2.5 *Strong Dependence of Contraction-Delaying Activity on Structure of ECM Analogs*

In dermis-free defects, ECM analogs typically delay the onset of contrac-tion, leading to a delay in contraction half-life, Δt, that varies sensitively with their structure (Chen, 1982). The data in Table 8.3 are arranged in terms of the three major homologous series of ECM analogs that were studied. As mentioned above, such a series comprises members that differ from each other in only one structural characteristic (i.e., variation in chemical com-position, average pore diameter, and cross link density).

Inspection of the data in Table 8.3 shows that analogs lost their ability to suppress contraction following certain well-defined changes. In the first series, the activity was sharply diminished when the chemical composition was altered to delete the glycosaminoglycan (GAG) component from the collagen-GAG copolymer; furthermore, substitution of chondroitin 6-sulfate with aggrecan left the activity unchanged whereas substitution with either dermatan sulfate or decorin significantly increased the activity (Shafritz et al., 1994). Contraction-delaying activity significantly declined when the average pore diameter increased above 100 μm, with an apparent cutoff point at 125 ± 35 μm, or decreased below 20 ± 4 μm (Yannas et al., 1989) (Figure 8.5).

When other properties of a porous substance remain unchanged, the spe-cific surface, measured in mm^2/cm^3, decreases with an increase in average pore diameter. The sharp drop in activity of ECM analogs observed at an average pore diameter of 125 ± 35 μm (Figure 8.5, top) corresponded to a minimum level for the specific surface, estimated at $6,000 \pm 3,000$ mm^2/cm^3 (Chang, 1988). An example illustrates the magnitudes involved. It has been observed that, following grafting of an ECM analog with average pore diameter of 10 μm, corresponding to an estimated specific surface of $80,000$ mm^2/cm^3 porous matrix, the fibroblast volume density inside the dermis-free defect is 10^7 cells/cm^3 matrix. The calculated surface density of bound cells is 125 cell/mm^2 matrix and hypothetically does not vary with pore diameter provided that the chemical composition of the matrix is unchanged. An increase in pore diameter of the ECM analog to 300 μm, corresponding to an estimated specific surface of only $3,000$ mm^2/cm^3, leads to a calculated cell volume density of 3.75×10^5 cells/cm^3 matrix. Accord-ing to this simple calculation, the volume density of captured cells becomes approximately 27 times lower when the average pore diameter is increased from 10 to 300 μm (Yannas, 1997).

An increase in degradation rate of ECM analogs, measured in enzymatic units (e.u.), in the range 3.5 to 90 e.u., left the activity relatively unchanged; however, the activity dropped sharply when the degradation rate increased

TABLE 8.3. Effect of structural features of ECM analogs on delay in contraction half-life.

Treatment of dermis-free defect	Contraction delay,[1] Δt, d
1. Identity of ligands[2]	
A. Deletion of GAG[3,4]	
Untreated dermis-free defect (control)	0
Silicone sheet, 0.125 mm thickness	2 ± 0.5
Collagen, 160 ± 26	8 ± 2
Collagen-Chondroitin 6-sulfate, 150 ± 40	12 ± 3
B. Substitution of Chondroitin 6-sulfate (Ch6-S)[3,5]	
Collagen-Ch6-S, 91 ± 12	14 ± 1.4
Collagen-Aggrecan, 99 ± 23	13 ± 0.6
Collagen-Dermatan sulfate, 102 ± 26	17 ± 0.8
Collagen-Decorin, 94 ± 23	16 ± 1.3
2. Variation in pore diameter[3,6]	
Collagen-Ch6-S, <1	2 ± 1.5
Collagen-Ch6-S, 6 ± 1	5 ± 2.5
Collagen-Ch6-S, 20 ± 5[7]	20 ± 3
Collagen-Ch6-S, 50 ± 13 (DRT)[7]	19.5 ± 2.5
Collagen-Ch6-S, 77 ± 20 (DRT)[7]	19.5 ± 4
Collagen-Ch6-S, 100 ± 25 (DRT)[7]	17.5 ± 3.5
Collagen-Ch6-S, 145 ± 35	13.5 ± 2.5
Collagen-Ch6-S, 150 ± 40	12 ± 3
Collagen-Ch6-S, 200 ± 50	11 ± 4
Collagen-Ch6-S, 450 ± 100	9 ± 3
Collagen-Ch6-S, 850 ± 200	8.5 ± 2.5
3. Variation in degradation rate[8]	
Collagen-Ch6-S, 2.5 e.u.	8 ± 1.5
Collagen-Ch6-S, 3.5 e.u.	13 ± 2
Collagen-Ch6-S, 10 e.u.	10 ± 2
Collagen-Ch6-S, 15 e.u.	12 ± 3
Collagen-Ch6-S, 90 e.u.	12 ± 1.5
Collagen-Ch6-S, 120 e.u.	6 ± 1.5
Collagen-Ch6-S, 200 e.u.	4 ± 1.5
Collagen-Ch6-S, 210 e.u.	3 ± 2
4. Seeded with keratinocytes[9]	
Collagen-Ch6-S seeded with KC	13.5 ± 1.5

[1] Contraction delay, Δt, is the difference in days between the half-life of the treated minus the half-life of the untreated dermis-free defect in the guinea pig model.

[2] Average pore diameter or cross-link density were not sufficiently different between ECM analogs to affect significantly the value of Δt.

[3] Pore diameter, in μm, is indicated.

[4] Degradation rate maintained at approx. 12 e.u. (enzyme units) for ECM analogs (silicone not degradable) (Flynn, 1983; Yannas et al., 1989).

[5] Degradation rate maintained between 8.0 and 38.6 e.u., a range inside which contraction delay was not significantly affected by degradation rate (Shafritz et al., 1994).

[6] Degradation rate of analogs maintained constant at average level 11 ± 4.7 e.u. in the series (Yannas et al., 1989).

[7] DRT, dermis regeneration template, an ECM analog that shows maximal contraction-delaying activity. Maximum activity observed in the pore diameter range 20–125 μm (Yannas et al., 1989).

[8] Degradation rate increases with indicated magnitude of enzyme units (e.u.). Average pore diameter maintained constant at 450 ± 100 μm in the series (Yannas et al., 1989). Values of Δt were consistently low in this series because of the relatively high value of average pore diameter.

[9] Seeded with 500,000 uncultured keratinocytes per cm^2 graft area; average pore diameter, 50 μm; degradation rate, 12 e.u.) (Yannas et al., 1989).

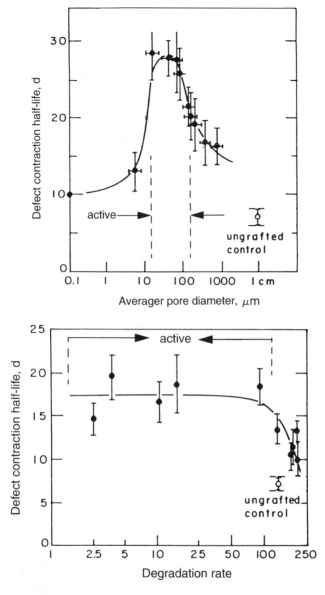

FIGURE 8.5. Contraction-delaying activity depended strongly on the structure of the nondiffusible regulator. The range of maximum activity is indicated by broken lines. The rate of contraction is characterized by the half-life, $t_{1/2}$ d, of the initial defect area. The half-life of the ungrafted control is shown. *Top* (Figure 8.5): A region of maximum contraction-delaying activity was observed when the average pore diameter of the regulator was between 20 and 120 μm. *Bottom* (Figure 8.5): Contraction delaying activity was maximal when the degradation rate was maintained between the two levels indicated in the diagram. Degradation rate in standardized collagenase solution (in vitro test) is reported in arbitrary enzyme units. When the degradation rate was controlled to levels below about 2.5 enzyme units, synthesis of scar resulted. (From Yannas et al., 1989.)

above 90 e.u., with an apparent cutoff point of 140 ± 25 e.u. (Figure 8.5, bottom). It was estimated that the critical level of the degradation rate corresponds to a maximum level of the average molecular weight between crosslinks for the network of 20 to 30 kDa (Yannas et al., 1975a, 1982a; Yannas, 1981). When other structural features of the degradable macro-molecular network remained constant, an increase in crosslink density was accompanied by increase in resistance to degradation both in vitro (in a standardized solution of collagenase) and in vivo (subcutaneous implantation). Based on data relating in vitro with in vivo degradation rates (Yannas et al., 1975b; Yannas, 1981) it can be estimated that the optimal degradation rate corresponded to a half-life of 10 to 15 d for the degrading analog implanted in the dermis-free skin defect.

In conclusion, the data in Table 8.3, as well as in Figure 8.5, show that contraction-delaying activity is lost unless the chemical composition, specific surface, and degradation half-life of the series of ECM analogs have all been maintained within relatively narrow limits. The critical dependence of activity on network structure identifies an insoluble, developmentally active factor, referred to as dermis regeneration template (Yannas et al., 1989). This insoluble regulator is the only reactant required for synthesis of the dermis in a dermis-free defect (Chapter 7).

8.3 Summary

Data were presented showing that induced regeneration of skin, a peripheral nerve trunk, and the conjunctival stroma coincided with significant reduction in extent of contraction as a mode of closure of the respective defects. Not only the extent of contraction but its rate as well was observed to be reduced during certain instances of induced regeneration. Two examples of spontaneous healing provided further support to the hypothesis that closure of a defect by contraction and by regeneration were antagonistically related processes. Scar was apparently entirely blocked when contraction was reduced, even moderately, under conditions of induced regeneration, suggesting that scar synthesis is a byproduct of defect closure by contraction. Suppression of contraction by pharmacological agents, or in certain cases of impaired healing, was not accompanied by regeneration, showing that suppression of contraction alone did not suffice to induce regeneration. A theory was proposed that describes selectively suppressed contraction in adult defects as a requirement for induced regeneration.

Several nondiffusible (insoluble) regulators have shown evidence of regenerative activity. All are insoluble macromolecular networks. Several well-defined members of a family of ECM analogs have inhibited contraction and have been used as probes of the mechanism of induced regeneration. Use of these ECM analogs has led to recognition of certain requirements for selective suppression of contraction, such as a minimum density of ligands for binding with cell receptors and optimal persistence of the regulator in a nondiffusible state. Nondiffusible regulators widely vary in regenerative activity; among these, certain ECM analogs have shown particularly high activity in skin, peripheral nerve, and conjunctival defects (regeneration templates).

9
Kinetics and Mechanism I: Spontaneous Healing

9.1 Mechanism versus Final State of Spontaneous Healing

In preceding chapters we inspected data from a large number of independent investigations which describe the phenomenon of induced regeneration in terms of the final state of the healing process. We considered studies conducted in the presence or absence of various reactants, both in vitro and in vivo. Very little mention, if any, was made of the pathway that led to the final state. The deliberate separation of a description of the final state from a discussion of the hypothetical mechanism for the process emphasized the distinction between two bodies of information: The first is the totally factual part of induced regeneration, embodied in the rather dry collection of empirical data from several investigators on the relation between reactants and final state; the second, the hypothetical part, addresses the most probable cell and molecular mechanisms that lead from reactants to final state. First the facts, then the hypothetical explanation.

In this chapter, as well as the next, we finally focus on mechanism. What happens first? Which signals start the healing process? Which signals call it off? What do the cells do? What is the role of the various regulators? How do defects close? In order to provide a basis for discussion of induced regeneration in the next chapter, we will first discuss in this chapter the mechanism of spontaneous healing.

9.2 Cell Phenotypes Exhibited During Spontaneous Healing

Healing of the dermis-free and transected nerve defects will be considered in terms of a cycle that starts with the injury and proceeds to closure through a large number of steps. Several classes of contributors to the spontaneous healing process have been identified; they include various cell types, cytokines, growth factors, integrins, and matrix components. As soon as the defect is generated, these factors are recruited by use of molecular signals calling for urgent action. When closure is eventually complete, the signals are systematically turned off and all healing processes, except for long-term remodeling, are shut down.

We are interested here in tracking the most probable path through which the freshly opened defect eventually closes spontaneously. This track will be pursued by following three lines of thought that have crystallized in preceding chapters; namely, the different phenotypes in which cells in the defect can be classified; a classification of such cells according to the regenerative or nonregenerative character of the adult tissues which they participate in synthesizing; and the signaling between cells and matrix components (nondiffusible regulators) that appears to be required for defect closure.

Keratinocytes and Schwann cells were each described as capable of expressing two phenotypes (Chapter 2). The stationary phenotype is characterized by lack of locomotion, secure adhesion to the basement membrane, and participation in a process of differentiation that leads to synthesis of a specialized tissue (epidermis, myelin sheath). The migratory phenotype of either cell type is characterized by loss of adhesion to the basement membrane, proliferation, transient adhesion to matrix, and locomotion. Another cell type that has been shown to exhibit these two phenotypes is the endothelial cell (Madri et al., 1996; Gerwins et al., 2000). In its migratory state, the microvascular endothelial cell proliferates, digests its basement membrane, and moves about; in its stationary state, it synthesizes a new basement membrane, adheres to it, and participates in angiogenesis. The fibroblast expresses even more phenotypes: In a typical scenario following injury, fibroblasts in intact tissues surrounding the defect proliferate for about 3 days; on day 4 they migrate into the defect, where they synthesize type I procollagen and other ECM molecules; on day 7 they express the myofibroblast phenotype by synthesizing thick actin bundles and behaving as contractile cells; eventually, as the defect closes up, myofibroblasts undergo apoptosis (Clark, 1993). This wealth of phenotypic expression suggests that the fibroblast is involved in almost every aspect of spontaneous healing.

A second theme is the identification of cell types that are required to synthesize regenerative tissues, as well as those that fail to synthesize nonregenerative tissues, in the spontaneously healing defect. In Chapter 2 it was recognized that epithelia (epidermis in skin, myelin sheath in peripheral nerves) are spontaneously regenerative tissues while the stroma of each organ (dermis and endoneurium, respectively) is not. In Chapter 7, it was concluded that an epidermis and a myelin sheath can be synthesized in vitro; the presence of cells from the stroma (endothelial cells, fibroblasts) was not required in these protocols (Tables 7.1 and 7.2). Although clearly not required for in vitro synthesis, it is likely that stromal cells make a finite contribution to the synthesis of epithelia in vivo. For example, an epidermis synthesized in vitro matures faster and to a greater extent after it has been grafted than would be the case if in vitro culture was prolonged over an equivalent period (Chapter 5); in this case, it is likely that the interaction between stromal cells and the cytokine field, described in Chapter 7, contributes significantly to the kinetics and extent of epithelial tissue synthesis. Furthermore, in the stroma of the adult skin defect, fibroblasts synthesize granulation tissue that eventually becomes scar. When the skin defect is relatively large, granulation tissue that has been synthesized near the center of the defect is clearly separated from keratinocytes migrating from the edges; in these cases, it can be readily concluded that the new, highly vascularized tissue has been synthesized primarily by endothelial cells and fibroblasts in the absence of keratinocytes. (A hypothetical peripheral nerve defect in which fibroblasts and endothelial cells have been separated from Schwann cells is the analog of such a defect in skin.) On the whole, it is clear that epithelial cells in a skin defect can engage in a great deal of tissue synthesis, both in vitro and in vivo, in the absence of interactions with stromal cells; and fibroblasts can likewise synthesize granulation tissue in vivo in the absence of interactions with keratinocytes.

A third theme concerns the extracellular matrices (ECMs) that are synthesized and participate in spontaneous closure of a defect. Following skin injury, the earliest matrix synthesized is a "provisional" matrix, consisting primarily of clotted fibrin, fibronectin and hyaluronic acid (Clark, 1996b). Later, the provisional matrix is replaced by granulation tissue, a richly vascularized tissue consisting mostly of collagen fibers. Although several cells (e.g., neutrophils, monocytes and macrophages) enter the defect and get involved in signaling and protein synthesis, synthesis of most ECM components is carried out by fibroblasts. In addition to this major role in ECM synthesis, fibroblasts also play a unique role in defect closure by organizing contraction; they do this by adopting the contractile phenotype and by exerting sufficient stress on the ECM near the edges (see below) to induce centripetal movement of the edges, eventually leading to closure of most of the initial defect area. Contractile fibroblasts also participate in closure of defects in transected nerves (Chapter 4). Although epithelial cells (i.e., keratinocytes, Schwann cells and microvascular endothelial cells) also synthesize ECM, it appears that this activity consists most prominently in synthesis of a basement membrane; furthermore, there is no evidence that epithelial cells adopt the contractile phenotype during closure either of skin or peripheral nerve defects.

In conclusion, consideration of the phenotypic expression by epithelial and stromal cells inside a defect, the nature of tissue synthesized, as well as the cell type primarily responsible for contraction, leads to a somewhat approximate but useful view of spontaneous defect closure. Following injury, epithelial cells become migratory, synthesize their respective regenerative tissues (epidermis, myelin sheath and associated basement membranes) and eventually resume their stationary phenotype, mostly with little requirement for interaction with stromal cells. The fibroblast is the main cell type involved in synthesis of stroma, a nonregenerative process leading to repair; it is also the cell type involved in closure of the defect by contraction. It follows that, in order to understand the nature of irreversible injury that characterizes the spontaneous healing of adult defects, we need to focus on the complex phenotypic expression of the fibroblast.

9.3 Go-Stop Signals for Skin Defect Closure in Adults

The sections below discuss these aspects of the healing process that appear to contribute most to an understanding of skin defect closure by contraction and scar synthesis.

For a much more extensive discussion of healing of skin defects, the reader is referred to a richly detailed treatise of the several steps of the inflammatory response following skin injury, as well as its resolution (Clark, 1996b). Reviewers of the wound healing process in skin have increasingly focused on the detailed cellular functions and molecular biological switches that control individual steps. Healing processes have been classified into major groups, such as inflammation, tissue formation, and tissue remodeling; in this context, the ligands of some 18 integrins have been identified (Clark, 1997; Xu and Clark, 2000). In another approach, the phases of wound healing have been identified as proliferation, migration, matrix synthesis, and contraction, and the behavior of each of several contributing cell types has been described; over 15 growth factor signaling systems, including the source of signal as well as the primary target cells and effect on them, have been identified (Martin, 1997). The discussion below deviates from these useful reviews by focusing almost entirely on the expression of irreversibility following injury.

9.3.1 Injury to the Dermis: A Signal for Generation of the Cytokine Field

In this volume we are primarily concerned with irreversible defects; accordingly, we wish to identify the signal that notifies organ and organism that this type of defect has been inflicted. Clearly, rupture of the epidermis alone does not qualify. An injury that is restricted to the epidermis is reversible: The final state is a spontaneously synthesized physiological epidermis, as discussed in detail in Chapter 2. In contrast, a defect that penetrates the basement membrane and extends into the dermis is an unmistakable go signal for an irreversible repair process in adult skin. The line of demarcation between reversible and irreversible injury in skin has been identified with a resolution of about 50 nm, close to the plane of the lamina lucida of the basement membrane (Uitto et al., 1996).

Injury of the vascularized dermis immediately causes release of blood, a tissue replete with diffusible regulators of cell function, including growth factors, cytokines, and clotting factors; for brevity, these soluble molecules that regulate cell function will be collectively referred to as cytokines. An additional, almost equally instant, source of cytokines is the platelet that releases them by degranulation; this process follows contact with a thrombogenic surface, such as fragments of collagen fibers. Clotting of blood results in formation of a scaffold primarily comprising fibrin, the product of polymerization of fibrinogen in blood that has invaded the defect. The fibrin matrix is traversed by several cell types: cells that release collagenase, elastase and other enzymes, allowing them to penetrate through the basement membrane of blood vessels and other extracellular matrix (ECM) and eventually digest bacteria (neutrophils); cells that bind on ECM proteins through integrin receptors and initiate processes that lead to further ECM degradation (monocytes, macrophages); and later, cells that synthesize new ECM (fibroblasts), new blood vessels (endothelial cells), and a new epidermis (keratinocytes).

Mechanical injury also induces release or uptake of cytokines by cells through disruptions in the cell membrane, as has been demonstrated with epithelial and endothelial cells (McNeil et al., 1989). Even though these disruptions can be eventually resealed by vesicle-vesicle fusion (McNeil et al., 2000), mechanical injury leads to instantaneous cytokine traffic between the cytoplasm and the tissue exudate and probably contributes to an increase in the rate with which the inflammatory response is established in the fresh defect.

The cytokine field consists of signals that cells send to each other and has been referred to as "crosstalk" (Xu and Clark, 2000). The signals are diffusible (soluble) polypeptides that are synthesized and secreted by a cell, typically in response to a signal received from another cell or matrix component. A cell conveys its message by secreting the appropriate cytokine in the medium, thereby allowing it to diffuse away and eventually bind on a receptor molecule located on the membrane of a neighbor cell (paracrine), a cell in a different organ (endocrine), or even the originating cell (autocrine). The latter pathway essentially describes a cell that "talks to itself" and amplifies greatly the effect of the message in this manner. Diffusible regulators provide signals for a variety of activities; among them are providing cells with a direction along a concentration gradient (chemotaxis), inducing mitosis that leads to cell proliferation, and inducing differentiation, including the process that converts the fibroblast into a vigorously contractile phenotype (myofibroblast). Individual regulators display characteristic behavior in vivo; yet, there is also evidence of substantial overlap in activity of different regulators as well as some antagonistic activity. Several well-studied growth factors have been exogenously supplied to various types of skin defects and have been shown to play distinct roles during the healing process (Mustoe et al., 1991; Pierce et al., 1992).

Below we review very briefly the function of several important regulators. The evidence supports a role for platelet-derived growth factor BB

(PDGF-BB), the isoform studied most extensively in skin wound healing studies, in which the exogenously supplied regulator accelerates influx of neutrophils as well as deposition of granulation tissue rich in fibroblasts, glycosaminoglycans, and fibronectin (Ross and Vogel, 1978; Mustoe et al., 1991; Pierce et al., 1991, 1992; Heldin and Westermark, 1996). PDGF-BB receptors are largely limited to cells of mesodermal (mesenchymal) origin, such as fibroblasts (Mustoe et al., 1991). An important conclusion from a review of these studies is that PDGF-BB does not alter the normal sequence of repair, but simply increases its rate (Heldin and Westermark, 1996). TGF-β_1, the isoform of transforming growth factor-β most studied, differs from PDGF in its distinctive role in enhancement of synthesis and remodeling of the extracellular matrix, particularly of collagen (Roberts and Sporn, 1996; Yang et al., 1999). Basic fibroblast growth factor, bFGF (FGF-2), has shown an angiogenic response as well as a collagenolytic activity (Davidson et al., 1985; Pierce et al., 1992; Abraham and Klagsbrun, 1996). Modulation of the healing process by several members of the fibroblast growth factor family has been described in detail (Abraham and Klagsbrun, 1996). In particular, keratinocyte growth factor (KGF or FGF-7) has been shown to lead to synthesis of a significantly thicker neoepidermis with a deeper rete ridge pattern than in untreated wounds (Staiano-Coico et al., 1993). Macrophage-colony stimulating factor (M-CSF) has been reported to be the first growth factor studied that has a stimulatory effect on granulation tissue but none on epithelial regrowth (Wu et al., 1997). Epidermal growth factor (EGF) (Brown et al., 1986; Nanney, 1990; Nanney and King, 1996) and transforming growth factor-alpha (TGF-α) (Clark, 1996b) have also been implicated in cell regulation during defect healing.

The cytokine field consists of the time-dependent and space-dependent concentrations of the diffusible regulators during healing in a given defect. Although the identity and major functions of several signals have been recognized, the cooperative interplay among cells that eventually orchestrate the inflammatory response is still largely unknown at present.

9.3.2 Synthesis of a Provisional Matrix and of Granulation Tissue

Soon after injury, at about the same time that a blood clot has been formed in the defect, fibronectin also appears from the circulation; a few days later, when the fibrin clot has been degraded by proteolytic enzymes, fibronectin is synthesized by fibroblasts and other cells (Clark et al., 1983; Clark, 1996b).

Fibroblasts migrate into the defect from neighboring intact tissues and are present in the defect as early as two to three days after injury (Rudolph et al., 1992). The migratory phenotype of fibroblasts appears to be upregulated by PDGF; the latter induces fibroblast surface receptors $\alpha_3\beta_1$ and $\alpha_5\beta_1$, which bind to fibronectin following enhancement by fibrin matrix (Xu and Clark, 2000). In addition to these two integrins, fibroblasts also express $\alpha_v\beta_1$,

$\alpha_v\beta_3$, and $\alpha_v\beta_5$; all five of these receptors bind on the Arg-Gly-Asp-Ser (RGDS) tetrapeptide located in the cell binding domain of fibronectin (Pierschbacher and Ruoslahti, 1984a,b; Hynes, 1990). Another receptor, $\alpha_4\beta_1$, recognizes the IIICs domain of fibronectin (Xu and Clark, 2000). Fibronectin receptors control, not only the onset, but the speed of migration as well (Xu and Clark, 2000). Fibroblast-fibronectin binding is accompanied by a series of cytoskeletal changes that have been described (Hynes, 1990; Xu and Clark, 2000). Following migration into the defect via the fibronectin path, fibroblasts gradually step up protein synthesis (Welch et al., 1990) and synthesize fibronectin in large quantity (Welch et al., 1990; Grinnell, 1992, 1994) as well as hyaluronan (hyaluronic acid) (Bently, 1967; Clark, 1996b). The detailed sequence leads to synthesis of a provisional matrix that facilitates migration of cells, including fibroblasts, into the defect (Clark et al., 1983; Clark, 1996b; Xu and Clark, 2000). It follows that, fibroblasts that have migrated into the defect are at first in contact with fibronectin and hyaluronan, not with collagen.

Although fibronectin continues to be present inside the defect for several days, probably until the termination of contraction (see below), hyaluronan concentration reaches a peak by 2 to 4 days (Balazs and Larsen, 2000) or, in another report, by 5 to 10 days (Bently, 1967) after injury and then drops significantly. Loss of hyaluronan from the defect has been attributed to degradation by hyaluronidase (Bertolami and Donoff, 1982; Clark, 1996b). An analysis of the potential function of hyaluronan during healing has led to the suggestion that its accumulation leads to loss of cell-matrix adhesion (abhesion) and promotion of cell proliferation (Clark, 1996b).

The onset of synthesis of granulation tissue can probably be placed at the time when the fibroblast, continuing its phenotypic modulation, eventually switches to a profibrotic phenotype, characterized by synthesis of collagen fibers (Welch et al., 1990). However, fibroblasts also synthesize TGF-β (Clark et al., 1995), itself a promoter of collagen synthesis (Ignotz and Massagué, 1986; Roberts et al., 1986); a positive feedback loop is thereby established. Synthesized collagen, primarily types I and III, eventually activates a negative feedback loop, by attenuation of the response of fibroblasts to TGF-β, and collagen synthesis ceases (Clark et al., 1995). Contact with collagen also induces a modification of the fibroblast phenotype to a primarily stationary one (Grinnell, 1994). We conclude that cell-matrix interactions are powerful at this point of the healing process, leading to a continuously evolving ECM, itself mediating phenotypic changes in the fibroblast. These interactions depend once more on utilization of a number of integrins: $\alpha_5\beta_1$ for the fibroblast-fibronectin interaction, as well as $\alpha_1\beta_1$ and $\alpha_2\beta_1$ (fibroblast-collagen) (Clark, 1996b).

9.3.3 Identity of Contractile Cells

Both undifferentiated and differentiated fibroblasts have been implicated in generation of contractile forces in defects.

The majority of investigators have focused their attention on the role of the myofibroblast, a differentiated fibroblast. The ultrastructural and biochemical features of this cell type that distinguish it from fibroblasts include a well-developed actin microfilamentous system, with microfilaments typically arranged parallel to the long axis of the cell (stress fibers), as well as a nucleus that consistently shows multiple indentations or deep folds (Desmoulière and Gabbiani, 1996). In addition, two cell-matrix adhesion macromolecules (vinculin and fibronectin) have been identified in myofibroblasts (Vaughan et al., 2000). The feature that provides the most useful operational distinction of differentiation is expression of the α-smooth muscle (α-SM) actin phenotype (Gabbiani, 1998). However, myofibroblasts are derived from fibroblasts, not smooth muscle cells (Grinnell, 1994).

Studies of induction of α-SM actin expression in vitro and in vivo have implicated TGF-β_1, TGF-β_2 and granulocyte-macrophage-colony stimulating factor (GM-SCF), as well as heparin; however, neither PDGF, bFGF, nor tumor necrosis factor-α (TNF-α) induced differentiation to the α-SM actin phenotype (Desmoulière and Gabbiani, 1996; Gabbiani, 1998; Schürch et al., 1998).

Since fibroblast differentiation to the contractile phenotype is upregulated by TGF-β but not by several other cytokines that were studied (Desmoulière et al., 1993), investigators have pursued relations between TGF-β concentration, fibroblast differentiation and its effects on healing. For example, it was reported that TGF-β_1 promoted in vitro a dose-dependent increase in the generation of contractile force in myofibroblasts and a concomitant increase in the expression of α-SM actin (Vaughan et al., 2000). In studies with fetal models, significant positive relations have been observed between the presence of exogenously supplied TGF-β_1 and scar synthesis (fibrosis) (Krummel et al., 1988); the level of secretion of TGF-β by fibroblasts and contraction (Coleman et al., 1998); myofibroblast presence and scar synthesis (Cass et al., 1997); as well as among TGF-β_1 presence, myofibroblast presence, increased contraction, and scar synthesis (Lanning et al., 1999, 2000). Evidence from healing processes in several organs has implicated the myofibroblast both in contraction and scar synthesis (Rudolph et al., 1992). As mentioned above, differentiation of fibroblasts in response to TGF-β is suppressed in the presence of collagen matrix (Clark, 1996b; Xu and Clark, 1996).

The presence of TGF-β in tissue fluid does not appear to be sufficient to induce fibroblast differentiation; it appears that the myofibroblast must also be at an appropriate mechanical state. TGF-β activity depends on the resistance of the substrate to deformation; apparently, the presence of intracellular tension is required for expression of the contractile cytoskeletal gene (Grinnell, 1994; Arora et al., 1999). Another study has shown that the force generated by individual fibroblasts was canceled when cell-matrix adhesion was suppressed by use of a serum-free medium; furthermore, force generation dropped when the cells became motile, suggesting that contractile force generation requires the presence of nonmotile fibroblasts (Roy et al., 1999).

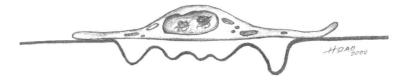

FIGURE 9.1. Fibroblasts apply traction to substrates. In this study, fibroblasts were placed on top of a thin silicone film in culture medium. Cells deformed the thin, flexible substrate, causing buckling. (Reprinted with permission from Harris et al., 1980. Silicone rubber substrate. *Science* 280:177–179. Copyright 1980, American Association for the Advancement of Science.)

Myofibroblasts are not the only cell type that contributes to contraction; undifferentiated fibroblasts also play a role. There is clear evidence that undifferentiated fibroblasts are present in rodent skin defect models as early as two to three days after injury, approximately at the time when contraction starts and a few days before myofibroblasts could be detected (Rudolph et al., 1992). Fibroblasts develop contractile forces by applying traction to the substrate underneath; these traction forces have been clearly implicated in cell migration (Harris et al., 1980, 1981; Stopak and Harris, 1982; Ehrlich, 1988; Ehrlich and Rajaratnam, 1990; Rudolph et al., 1992) (Figure 9.1). The mechanism of contraction will be discussed below in terms of these two types of contractile cells, both those that express the α-SM actin phenotype (myofibroblasts) and those that do not (fibroblasts).

Detailed studies of wound contraction in the rat and rabbit showed that there was an early, almost immediate, contraction following injury that occupied the first 50 to 60 h. This "early closure phase" accounted for about 20% reduction in wound area in the rat and about 40% in the rabbit. Early contraction was followed by a stationary phase during which contraction was essentially stalled between 60 and 120 h after wounding. This phase was then followed by rapid contraction, characterized by a logarithmic rate, which extended from 120 h to about 20 days, at which time defect closure was complete. The contraction kinetics in the guinea pig lacked an early closure phase (<60 h after wounding), a difference attributed to the relative lack of mobility of guinea pig skin; in this model, a significant decrease from the initial wound area was observed as late as 150 h after wounding (Kennedy and Cliff, 1979). A study of the appearance of cells that stain for α-SM actin during healing of full-thickness skin wounds in the guinea pig showed that, on day 6 (about 150 h after wounding), clearly after wound contraction was observed to have started, the vast majority of fibroblasts in the wound bed did not stain for α-SM actin; intense staining for α-SM actin was observed by day 8, during the rapid phase of contraction (Troxel, 1994). The combined data suggest that, at least with rodent models, the earliest evidence of contraction can be accounted for by undifferentiated fibroblasts while the rapid phase, which occurs later, is due to myofibroblast action; if so, the intermediate "stationary" phase described with the rat and rabbit models (Kennedy and Cliff, 1979) may hypothetically be the period required for a transition between the two cell types (i.e., the period required for expression of the α-SM actin phenotype).

Undifferentiated fibroblasts do not appear to require specific signaling in order to exert contractile forces on the matrix; their contractile activity has been referred to as traction locomotion (Rudolph et al., 1992; Ehrlich, 2000). In contrast, the data reported above have shown that TGF-β_1 and TGF-β_2, as well as an increase in mechanical resistance of the contracting wound, are primarily responsible for differentiation to the myofibroblast phenotype. There is substantial evidence, however, that migrating fibroblasts at the edges of the defect generate sufficient force to initiate contraction; as contraction proceeds and mechanical resistance increases, these migrating fibroblasts eventually differentiate to myofibroblasts (Grinnell, 1994).

In summary, undifferentiated fibroblasts appear to be responsible for early contraction of the defect while fibroblasts that have expressed the contractile phenotype (myofibroblasts) take control later on and continue until contraction has been arrested. TGF-β upregulates differentiation of fibroblasts to the myofibroblast phenotype, characterized by expression of α-SM actin; the presence of intracellular tension appears to be required as well for phenotypic expression. The functional significance of α-SM actin in fibroblasts in the adult dermis-free defect is partly understood. Extensive evidence has implicated the myofibroblast both in contraction and scar synthesis.

Fibroblasts that hypothetically participate in defect contraction will generally be referred to below as contractile cells, unless there is specific evidence that they have differentiated into the myofibroblast phenotype.

9.3.4 Generation of Local Stress by an Individual Contractile Cell

Development of a local contractile stress in a matrix by an individual cell requires secure adhesion of the contractile cell to the matrix. A specific link between fibroblasts and ECM components, referred to as fibronexus, has been identified (Singer, 1979; Singer et al., 1984). It consists of a transmembrane link that connects cytoskeletal structures, such as actin, to ECM components, primarily collagen and fibronectin, through integrin receptors. During defect contraction, linkage of fibroblasts to the collagenous component of the matrix occurs through the $\alpha_2\beta_1$ integrin receptor (Schiro et al., 1991) and the $\alpha_1\beta_1$ receptor (Clark, 1996b; Xu and Clark, 2000); and to fibronectin, probably through the $\alpha_5\beta_1$ receptor (Welch et al., 1990) as well as through other receptors (Xu and Clark, 2000). The fibronexus appears to anchor fibroblasts together, generating a network that transmits the force of the entire contractile cell population across the defect (Hynes, 1990; Eyden, 2001).

The relative importance of $\alpha_1\beta_1$ and $\alpha_2\beta_1$ integrin receptors during contraction was further studied in a quantitative comparison of expression of integrin subunits, during in vivo injury as well as in vitro contraction of collagen gels. The study focused on the relative extent of expression of alpha1 and alpha2 integrin subunits in these two media. The study conducted in vivo showed that alpha1 expression was maintained throughout and that alpha2 was expressed at all times during injury at a level less than 8% of alpha1. In culture, however, contraction of collagen gel was blocked 70% by anti-alpha1 and as much as 30% by anti-alpha2. It was concluded that alpha1beta1 is the sole integrin utilized by myofibroblasts during contraction in vivo; and that expression of alpha2beta1 by myofibroblasts is a response to culture (Racine-Samson et al., 1997).

The mechanism of generation of local traction appears to depend on the detailed cell-matrix interactions in the immediate vicinity of a contractile cell. Fibroblasts, which may not have expressed the myofibroblast phenotype, are known to pull at the matrix to which they are bound, inducing formation of wrinkles (buckling) in the matrix that extend over several cell diameters to other cells (Harris et al., 1980, 1981; Stopak and Harris, 1982; Ehrlich, 1988). The cells themselves do not contract. These relatively large ECM deformations amount to a mechanical signal that is transferred to nearest-neighbor cells. Such a signal may hypothetically induce nearest-neighbor cells to exert their own traction forces on the matrix to which they are bound, thereby propagating the signal to their own neighbors.

9.3.5 Mechanisms of Closure by Contraction

How does the contractile force of a single cell eventually become a macroscopic force that leads to closure of the defect? This question has led to some controversy about the relative role of contractile cells in two locations: the center and the edges of the defect.

Movement of the edges of the defect toward each other has been historically assumed to result from transfer of forces across the entire defect, via the granulation tissue. In an early study, dermis-free rabbit defects were mechanically splinted; later, incisions were made in the granulation tissue, in such a way as to mechanically isolate, down to the *panniculus carnosus*, a central area of granulation tissue accounting for two-thirds of the total tissue (Abercrombie et al., 1960). Following isolation, the central granulation tissue rapidly contracted into a button of tissue conspicuously projecting above the skin surface, while the rim of granulation tissue remaining at the edges retracted away from the center. This finding demonstrated the intrinsic contractility of granulation tissue, although it did not constitute adequate proof that the contractile forces it develops at the center are either necessary or sufficient to initiate or complete the process of contraction. The subsequent demonstration of myofibroblasts inside the granulation tissue led to the hypothesis that these cells play a major role in contraction of granulation tissue; the latter, therefore, was viewed as the "organ" responsible for contraction across the wound bed (Gabbiani et al., 1971, 1972; Majno et al., 1971). The clear inference from these studies was that granulation tissue, which covers most of the defect following the early phase of healing, serves as the continuous medium that transfers the contractile force across the entire defect area.

The hypothesis that contraction forces are acting across the entire defect and are driven entirely by the granulation tissue was not supported by the results of a study in which tissue was excised either from the center or from the edges of the dermis-free defects in the guinea pig. Contraction was suppressed when strips of granulation tissue, located very close to the contracting wound edges, were surgically excised but not when granulation tissue from the center of the wound was excised; if granulation tissue from the center was responsible for pulling the defect edges together, excising it from the center of the defect should have led to suppression of contraction, contrary to observation (Watts et al., 1958). Similar results were obtained in a study of dermis-free defects in the swine, in which the skin is tethered more securely than in the guinea pig; once more, excision of the granulation tissue from the center of the defect, repeated daily to ensure that newly synthesized tissue would be removed in timely fashion, had no effect on rate or extent of contraction. These observations were clearly at odds with the hypothesis of a closure process driven by central granulation tissue (Gross et al., 1995).

The location of contractile forces in the dermis-free defect in the guinea pig was explored in a study in which thin strips of the dermis regeneration template (DRT), a known suppressor of contraction (Yannas, 1981; Yannas et al., 1989), was grafted alternatively at the center or at the two contracting edges of the defect. When DRT strips were grafted at the edges, the delay in onset of contraction observed was as strong as when the entire defect surface had been grafted with DRT; however, the rate of contraction was slightly higher than when the entire defect had been grafted. When DRT strips were grafted in the center of the defect, at least 5 mm away from the contracting edges, there was almost no delay in the onset of contraction; however, about 10 d after contraction had started, the rate of contraction slowed down to that observed when the entire defect had been grafted with DRT (Troxel, 1994) (Figure 9.2). These results supported the hypothesis that contraction was initiated at the edges, but left open the possibility that the central granulation tissue participates to some extent in the rate of the closure process that eventually develops.

Morphological observations at the edges of the dermis-free defect in the same model showed the presence of a thick cell cluster; the cluster thickness, δ, measured along a direction perpendicular to the defect surface (defect base), comprised about 30 cells and measured about $100\,\mu m$ at the time of onset of contraction, t_o. The first evidence of contraction of the defect area was observed at 3 ± 1 d after the injury. One day before con-

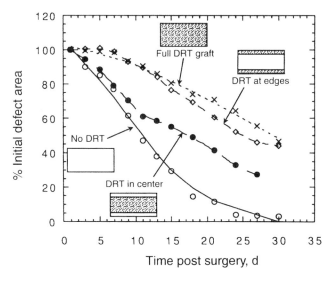

FIGURE 9.2. Probing for the site where contraction is initiated in a skin defect. Strips of dermis regeneration template (DRT), a known inhibitor of contraction, measuring 5 mm in width, were grafted at the edges (DRT at edges) or at the center (DRT in center) of the dermis-free defect that measured 20 m × 30 mm. DRT grafts were also used to cover the entire defect area (full DRT graft). Ungrafted defects (no DRT) were also studied. Measurement of contraction kinetics showed that the onset of contraction was delayed when DRT strips were placed at the edges rather than at the center. However, grafting at the center led to a delayed decrease in contraction rate after about 10 d. (From Troxel, 1994.)

traction started, at $t_o - 1$ d, there was negligible accumulation of cells at the edge; however, the thickness of the cell cluster δ became approximately 100 μm at $t_o + 1$ d, increasing to 300 μm at $t_o + 2$ d, to 500 μm at $t_o + 5$ d as well as at $t_o + 7$ d, and reaching 650 μm several days later (Troxel, 1994) (Figure 9.3).

The presence of this proliferating, and apparently active, cell cluster at the edges supported the hypothesis of a "picture frame," comprising cells at the edges of the defect that pull the dermal edges centripetally, without requirement of a centrally located contractile force (Watts et al., 1958; Gross et al., 1995). However, the active cluster did not remain isolated at the edges, as expected from this simple model: about nine days after the injury, when contraction was fully underway, the thick cell cluster at the edges had become continuous with a cell layer that spanned the entire defect, becoming thinner toward the center where it measured only about 15 to 30 μm in thickness (about 5–10 cell layers). The entire cell assembly, extending from the edges across the entire defect, stained positively for α-SM actin, the myofibroblast marker (Troxel, 1994) (Figure 4.4).

Summing up these observations, we conclude that there is evidence for two, not one, locations for development of contractile activity in the dermis-free defect. In what follows, we will retain the working hypothesis of two spatially distinct loci of contraction activity in the defect that are activated at different times. Focusing on the data from the guinea pig model presented above, the hypothesis describes the observed onset of inward movement of the edges at 4 d as a result of activity developed by a cell cluster, about 100 μm in thickness at the onset of contraction and becoming thicker later, that is located at the edges of the defect. The hypothesis further describes a cell layer, about 15 to 30 μm in thickness and extending through

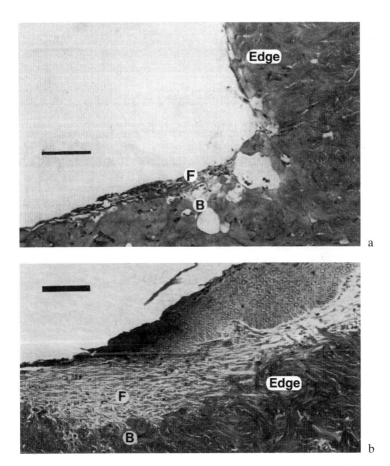

FIGURE 9.3. The size of the cell cluster δ at the edge of the ungrafted skin defect increases during onset of contraction. *Top* (Figure 9.3a): Cell cluster (F) shown at 2 d post injury. *Bottom* (Figure 9.3b): Cell cluster (F) at 6 d postinjury. Contraction of defect edges was first observed at 3 d. Observed where the inclined plane of the defect edge (Edge) intersects the defect base (B). Bar: 100 μm. (From Troxel, 1994.)

the entire defect area, including the defect center, that displays its activity approximately 9 d after injury and maintains by itself, or assists the cell cluster at the edges in maintaining, movement of the edges inward until its activity ceases at about 30 d.

9.3.6 Directional Closure of Defects; Translation of Perilesional Dermis

The defect edges have been observed to become displaced along a major direction of closure in a defect with square or rectangular shape (Peacock, 1971, 1984; Peacock and Van Winkle, 1976; Kennedy and Cliff, 1979). The observed direction of defect closure will be referred to as the principal (major) contraction axis. A principal axis can hypothetically become established inside a defect provided that the latter responds to a mechanical field differently along major directions (anisotropically). Such a defect could result either if the applied contractile force was not equally applied in all directions in the plane of the defect or if the compliance of the defect was greater along a preferred direction, leading to increased deformation along this direction.

Evidence has been presented supporting random orientation of contractile cell axes in the plane of the epidermis in dermis-free defects in the guinea pig (Murphy et al., 1990). This observation is inconsistent with presence of a preferred axis for the contractile force. However, a difference in compliance (deformability) of the skin surrounding the defect (perilesional skin) along the two major directions in the plane of the defect, typically arising from differences in tethering of the dermis to subcutaneous tissues, has been noted in several anatomical sites in rodents (Kennedy and Cliff, 1979). These observations suffice to account for the frequently observed directional closure of defects: Even though the cells hypothetically exert tractions randomly along all directions in the plane of the epidermis, the mechanical anisotropy of tethered perilesional skin induces, in many anatomical sites, the dermal edges to deform preferentially along an axis.

The deformation of skin immediately outside the defect edges during contraction appears to be much more limited than previously thought. In early studies of contraction, tattoo marks were placed at the defect edges but not at a distance from the edges; during contraction, the tattoo marks were shown to be displaced toward the interior of the defect, suggesting that the tissue surrounding the defect was stretched, thinned, and under tension (Peacock and Van Winkle, 1976). However, in a later study of contraction of rectangular, 2 cm × 3 cm, dorsal dermis-free defects in the guinea pig, tattoo marks were placed at two distinct levels away from the dermal edge (i.e., at a distance of 1 mm and 1 cm away, respectively). The displacement between marks at these two levels was used as a measure of mechanical strain in the perilesional skin. The data clearly showed that the perilesional dermis was not stretched to cover the defect during the greater part of the contraction process in the guinea pig model; instead, it was simply translated. In contrast, study of the tissues underneath the dermis by polarized optical microscopy, together with use of strategically placed suture marks to measure displacement subcutaneouly, showed that the tissue layer attached underneath the dermis (*adiposus carnosus*) had undergone substantial shear deformation toward the center of the defect during the period when the relatively unstrained dermis was being translated along the same direction. The adiposus layer remained deformed underneath the scar that eventually was formed at the end of defect contraction (Troxel, 1994). These observations suggested that, during most of the contraction process, the defect area was not reduced by stretching of dermis at the defect edges but by its translation, ferried by a layer of adipose tissue, to which the dermis was attached; however, the subdermal tissue layer underwent significant shear deformation in the process (Figure 9.4).

9.3.7 Synthesis of Scar

Observation of the long axes of cells that had expressed the α-SM actin phenotype and were classified as myofibroblasts showed that they were oriented in the plane of the defect surface; out-of-plane orientation of axes of contractile cells was negligible (Murphy et al., 1990). With all contractile forces inside the relatively thin layer of granulation tissue, the stress distribution corresponds to conditions of stress entirely in the plane (plane stress). Fibroblasts that are present in the contracting defect align themselves along the direction of maximum deformation (Ryan et al., 1974). Since fibroblasts deposit newly synthesized collagen fibers in a direction parallel to their orientation (Birk and Trelstad, 1985), new collagen fibers end up aligned in the plane of the defect and, to the extent that a principal deformation axis exists in the contracting defect, these fibers hypothetically align themselves along that direction.

When contraction has run its course, a fraction of the initial defect area has been covered by epithelialized scar while additional scar is present underneath the extended perilesional skin, as discussed in Chapter 4 (Luccioli et al., 1964; Peacock and Van Winkle, 1976; Horne et al., 1992) and shown in Figure 9.4. The collagen fibers comprising scar are highly oriented in the plane of the epidermis (Hunter and Finlay, 1976; Knapp et al., 1977). A quantitative study of collagen fiber orientation in guinea pig tissues by laser light scattering has shown that the orientation of fiber axes in scar was very prominent along the direction of the major contraction axis and almost totally absent at right angles to the contraction axis (Table 4.1) (Ferdman and Yannas, 1993). The combined evidence strongly suggests that the collagen fibers in scar are aligned principally, but perhaps not totally, along the major contraction axis as the direct result of the mechanical field that is active during contraction along this axis.

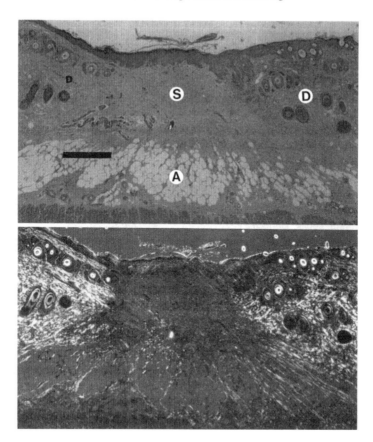

FIGURE 9.4. Deformation of subdermal tissues following closure of an ungrafted dermis-free defect in the guinea pig by contraction and scar synthesis. *Top*: Micrograph, obtained with natural light, shows scar synthesis (S) adjacent to the dermis (D) and over adipose tissue (A). *Bottom*: Polarized light micrograph of same tissue section as above shows highly deformed tissues in scar and adipose layer underneath scar. Bar: 500 μm. (From Troxel, 1994.)

9.3.8 Mechanism of Contraction Arrest

What is the stop signal for contraction? One hypothetical mechanism is based on the premise that epidermal confluence signals the onset of defect closure; since defect closure typically occurs largely by contraction, the latter process is also turned off at the time of epidermal confluence. Let us examine the evidence for and against this hypothesis.

Approximately at the time of confluence, migratory epithelial cells are transformed into the stationary phenotype. The synthesis of laminin, the main component of lamina lucida of the basement membrane, has been described as the "brake" for keratinocyte motility (Woodley et al., 1988b,

1991). This model is supported by the observation, among others, that laminin did not consistently appear until the migratory epithelium had almost completed its migration and was becoming stationary (Clark et al., 1982). Keratinocytes in contact with collagen attach and then begin to migrate; in contrast, addition of laminin inhibits keratinocyte migration in a concentration-dependent fashion (Woodley, 1996). In addition, an isoform of laminin, laminin 5, that has been localized inside the lamina lucida also inhibits keratinocyte migration, strongly promotes keratinocyte attachment, and is thought to anchor the keratinocytes to the substrate (Woodley, 1996). The integrin receptor for laminin 5 is $\alpha_3\beta_1$ (Kim et al., 1992). Eventually, following cessation of lateral movement, keratinocytes settle down to commence their terminal differentiation program that leads to synthesis of a keratinizing epidermis. The data support a model of epidermal confluence in which the stop signal for migrating epithelial cells is supplied by synthesis of one of the components of the nascent basement membrane.

We now look for direct evidence relating arrest of contraction with the timing of epidermal confluence. A continuing reduction in volume of granulation tissue directly underneath its newly formed epidermal cover was evident in immunohistochemical or histological data for several days after epidermal confluence had been reached in dermis-free defects in rodents (ffrench-Constant et al., 1989; Troxel, 1994). Histological data of defect healing in the fetal sheep model showed that contraction of granulation tissue underneath the newly formed epidermal cover also continued for at least seven days after epidermal confluence had been reached (Horne et al., 1992). In the swine model of the spontaneously healing dermis-free defect, reepithelialization data were obtained up to day 21 while detailed contraction data, based on tattoo marks, were obtained to day 43 (Leipziger et al., 1985). If the reepithelialization data reported by these investigators are linearly extrapolated beyond day 21, epidermal confluence appears to have been reached between 25 and 30 days; in contrast, direct observation of dermal edge contraction by use of tattoo marks showed that contraction continued much longer, to about day 43, when the study was terminated (Leipziger et al., 1985). Data from two other studies of the same defect model in the swine showed that contraction clearly continued beyond day 30 and was eventually arrested after day 80 (Rudolph et al., 1977; Rudolph, 1979). Additional data with the swine model showed that in defects that became reepithelialized in 7 to 9 d, contraction continued for approximately 7 d longer (Clark et al., 1982).

Epidermal confluence clearly precedes arrest of contraction by at least several days. This conclusion is directly supported by data, presented above, both from animals with a so-called mobile integument (rodents) and those in which skin is more tightly tethered to subdermal tissues (swine). The data do not support the hypothesis that epidermal confluence is the direct switch that turns off contraction. However, it is possible that epidermal confluence sets in motion another process that develops with some delay and that may be responsible for the lagging arrest of contraction. For example, it is known that, as keratinocytes stop migrating, first type IV collagen and then laminin, two major macromolecules of the basement membrane, are synthesized at the defect edges and eventually toward the center of the defect (Clark et al., 1982). Does the synthesis of basement membrane turn off contraction?

There is convincing evidence that basement membrane in skin defects is synthesized by the migrating keratinocytes and is completely restored only after epidermal confluence has been reached (Woodley and Briggaman, 1988; Stenn and Malhotra, 1992; Uitto et al., 1996). The evidence presented above supported the hypothesis that the stop signal for transformation of migratory epithelial cells to stationary ones is synthesis of laminin, one of the components of the basement membrane. Since synthesis of laminin appears to coincide with epidermal confluence, itself reached several days before arrest of contraction, it would appear that synthesis of basement membrane is a process that precedes contraction arrest by a significant interval. However, it is conceivable that the required signal for arrest of contraction is not the initiation of membrane synthesis but the completion of the process. How long does the entire process for synthesis of the basement membrane last?

Estimates of the time required for the completion of synthesis of the basement membrane following conclusion of epidermal confluence depend sensitively on the defect model used. For this reason, it is necessary to compare the time for completion of basement membrane synthesis and arrest of contraction in the same model. A relatively rare opportunity to directly compare the kinetics of basement membrane formation with the kinetics of contraction emerges from the combined data of two studies performed in the same laboratory using the identical defect model (Carver et al., 1993a,b). In the first study, the investigators studied healing of defects that either were ungrafted or were grafted with cultured keratinocyte sheets; they observed that the contraction kinetics of the two defects were identical (Carver et al., 1993a). In the second study, they reported, among other observations, on the kinetics of synthesis of basement membrane components of the grafted defect (Carver et al., 1993b). Although the authors' data with the grafted defect fall strictly outside the scope of a chapter that focuses on spontaneously healing (ungrafted) defects, their observations of the kinetics of synthesis are pertinent in this discussion and will be pursued.

The combined data from these two studies (Carver et al., 1993a,b) showed that certain components of the basement membrane (continuous lamina lucida and lamina densa) had already been synthesized with normal structure at a time when contraction was still vigorous (day 10); however, synthesis of other attachment structures (hemidesmosomes and sub-basal dense plates) was delayed and was still undergoing significant remodeling at the time that contraction stopped (days 20–25). Cessation of contraction occurred at least 10 d after certain important components of the basement membrane (laminin, type IV collagen) had been synthesized but during the time when other components (hemidesmosomes and sub-basal plates) of the membrane were undergoing synthesis. Furthermore, synthesis of anchoring fibrils was occurring between 13 and 27 d (Carver et al., 1993a,b). The data clearly show that synthesis of certain components of the basement membrane had not been completed at the time that contraction was arrested but provided no further information that could be used to test the hypothesis that the synthetic events constituted a signal for arrest of contraction.

Up to this point, we have been looking at hypothetical locations of the stop signal for contraction either in the epidermis or in the basement membrane. However, we need to recall that contraction is essentially a mechanical phenomenon, driven by unbalanced tractions generated by the contractile cells; it must therefore be arrested by a process that somehow cancels these tractions. This view suggests the possibility that the required stop signal must either be transferred through or reside in the stroma (i.e., in the scar) rather than in the epidermis or the basement membrane. Although the discussion on the mechanism of contraction above referred to two distinct locations for contractile activity, namely, the edges of the defect and its center, the hypotheses discussed below are not specific enough to distinguish between these two locations.

At least four hypotheses for the mechanism of contraction arrest are entirely located in the stroma and each qualitatively accounts for the available data. In the first, contraction is suppressed by downregulation of fibronectin synthesis, leading to loss of cell-ECM adhesion and cancellation of traction ("grip to slip" mechanism). In the second mechanism, granulation tissue becomes critically degraded by collagenases, losing its structure as a three-dimensional stress-supporting network and allowing the tractions to relax to zero (matrix relaxation mechanism). In the third mechanism, loss of traction is the result of depletion of contractile fibroblasts, either following inhibition of expression of the contractile phenotype or following apoptosis; either of these presumptive instances of fibroblast depletion can result from synthesis of a significant mass of collagen (cell depletion mechanism). In a fourth hypothetical mechanism, contraction stops when the perilesional skin that covers the defect has been stretched to a limit beyond which additional extension becomes difficult. The evidence supporting or detracting from each hypothetical mechanism is discussed below.

Although fibronectin synthesis continues after epidermal confluence has been reached, it appears to have become significantly suppressed about seven days later (ffrench-Constant et al., 1989). Furthermore, there is evidence that the appearance of laminin and type IV collagen in the newly formed BM in skin defects coincides with decrease in intensity of staining for fibronectin and fibrinogen (Clark et al., 1982). In corneal defects, where distribution of fibronectin is similar to that in skin defects, it was shown that, following resynthesis of the basement membrane, the level of fibronectin in corneal stroma (analogous to granulation tissue in deep skin defects) was reduced to the lower, normal level (Grinnell, 1992). In dermis-free rabbit defects, seeded with freshly isolated keratinocytes, it was observed, during resynthesis of the basement membrane, that keratinocytes stopped expressing the fibronectin receptor function by 10 d after seeding, at the same time that a normal basement membrane had been synthesized (Takashima et al., 1986). Circumstantial evidence links, therefore, the synthesis of basement membrane with suppression of synthesis of fibronectin or fibronectin receptor function. A defect that becomes relatively depleted in fibronectin would be expected to show evidence of suppressed formation of fibronexi with a resultant change from contractile cell gripping to slipping on the ECM; loss of traction should follow and contraction should stop.

A quite different type of signal that may turn off contraction is hypothesized to result from degradation of the ECM network by matrix metalloproteinases (MMP), such as collagenase (MMP-1). Hypothetical enzymatic degradation of granulation tissue to the point where it ceases to behave as a continuous, three-dimensional collagenous network should rapidly cancel its ability to support a macroscopic stress (Yannas et al., 1975a; Huang and Yannas, 1977); the resulting rapid stress relaxation across the ECM should render it ineffective for supporting contractile forces. Collagenase is localized in the papillary dermis (i.e., in the region of dermis closest to the epidermis) (Bauer et al., 1977). A study of collagen metabolism in the dermis-free defect in the rat led to the conclusion that in the early stages of healing, collagen degradation occurred slowly; in contrast, after contraction had proceeded and scar was being formed, collagen degradation was accelerated (Zeitz et al., 1978). Collagenase is synthesized and released by keratinocytes (Woodley et al., 1986; Petersen et al., 1989, 1990), as well as by fibroblasts and other cell types; furthermore, it has been observed that much more collagenase was synthesized by migratory keratinocytes apposed to type I collagen than by nonmigratory keratinocytes apposed to laminin (Petersen et al., 1989). In human skin defects, collagenase expression stopped when reepithelialization was complete (Inoue et al., 1995). Although the kinetic data are insufficient, they suggest that the degradation rate of collagen remains at a relatively low level in the early part of defect healing; it then increases and goes through a maximum when contraction is almost completed, until it is eventually reduced to a very low level. Although the evidence is incomplete, the hypothesis of matrix degradation is inconsistent with the observed eventual transformation of granulation tissue into a stress-bearing dermal scar. This hypothesis will not be pursued further.

Evidence was presented above showing that fibroblasts express the contractile phenotype primarily in response to TGF-β. However, fibroblast response to TGF-β has been also shown to depend on contact with collagen. For example, contact with collagen has been shown to induce a modification of the fibroblast phenotype to a primarily stationary one (Grinnell, 1994). Furthermore, differentiation of fibroblasts in response to TGF-β is suppressed in the presence of collagen matrix (Clark, 1996b; Xu and Clark, 1996). It is suggested that continuing fibroblast differentiation to the contractile phenotype may become inhibited by a sufficiently extensive mass of newly synthesized collagen. Contractile cells eventually become depleted through apoptosis (Desmoulière et al., 1995, 1997); it is conceivable, therefore, that apoptosis could become a significant cause of contractile cell depletion. It has been hypothesized that the observed death of at least a subpopulation of myofibroblasts could be attributed to withdrawal of cytokines at the later stages of healing (i.e., during transformation from granulation tissue to scar) (Desmoulière et al., 1995).

The fourth hypothetical mechanism mentioned above is based on the mechanical behavior of skin, characterized (as is true of most soft supporting tissues) by a positive curvature of the stress-strain curve. Such behavior is consistent with a rapidly increasing resistance to additional deformation at large strains. According to the hypothesis, contraction is arrested simply due to the inability of contractile cells in the defect to marshal the high stresses required to extend skin further. This hypothesis appears to be contradicted directly by the observation, described in detail in an earlier section, that the skin immediately surrounding the defect in a rodent (perilesional skin) suffers very little extension during closure of the defect by "contraction"; instead, closure occurs primarily by translation of a relatively starin-free perilesional skin (Troxel, 1994).

Of the four hypothetical mechanisms for loss of cell-matrix traction (or for the presence of a limiting traction) that presumably account for eventual cancellation of net contractile forces in the defect, leading to arrest of contraction, the second and fourth are indirectly or directly contradicted by evidence. The hypotheses that were rejected were based on the presumption that the newly synthesized matrix eventually loses its ability to support stresses due to degradation by matrix metalloproteinases; or that stretching of the perilesional skin to cover the defect is stopped due to a requirement for marshaling of stresses too high to be supported by the contractile cells. The remaining two hypothetical mechanisms depend on critical depletion in the defect either of fibronectin or of myofibroblasts.

The discussion in this section has served to identify two major events that are hypothetically connected closely to contraction arrest. The first is closure of the defect by epidermal confluence and synthesis of basement membrane, and the second is loss of cell-matrix traction by depletion either of fibronectin or myofibroblasts. In retrospect, it appears that defect closure may give out the signal that eventually induces loss of cell-matrix traction. If so, arrest of contraction hypothetically involves an interaction between epithelial and mesodermal tissues.

9.3.9 *Summary of Mechanisms for Initiation, Propagation, and Termination of Skin Defect Contraction*

An irreversible healing response in adult skin, leading to repair rather than regeneration, is generated by an injury that penetrates the basement membrane and enters into the dermis. The healing response is essentially turned off when the defect has been closed, partly by contraction and partly by epithelialization of granulation tissue (scar synthesis). Many complex pathways can be traced to describe spontaneous healing; in this chapter, emphasis has been placed on the track that leads to healing of the injured dermis, the nonregenerative tissue in skin.

Contraction is driven by two cell types, the undifferentiated fibroblast and a fibroblast that has expressed the α-smooth muscle actin phenotype (myofibroblast). In the rodent model, the first type appears to be responsible for contraction approximately during the first five days while the myofibroblast appears to take over seven to nine days after injury. There is evidence that expression of the myofibroblast phenotype requires the presence of TGF-β and of a minimal level of mechanical stress. Local traction in the immediate vicinity of an individual cell is generated by pulling against the ECM of granulation tissue through fibronexi, transmembrane links that connect the cytoskeleton to the ECM (mainly fibronectin and collagen) via integrin cell receptors. There is evidence, however, that alpha1beta1 is the sole integrin utilized by myofibroblasts during contraction in vivo.

Reduction in area of the defect appears to be due to the activity of contractile cells in two locations. Contraction is hypothesized to start following activity of a 100-μm cell cluster at the edge and then continues with traction forces exerted by a layer of myofibroblasts that extends through the entire defect area. Contractile cells are randomly oriented in the plane of the epidermis; since, however, the perilesional dermis is displaced more easly along one of the two major axes in the plane of the defect in most anatomical sites, cell tractions leads to establishment of a major axis of contraction. During most of the contraction process, the perilesional dermis that is immediately adjacent to the defect edges (about 10 mm away from the wound bed) is stretched very little during most of the contraction process; instead, it is translated in a relatively strain-free state.

Contraction of granulation tissue proceeds for several days after epidermal confluence has been reached and after major components of the basement membrane (laminin, type IV collagen) have been synthesized. However, contraction is arrested before synthesis of basement membrane has being completed. It is conjectured that contraction is arrested by a signal associated with the synthetic events in the nascent basement membrane; and that this signal is transferred to the stroma, inducing loss of traction between contractile cells and matrix. Specifically, it is hypothesized that traction of matrix by contractile cells is cancelled either when fibronectin becomes critically depleted (leading to a "slip to grip" conversion in cell-matrix interactions) or that the contractile cells become critically depleted due either to loss of the contractile phenotype or to apoptosis.

9.4 Skin Defect Closure in Fetal Models

Healing of fetal skin defects has been often considered to be free of contraction and scar synthesis, eventually leading to regeneration; however, generalities are difficult to establish because the experimental problems of a study on an injured fetus are significant. The traditional advantage of studies of defect healing in the adult skin has been ready experimental access to the injured site and the associated ability to directly monitor the healing process. This advantage is lost when the injured site is on a fetus. For this reason, kinetic studies of the developmental transition from fetal to adult wound healing have been rare. In this section we review the major differences between fetal and adult healing that have been observed so far.

A relative lack of inflammatory response in the fetus has been suggested as a fundamental difference with adult healing (McCallion and Ferguson, 1996; Martin, 1997). Fetal defects have been shown to contain a smaller number of monocytes and macrophages (Adzick and Lorenz, 1994; Cowin et al., 1998), to lack a fibrin clot, and to exhibit poor platelet degranulation; furthermore, PDGF was cleared in fetal defects much earlier than in adult defects (McCallion and Ferguson, 1996). All these observations suggest the presence of a cytokine field in the fetal defect that is significantly different from that in the adult.

An increasing amount of attention has been paid to the regulation of TGF-β in fetal defects. There has been wide interest in the suggestion that synthesis of TGF-β, or at least certain of its isoforms, is downregulated in fetal defects; and that the resulting depletion of TGF-β may account both for lack of contraction and for scarless healing in models of fetal healing during early gestation. Somewhat conflicting observations of TGF-β concentration levels have been made in fetal defects, probably reflecting differences in the interpretation of assay data (Whitby and Ferguson, 1991; Longaker et al., 1994; Nath et al., 1998; Chin et al., 2000). Another approach has focused on modifications in adult defect healing brought about either by adding antibody to TGF-β or by adding its isoform-specific neutralizing antibodies. There is evidence from studies with incisional defects that specific antibodies for TGF-β may prevent scarring in the adult defect (Shah et al., 1992, 1994, 1995; McCallion and Ferguson, 1996). Another approach has been based on providing for continuous release of exogenous TGF-β to the dermis-free defect in the fetal rabbit, which expands rather than contracts after injury. As a result of TGF-β release, it was observed that the normally contraction-free rabbit defect actually contracted, showing also an increased number of inflammatory cells and a greater amount of fibrosis (Lanning et al., 1999). In another study, it was shown that release of

TGF-β to the dermis-free defect in the fetal rabbit induced expression of α-SM actin as well as contraction (Lanning et al., 2000). Inhibition of fibroblast differentiation was suggested as the marker of fetal wound healing in a study of RNA differential display (Stelnicki et al., 2000).

There is little disagreement about the finding that hyaluronan (HA; hyaluronic acid) is present in fetal defects at much higher concentration and over a much longer period of time than in the adult defect (Clark, 1996b; McCallion and Ferguson, 1996; Sawai et al., 1997; Chin et al., 2000). Specifically, hyaluronan is continuously present at high concentration in the fetal defect for at least 21 d after injury; in the adult defect, hyaluronan reached a peak concentration at 3 d and fell sharply thereafter, dropping to near zero by 7 d (Longaker et al., 1991c; Chin et al., 2000). Degradation of HA by addition of the enzyme hyaluronidase to the fetal defect drastically modified the healing response, leading to increased fibroblast infiltration, collagen deposition, and capillary formation (Mast et al., 1992b). It has been suggested (see above) that HA promotes cell movement by weakening adhesion between cells and matrix. Furthermore, since HA immobilizes a mass of water more than 1000 its own, it has been suggested that HA expands interstitial space, providing for increased cell movement (Clark, 1996b).

The ontogenetic transition from fetal to adult healing has been monitored in a few studies. The fetal lamb model, with a size large enough for controlled surgical manipulation, has a term of 145 to 150 d and has been quite useful in studies of this developmental transition. In one study, dermis-free defects in fetal lambs were made between 75 and 120 d gestation and it was observed that a defect made at 100 d gestation healed by contraction (Longaker et al., 1991a). In another study it was observed that α-SM actin was absent in defects made at 75 d gestation but was present in progressively larger amounts in defects made at 100 and 120 d gestation (Estes et al., 1994). In a third study with the same animal model, it was observed that all defects studied at 75, 90, and 120 d gestation closed by contraction and scar synthesis (Horne et al., 1992). Levels of hyaluronic acid were monitored in the fetal lamb at 75 and 100 d gestation, where it was observed that the HA level was elevated for up to 2 wk after injury; in contrast, HA level was significantly lower in 120-d gestation fetuses and was similar to those in the adult lamb (Estes et al., 1994). The combined data from these kinetic studies in the lamb model described an ontogenetic transition in healing in terms of increasing expression of α-SM actin and reduced levels of HA; however, closure of dermis-free defects occurred by contraction and scar synthesis as early as 70 d gestation.

Contraction of fetal dermis-free defects has been studied in several species other than sheep. Failure to close by contraction has been reported with defects in, among others, fetal monkeys (Sopher, 1975) and fetal rabbits (Krummel et al., 1987, 1989).

Although it has been frequently suggested that fetal wound healing is generally free of contraction and scar synthesis, the experimental problems currently associated with quantitative study of defects in fetal models conspire to undermine the validity of such a generalization. There are also problems of interpretation of data. One of these derives from general lack of information on the timing of the transition from fetal to adult healing in a given species. Evidence suggesting either that the transition is sharp or gradual depending on the species has been reviewed (Martin, 1996). The second problem stems from wide differences in length of gestation period among species (e.g., 21 d in mice, 150 d in sheep) that make it difficult to generalize. In conclusion, the available evidence provides useful information on the healing response of certain species at certain gestation times but it is insufficient to enable reaching sound generalizations about the incidence or absence of contraction or scar synthesis as a function of (say) fractional gestation time in fetal models.

The experimental difficulties associated with monitoring the kinetics of healing in the mammalian fetus practically disappeared in a study of the developmental transition in a frog (Chapter 8). Although this amphibian is phylogenetically quite apart from the mammal, it shows a well-defined developmental transition from regenerative healing of an amputated limb to closure by scar synthesis at the stage of metamorphosis from tadpole to frog (Wallace, 1981). In a study of healing of the dermis-free defect with the North American bullfrog, it was confirmed that the transition from regenerative closure to closure by scar occurred at metamorphosis for this frog species as well. The study was focused on healing behavior in four, well-defined developmental stages of the larva (tadpole), as well as at the frog stage (i.e., post-metamorphosis). The results showed that contraction and regeneration alone, without contribution from scar synthesis, accounted for defect closure at all four developmental stages of the tadpole. However, during tadpole development, contraction gradually became an increasingly important process for closure while regeneration correspondingly declined in importance. Following metamorphosis to the adult frog, contraction persisted as the major mode of defect closure while regeneration disappeared; instead, scar synthesis was observed. The data suggested that contraction and regeneration were mutually exclusive phenomena and that, during development, closure by contraction gradually dominated (Yannas et al., 1996).

In summary, the ontogenetic transition in defect healing from fetal to adult defect closure is characterized by increased expression of the fibroblast phenotype associated with contraction of granulation tissue and decreasing levels of hyaluronic acid synthesis. There is also evidence that, with increase in gestation time, there is increasing importance of closure by contraction and scar synthesis rather than by regeneration.

9.5 Spontaneously Healing Defects in Peripheral Nerves

Injured peripheral nerves have historically not been regarded as healing wounds by most investigators, as has been the case with injured skin. Instead, with very few exceptions, authors have focused on studies of tubulated nerves that, as explained in detail above, do not spontaneously heal. Healing following tubulation of a transected nerve is not a spontaneous process; for this reason, its mechanism will not be discussed in this chapter. Instead, the discussion will focus on a hypothetical pathway for conversion of a transected stump into a neuroma.

9.5.1 Signal for Irreversible Healing Response of a Peripheral Nerve

A comparison of the response of the nerve to various types of injury sheds useful light on the extent of structural damage that signals the onset of an irreversible healing process. The evidence will be reviewed by picturing the injury as a mechanical crack that hypothetically propagates along the radial direction in the nerve, from the centrally located axon to the epineurial sheath at the periphery. In these terms, a crushing injury is the equivalent of a tiny crack, roughly 1 to 5 μm long, located at the axoplasm; at the other extreme, transection of the nerve trunk is a very large crack, say 500 μm long, that has propagated along the entire fascicular diameter. (Use of a crack propagation model is made only for convenience of presenting the evidence not because it is a realistic model for actual nerve injury.)

We recall from Chapter 2 that, following removal of the crushing force that had led to loss of axonal continuity but had left the basement membrane intact, structural and functional recovery had ensued (Haftek and Thomas, 1968; Madison et al., 1992). In another study, following crush injury of the mouse sciatic nerve, the endoneurial collagen became more abundant than in the uninjured nerve and formed large bundles; at 4 wk after the injury, however, the endoneurial stroma had recovered its original structure (Moss and Lewkowicz, 1981). In another study of the effect of crush injury, the focus was on the endoneurial blood flow pattern in the rat sciatic nerve. Endoneurial blood flow, oxygen tension, and pH were monitored at the site of a crush injury that was applied either over a short or a prolonged period. The length of crushing period did not affect the results. It was observed that, immediately following injury, a small fluctuation in endoneurial blood flow was observed; however, later observations showed that blood flow had been restored to normal level. Neither was evidence of loss in oxygen tension (hypoxia) or decrease in pH (acidosis) observed following crushing (Zochodne and Nguyen, 1997).

The above data suggested that neither separation of the axoplasm alone (i.e., without rupture of the basement membrane) nor deformation of the endoneurial sheath (presumably also without rupture of the basement membrane) were irreversible injuries. This evidence suggests that the injury becomes irreversible when the basement membrane, as well as the attached endoneurial stroma, has been ruptured. However, the possibility that irreversibility of healing response requires rupture of structures beyond the endoneurial sheath (e.g., the perineurium) is not addressed by the limited evidence.

Evidence on the nature of the anatomical site that must be reached along the radial direction before the injury becomes irreversible can be found in functional studies performed after gradual stretching of a nerve along its axis (Sunderland, 1990). During stretching, the nerve progressively lost the continuity of its structures, starting at the smallest scale and extending outward. First, the axoplasm became separated without loss of continuity of the endoneurial sheath (defined in this study as the combined basement membrane and the endoneurial stroma attached to it); at higher strain levels, the endoneurial sheath lost its continuity (intrafascicular injury) without causing separation of the fascicle itself or the perineurial sheath; at even higher strain, the fascicle lost its continuity but a strand of disorganized tissue maintained continuity of the trunk; finally, the entire trunk fractured. It was reported that hemorrhage, swelling (edema), an inflammatory response, and fibrosis were all first observed during this process of progressive rupture when the endoneurial sheath lost its continuity (Sunderland, 1990).

Even though somewhat limited, the combined evidence suggests that rupture of the Schwann cell basement membrane and the endoneurial stroma attached to it, rather than rupture of the perineurium, is the smallest injury along the radial direction that leads to an irreversible healing response in a peripheral nerve.

9.5.2 Proximal Stump; Traumatic Degeneration of the Myelin Sheath

One of the first events that follows transection of the sciatic nerve trunk is the gradual dismantling of the myelin sheath. A detailed study of this degenerative process was focused on the proximal stump (Morris et al., 1972a). The process started at the edge of the proximal stump, about 36 h after transection, and appeared in cross-sectional view as extensive splitting of the myelin laminae that gave the sheath a wrinkled appearance. Splitting first appeared in the inner laminae of the myelin sheath, but eventually propagated through the whole thickness of the sheath. This was followed by erosion of the circumferential laminae with subsequent loss of cohesion and fragmentation of the myelin sheath. While the myelin sheath surrounding axons was undergoing these changes, the sheath in the immediate proximity of the nodes of Ranvier appeared to have withdrawn from the node; following withdrawal, the recently denuded area became covered only by Schwann cell cytoplasm (Morris et al., 1972a).

In parallel with the above, Schwann cells associated with the degenerating myelin in the proximal stump started undergoing frequent mitoses, an event not often observed in Schwann cells associated with the intact nerve. Myelin debris was transiently observed in the cytoplasm of Schwann cells but eventually was digested; by 10 d, few Schwann cells contained myelin debris and by 18 d evidence of myelin digestion in the cytoplasm of Schwann cells had disappeared (Morris et al., 1972a). The basement membrane of many Schwann cells acquired a loosened appearance by 3 d; between 3 d and 10 d, lengths of basement membrane that were not associated with cells were occasionally seen in the endoneurium. Cells that were only partly covered by a basement membrane were identified as Schwann cells that had become unattached from axon processes and were digesting myelin (Morris et al., 1972a).

9.5.3 Sprouting of Axons from the Proximal Stump; Minifasciculation

The diameter of axons in the proximal stump became smaller as early as 30 min after transection of a peripheral nerve. The result was retraction of the axon circumference from the innermost lamella of the myelin sheath with which it was initially in contact, suggesting that the axon diameter had shrunk, leaving a gap. The longitudinal orientation of nerve fibers was maintained in its original highly aligned configuration during the first 24 h after transection; after that, nerve fibers at the edge of the stump became misaligned (Morris et al., 1972c).

Myelinated axons in the proximal stump produced collateral and terminal sprouts in the first 6 d. Axon sprouts were assembled in groups that included Schwann cells, the latter involved in extensive mitotic activity. The data suggested that such groups typically consisted of sprouts produced by a single myelinated axon that had become degenerated, shedding its basement membrane as described above. Synthesis of new basement membrane around many individual Schwann cells also appears to have been taking place; eventually, however, entire groups of sprouting axons became enveloped each in a single, occasionally fragmentary, cylindrical basement membrane (Morris et al., 1972b).

During the six-week period following transection, the one or two large fascicles typically comprising the rat sciatic nerve at the point of transection disappeared and were replaced by a large number of small fascicles (minifascicles), each with its own multilaminate perineurium (compartmentation). The number of perineurial layers in compartment walls varied from 1 to 5, compared with 5 to 7 layers for the normal control; all layers were encased in a basement membrane. The separation between layers was increased over that observed in the normal control. It was hypothesized that cells, identified as endoneurial fibroblasts, became circumferentially elongated around groups of axons and Schwann cells, eventually forming these layers (Morris et al., 1972d).

9.5.4 Long-Term Degenerative Processes in the Distal Stump

During the first several weeks after transection, axons in the distal stump that had been cut off from the proximal stump, as well as their associated myelin sheaths, underwent degradation by Schwann cells and macrophages (Wallerian degeneration). The outcome of such phagocytic activity was formation of endoneurial sheaths (endoneurial tubes) in the distal stump (i.e., cylindrical structures of basement membrane free of axons and myelin).

Following removal of axons and myelin from the endoneurial tubes, non-myelinating Schwann cells that had been deprived of axonal contact and had begun to proliferate formed linear structures (bands of Büngner) along the empty basement membrane of the endoneurial tubes (Cajal, 1928; Nathaniel and Pease, 1963; Fu and Gordon, 1997).

Over the course of several months, the endoneurial tubes shrank to about one-half their original diameter, became fragmented, and eventually were replaced by collagen fibrils (Salonen et al., 1987b; Röyttä and Salonen, 1988; Giannini and Dyck, 1990; Bradley et al., 1998). Eventually, the sites occupied by the original nerve fibers were filled by densely packed, longitudinally oriented collagen fibrils (Bradley et al., 1998).

9.5.5 Fibrosis and Angiogenesis in the Stump

Nerve transection resulted in significant increases in mass of fascicular collagen both proximally and distally to the transection site while nerve crush led to a much smaller increase in mass of fascicular collagen (Eather et al., 1986). Collagen accumulation was observed in the endoneurium and perineurium of the transected nerve (Salonen et al., 1985). In the distal stump of the transected nerve there was deposition of collagen fibrils, measuring one-half the diameter of those observed in normal endoneurium, around the Schwann cell columns (Büngner bands) (Salonen et al., 1987a,b)

A study of collagen types synthesized in the distal stump showed that expression of type I and type III collagens peaked 7 to 14 d after transection; however, expression of ECM genes, including the fibronectin gene, lasted much longer in the proximal stump (Siironen et al., 1992a). Type I collagen was expressed in the epi-, peri- and endoneurium, both in stumps that were reinnervated as well as in denervated stumps. These data showed that expression of the ECM genes occurred through the entire stump cross section and without requiring the presence of axons (Siironen et al., 1992a). A study of gene expression of basement membrane components in the proximal stump of the transected nerve showed that laminin and type IV collagen were both synthesized during the two-week period following injury (Siironen et al., 1992b).

Prior to formation of a neuroma in the proximal stump of a transected nerve, there was evidence of angiogenesis in the stump as early as 7 d after transection; the new microvessels were synthesized between layers of perineurial cells of former fascicles or in the epineurial connective tissue (Zochodne and Nguyen, 1997).

9.5.6 Presence of Myofibroblasts in Peripheral Nerve Stumps

A study was made of contractile cell presence following peripheral nerve trauma in humans. Myofibroblasts, identified as a component of the neuroma, were observed to increase in number during the period from 2 to

6 months following injury and to decrease thereafter (Badalamente et al., 1985).

A study of the connective tissue response in the transected peripheral nerve was focused on the presence of myofibroblasts in the two stumps. At the proximal neuroma, studied at 6 wk after injury, a thick, collagenous capsule, which resembled dermal scar in skin defects, surrounded the nerve tissue and converged to form a cap at the end of the neuroma. The tissue capsule around the nerve stump was about 20 to 50 μm thick. In the distal stump, a collagen capsule, about 50 μm thick, was also present and capped the distal stump. Cells staining with antibody to α-SM actin, indicative of the myofibroblast phenotype, were identified inside the tissue capsules capping the stumps. In addition to their presence in such circumferentially aligned layers, myofibroblasts were also observed within the bulk of the nerve, aligned parallel to the nerve axis. In some cases, these axially aligned myofibroblasts comprised as many as 20% of all nonneuronal cells (Chamberlain et al., 2000a).

In view of the strong evidence that fibroblast differentiation to the contractile phenotype is upregulated by TGF-β (Desmoulière et al., 1993) it is important to review the available evidence for the role of this regulator in peripheral nerve wounds. Presence of TGF-β isoforms was detected at the site of injury in transected peripheral nerves; TGF-β1 and −3, but not TGF-β2, were detected in the proximal stump by 12 h after injury but only after 48 h at the distal stump (Nath et al., 1998). Treatment of injured nerves with antibody to TGF-β was reported to have neutralized TGF-b activity and to have resulted in improved regeneration (Nath et al., 1998; Davison et al., 1999).

9.5.7 Mechanism of Closure of Nerve Stump

The presence of myofibroblasts both in the capsule formed around the proximal and distal stumps of the transected nerve, as well as axially aligned inside the nerve trunk, as described above, suggests a hypothesis for closure of a stump following transection. Closure of the defect (capping) is hypothetically controlled by the interplay among three forces. The first two lead to closure and include circumferential forces generated by myofibroblasts in the capsule surrounding the nerve trunk as well as axial forces developed by myofibroblasts aligned parallel to the nerve axis inside the nerve trunk. The third force opposes the first two, and leads to outflow of endoneurial fluid due to the presence of a positive intrafascicular pressure.

According to this hypothesis, closure of the stump with formation of neuroma occurs when the circumferential and axial forces pulling tissues away from the plane of transection at each stump overcome the force that causes outflow of endoneurial fluid. If formation of a contractile capsule is suppressed by inserting the stumps inside a silicone tube, or even entirely blocked by use of a collagen tube, flow of endoneurial fluid occurs, according to the hypothesis, in spite of the continuing presence of the axial contractile force as has been observed (Chamberlain et al., 2000a).

The evidence supporting the presence of a positive intrafascicular pressure in the normal nerve is considerable and has been reviewed in some detail (Olsson, 1990). Spontaneous flow of intrafascicular fluid, leading to the well-known "endoneurial bulge," has been shown to cause bulging of each stump by as much as 1.0 to 1.3 mm beyond the cut edge of the perineurium 24 h after transection. Histological study of the fluid comprising the bulge showed that it comprised Schwann cells, fibroblasts, and axon sprouts (Archibald and Fisher, 1987). Flow of fluid from the transected stump has been observed to fill the tubulated gap in 1 to 2 d (Williams and Varon, 1985).

A speculative interpretation of minifascicle formation in the transected but untubulated proximal stump can be based on a decrease in the diameter of the stump due to the circumferential (hoop) stresses generated by the constrictive capsule surrounding it. Deformation along the radial direction of the healing stump should lead to contraction of the endoneurial space, resulting in the hypothetical unavailability of space for regeneration of endoneurial blood vessels and to eventual suppression of growth, leading to synthesis of structures that cannot extend much along the radial direction (minifascides).

Since the interaction between the myofibroblast and the matrix during contraction is regulated by one or more integrins, it is useful to review the evidence for expression of integrin subunits that have been shown, in studies with skin wounds, to be involved in contraction. A study of expression of the alpha1 integrin in the transected sciatic nerve showed that, by 24 h after transection, the subunit was expressed by endoneurial fibroblasts. The number of positively staining cells reached a peak at 4 wk and declined until no such cells could be detected by 8 wk. Expression of alpha1 seemed to start at the proximal stump and to appear at the distal stump with some delay (Taskinen et al., 1996). This study showed that a hypothetical mechanism of contraction induced by myofibroblast-ECM interaction in nerve wounds could be plausibly based on the utilization of the alpha1beta1 integrin. Evidence has been presented in an earlier section showing alpha1beta1 to be the integrin that is principally involved in contraction of skin wounds by myofibroblasts (Racine-Samson et al., 1997).

9.5.8 Healing of the Nerve Defect in the Fetal Model

Studies of nerve healing in fetal models have emphasized repair with sutures and do not appear to have included studies of spontaneous healing (Lin et al., 1994; Meuli-Simmen et al., 1997; Butler et al., 1999b). Suturing controls the geometry of the healing defect by imposing closure and preventing expression of endogenous processes that lead to closure in spontaneously healing defects.

9.6 Summary

Spontaneous healing of the dermis-free defect in skin models and of the transected peripheral nerve appear to proceed, at least in part, along somewhat similar pathways. The mechanism of defect closure has been studied much more extensively with the skin defect.

Closure appears to be initiated at the time of injury of a nonregenerative tissue in skin or nerve, when a host of growth factors and cytokines are released inside the defect, generating the cytokine field. This field, consisting of the time-dependent concentrations of several diffusible regulators, modulates phenotypic expression in several cell types. Keratinocytes, endothelial cells, and Schwann cells change from a stationary to a migratory phenotype, while fibroblasts go through the same change, while also expressing a contractile phenotype. Fibroblasts eventually close part of the defect area by contraction; keratinocytes and Schwann cells each contribute to healing by their own differentiation program, which leads to synthesis of an epidermis or a myelin sheath around axons, respectively. While the activities of fibroblasts in the adult defect lead to synthesis of nonregenerative tissues (scar or neuroma), those of keratinocytes and Schwann cells lead to synthesis of regenerative tissues. A mechanistic study of spontaneous repair of a defect in the adult is focused by necessity on the activities of the fibroblast since these are the pathways that lead to irreversible injury and that need to be altered during induced regeneration.

Fibroblasts migrate into a skin defect over a provisional matrix comprising fibrin, fibronectin and hyaluronic acid. The composition of the matrix soon changes due to loss of fibrin and hyaluronic acid; however, fibronectin persists until closure. Fibroblasts eventually begin to synthesize collagen and other ECM components; they also become attached to the ECM via integrins and undergo a change to the contractile phenotype. Contraction is initiated before fibroblasts go through such a phenotypic change; it is hypothesized that while undifferentiated fibroblasts are responsible for onset of contraction, differentiated fibroblasts eventually bring definitive closure by contraction. Contraction itself amounts mostly to translation, rather than stretching, of perilesional dermis, and frequently has a principal axis along which defect area decreases faster. Although there are unanswered questions about the importance of granulation tissue in contraction, there is evidence that contraction is initiated at the edges of the defect rather than at the center; furthermore, there is evidence, that a continuous stream of contractile cells propagates away from the edges to the center and participates in the intermediate and late stages of closure. Contractile cells appear, therefore, to be active both at the edges and center of the defect. Synthesis of scar amounts to elaboration of collagen fibers by fibroblasts inside a tensile field extending over the plane of the defect, generated by the contractile cells, which orients the new fibers along its principal axis.

Contraction of a skin defect is eventually arrested by a pathway that appears to be independent of epidermal confluence and of the early steps in synthesis of basement membrane. It is hypothesized that the signal for eventual arrest of contraction is initiated during maturation of the basement membrane and is transmitted to the contracting stroma, inducing loss of traction between contractile cells and matrix. Loss of traction is hypothetically induced either by depletion of fibronectin or of the myofibroblast population through apoptosis.

Fetal skin defect healing differs from healing in adults primarily in the persistence of high levels in hyaluronic acid in fetal defects. There is also evidence that there is relative depletion of TGF-β in fetal defects. Contraction was absent in some (monkey, rabbit) but was present in other species (lamb) at selected points of gestation time. Evidence from an amphibian healing model showed that contraction gradually displaced regeneration during development of the tadpole.

Spontaneous healing of nerve defects has been sporadically studied relative to studies of healing of skin defects. There are several similarities between healing processes in the two organs. For example, the fibrin cable that is formed following tubulation of the transected stump is an elongated fibrin clot, very similar, if not identical in composition, to that which forms in skin wounds. The clot that forms in skin wounds comprises fibrin and fibronectin, as well as several other glycoproteins; it acts as a provisional matrix for the influx of cells of various types and as a reservoir of cytokines that are released during the clotting process, before it eventually becomes degraded (Clark, 1996b). Unlike the exudate from skin wounds, however, that from a transected nerve contains endoneurial fluid (Myers et al., 1983); furthermore, fibrin fibers are highly oriented in a nerve clot (Williams et al., 1983; Williams, 1987), probably much more so than they are in a skin clot.

A completely transected peripheral nerve closes largely by contraction of a capsule of contractile cells that have expressed the α-SM actin phenotype. The capsule hypothetically imposes circimferential stresses around the stump and restricts flow of axoplasm outside the stump; eventually, connective tissue is synthesized around the stump, forming a thick cap that closes the stump. Contractile cells are also assembled along the nerve axis; their contribution to closure of the transected stump is less clear.

10
Kinetics and Mechanism II: Induced Regeneration

10.1 Induced Regeneration versus Spontaneous Healing

Having reviewed the cell-matrix interactions that dominate healing of spontaneous defects by repair in skin and peripheral nerves, we now turn to finding out how these elaborate controls are modified in favor of induced regeneration. Almost all discussion of induced regeneration has been limited to the empirical facts that describe in situ synthesis of skin, peripheral nerves, and the conjunctival stroma. We will now discuss in some detail both the sequence and timing of the synthetic events as well as the elementary cell and molecular biological steps that lead to the regenerated organs. This chapter is therefore devoted to a discussion of the kinetics and mechanism of induced regeneration.

The discussion will center on the irreducible reaction diagrams for synthesis of these organs. These simple reaction protocols were identified in Chapter 7.

10.2 Kinetics of Skin Regeneration

A collection of the protocols, presented in the form of reaction diagrams, for synthesis of the tissue components of skin as well as of the entire organ (minus appendages) appear in Table 7.1. Following a detailed description of these reaction diagrams (Dg.) in Chapter 7, it was concluded that synthesis of skin using the minimum number of reactants required the exogenous supply only of keratinocytes and the appropriate nondiffusible regulator (Dg. S30).

Looked at somewhat differently, the protocol required simultaneous supply of the keratinocytes (KC) that alone were required for synthesis of the epidermis with its basement membrane (Dg. S13 in vitro; Dg. S9 in vivo) and, in addition, the nondiffusible regulator (DRT, dermis regeneration template), alone required to synthesize the dermis (Dg. S19). Inspection of the diagrams gave an impression that synthesis of the entire organ, without appendages, could be accomplished simply by "adding" the reaction diagrams for separate synthesis of its two major tissue components (Dg. S30). Partial synthesis of skin (i.e., a complete epidermis, basement membrane, and dermis without appendages) was achieved under these conditions; a detailed morphological and functional description of the synthesized organ is presented in Chapter 5 and summarized in Table 5.2. A brief morphological summary of the partial synthesis of skin appears in Figure 10.1.

This simple protocol for synthesis of skin will form the basis of the discussion on kinetics and mechanism that follows. The kinetic data used to trace the synthetic pathway are taken mostly from two strictly morphological studies of skin synthesis, one based on the guinea pig model (Murphy et al., 1990), the other on the swine (Compton et al., 1998).

10.2.1 Kinetics of Synthesis of the Epidermis and Basement Membrane

Before grafting, the keratinocyte-seeded DRT consisted of a highly porous network, 0.5 mm in thickness, comprising thin collagen-GAG strands embedded in a lucent fluid filled with keratinocytes.

DRT was a graft copolymer of type I collagen and chondroitin 6-sulfate (97.4/2.6 w/w); pore volume fraction over 0.96; pore diameter $50 \pm 20\,\mu m$; pore channel orientation, random; degradation rate in standardized collagenase solution in vitro corresponding to half-life in vivo of about 10 d (guinea pig); average molecular weight between cross links $12.75 \pm 3.3\,kDa$; triple helical structure of collagen intact by infrared spectroscopy; banded structure of collagen selectively converted to amorphous state following treatment at pH 3 (Yannas, 1990). DRT was grafted as a bilayer membrane, comprising a proximal DRT layer and a distal layer consisting of a thin silicone elastomer (Yannas et al., 1982a).

Autologous keratinocytes were harvested by separating epidermis and dermis from a partial-thickness skin biopsy, following incubation in Dispase, dissociation of KC from the epidermis using trypsin and ethylenediamine tetraacetic acid, and, finally, placing the resulting single-cell suspension in Weymouth's medium supplemented with fetal calf serum and growth substances, as described by Regauer and Compton (1990).

Isolated KCs were seeded onto the porous side of the DRT-silicone bilayer at a density of 5×10^5 cells/cm^2 defect surface and were then centrifuged at 500 rpm at 15 min at 4°C while maintaining the centrifugal force vector perpendicular to the graft surface. With this procedure, the keratinocytes were centrifuged through the DRT thickness to a plane near the silicone interface. The seeded DRT was then grafted on a dermis-free defect in the guinea pig or swine. The seeding process lasted about 4 h (Yannas et al., 1982a,b, 1989; Orgill, 1983).

Distinct steps along the synthetic pathway are described below.

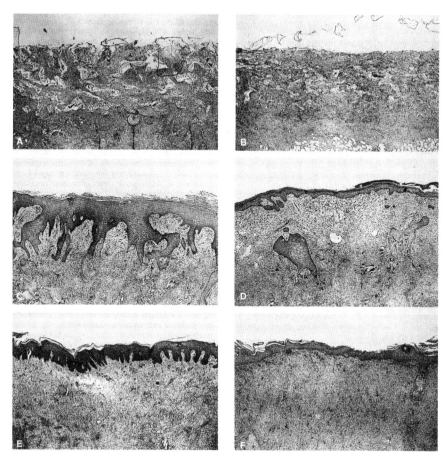

FIGURE 10.1. Kinetics of skin synthesis using two related protocols. A dermis-free defect in the swine was grafted with keratinocyte-seeded dermis regeneration template (DRT). The histological appearance of the regenerating skin is shown at 7, 14, and 20 d postgrafting. *Left* (photos A, C, E): Keratinocytes were cultured for 14 d before seeding into the porous DRT as a single-cell suspension prior to grafting. *Right* (photos B, D, F): Keratinocytes were dissociated from skin biopsy, but not cultured, before seeding into DRT. A thicker epidermis and a greater number of dermo-epidermal undulations (rete ridges) resulted following seeding of DRT with cultured keratinocytes. (From Butler et al., 1999a. Copyright 1999. Harcourt Publishers Ltd.)

Isolated Keratinocytes Inside the Defect (4 d)

Soon after the keratinocyte-seeded DRT was grafted on the dermis-free defect (guinea pig or swine), exudate had filled the inner (deep) one-third of its porous structure and was soon followed by cells migrating from the surface of the defect. All keratinocytes inside the DRT were identified as basal cells. Epidermal attachment specialization molecules, including laminin (lamina lucida of basement membrane), type VII collagen (anchoring fibrils), or $\alpha_6\beta_4$ integrin (hemidesmosomes) were not observed at this time.

Formation of Islands and Cords of Keratinocytes; Segmented Basement Membrane (8 d)

A greatly increased cell density caused an expansion in DRT thickness to about 1.5 mm. The keratinocyte population had significantly increased compared with 4 d. About 50% of the cell population inside DRT had formed irregularly shaped islands and cords of keratinocytes that interlaced and were outlined at the surface with basal-like cells. The proportion of proliferating cells was as great as on 4 d, consisting of roughly equal numbers of keartinocytes and stromal cells. No expression of keratin 1 (K1), the major cytoskeletal component of suprabasal cells, was observed at that time. Discontinuous linear segments of laminin, type VII collagen, and $\alpha_6\beta_4$ integrin were observed at the surface of epithelial cords, indicating local synthesis of lamina lucida, anchoring fibrils, and hemidesmosomes, respectively, but absence of a continuous basement membrane.

Partial Epidermal Confluence; Continuous Basement Membrane Synthesized (12 d)

Continuing cell proliferation and migration had by now increased the DRT thickness to about 2.75 mm. The islands and interlacing cords of keratinocytes showed well-defined basal layers at their surfaces and evidence of keratinocyte maturation in the direction toward the interior of the cords. A partly confluent epidermis now covered the DRT surface. Although immature, the epidermis showed the beginning of the epithelial differentiation program. A continuous basement membrane had been synthesized around all epithelial islands and cords, indicating maturity of hemidesmosomal and anchoring fibril attachments.

Keratin Cyst Synthesis (15 d)

No further expansion of DRT volume was observed. A large number of keratin cysts had formed inside the epithelial islands during the previous 3 d. Cysts were characterized by a maturation gradient pointing inside an island or cord (i.e., a basal cell layer outside and an increasingly keratinized interior). The basement membrane structure had remained unchanged.

Extrusion of Keratin Cysts (19 d)

Cysts had almost completely disappeared at this time point by extrusion through the fully confluent epidermis. The mechanism of appearance and disappearance of keratin cysts was not studied and will not be discussed further. The epidermis had become fully confluent whereas the basement membrane appeared unchanged.

Maturation of Epidermis (35 d)

The proportion of proliferating cells had approached the level present in the normal epidermis. The epidermis had become opaque and differed little from normal skin controls although not all of the epidermal keratin programs had yet become fully normalized. The basement membrane was continuous along the epidermal basal cell surface.

10.2.2 Synthesis of Rete Ridges and the Dermis

In this section, we describe the stages in the degradation of DRT, as well as the main events associated with synthesis of rete ridges and the dermis.

Cell Migration and Proliferation Inside DRT (4 d)

The top (distal) one-half of DRT was sparsely populated with cells, whereas the bottom one-half was densely infiltrated with cells that had either migrated from the surface of the defect or were products of very active proliferation. Cells infiltrating the highly porous structure of DRT included mononuclear cells, granulocytes, red blood cells, multinucleated giant cells, and cells with the shape of fibroblasts. Although about 30% of cells inside DRT were endothelial cells, they were not organized in histologically recognizable vascular structures. At 4 d, 30 to 50% of cells inside DRT were actively cycling. Cycling cells are rare in the dermis of normal controls. DRT strands, loosely aggregated fibrin, and mononuclear cells were arranged with no apparent pattern.

Cell Adhesion on DRT Fibers (8 d)

The DRT fibers were distinct and largely undegraded throughout the defect. A fibrin layer had formed on the surface of DRT fibers and was invariably present when mononuclear cells adhered to DRT fibers, typically by extending pseudopod-like processes toward the DRT surface. Occasionally, mononuclear cells were adherent onto the DRT surface in the form of a continuous cell layer along the fiber axis; however, no mononuclear cells were observed apposed to the surface of DRT fibers on which a fibrin coating was not visible. Although membranes of mononuclear cells arranged along a DRT fiber axis were very close to the fiber surface, pseudopods were still visible. Multinucleate giant cells were also observed to be intimately associated with DRT fibers. Cell-DRT associations were especially frequent in the proximal third of the DRT thickness. Such apparently organized cell-DRT assemblies stood in contrast to DRT-free control defects, in which macrophages were associated with the fibrin matrix in apparently random arrangements. There was no evidence inside the defect either of a foreign body reaction or a delayed hypersensitivity response to alloantigens.

Angiogenesis and Stroma Synthesis; DRT Degradation (12 d)

By 10 d, more than 50% of the DRT mass had been degraded (guinea pig), leaving small fragmented residues surrounded by numerous mononuclear cells, including the following cell types: phagocytic macrophages, often containing small fragments of DRT; fusiform fibroblast-like cells oriented at random axes; granulated cells suggestive of mast cells or basophils; and cells forming focally branching cords with small central lumens and confirmed to be blood vessels. Angiogenesis appeared to be initiated in the form of slender vascular structures penetrating DRT from the surface of the defect below and occasionally extending all the way to the distal DRT surface. By 12 d, newly synthesized stroma was visible between keratinocyte cords; it was highly heterogeneous, ranging from areas of abundant cellularity and extracellular matrix deposition, largely in the form of dense hyaline material, to extracellular matrix–poor areas containing many giant cells and residual DRT fibers but few repopulating stromal cells.

Random Alignment of Dermal Fibroblasts (15 d)

By 14 d, residual DRT fragments and associated giant cells were observed in a few locations. The axes of dermal fibroblasts were randomly aligned; less than 10% of them were identified as myofibroblasts. Dermal blood vessels formed a discrete, horizontally oriented subepidermal plexus by 14 to 17 d. A densely cellular connective tissue had formed within the deep (proximal) section of the DRT.

Intensified Synthesis of Dermis (19 d)

Rare, minute foci of residual DRT with associated giant cells were detected. There was a loss of sharp demarcation between proximal DRT and the defect surface. Collections of hyaline material, observed earlier in the neostroma amid epithelial cords, were no longer present. Increased deposition of dermal collagen was observed, accompanied by decrease in dermal cellularity. Small collections of lymphocytes surrounded blood vessels in the neodermis.

Synthesis of Rete Ridges (35 d)

Evenly spaced, newly formed rete ridges were seen. The neodermis appeared histologically homogeneous throughout; however, it was hypercellular and hypervascular. There were no discernible bilayers equivalent to those of papillary and reticular dermis. In contrast to scar tissue, the axes of collagen fibers in the neodermis had a three-dimensional orientation.

10.2.3 Synchronization Between the Processes for Synthesis of Epithelia and Stroma

Although the kinetics of synthesis of skin have been presented along two tracks (i.e., synthesis of an epidermis and a dermis), it is important to recall that there is evidence for synchronization between these two synthetic pathways. This becomes especially noticeable during the synthesis of rete ridges, a rather late synthetic event. This topological feature is described by the intimately interdigitating configurations of the two major tissues of skin. It is impossible to explain rete ridge synthesis on the basis of a mechanism that neglects a specific interaction between epidermis and dermis. An epithelial-mesodermal interaction, similar in scope to that which plays an important role in development of the embryo, appears, therefore, to be required for synthesis of rete ridges.

Support for a hypothesis that an epithelial-mesodermal interaction accounts for rete ridge synthesis is found by comparing the morphology of rete ridges synthesized by two processes, identical in all respects except in the extent of time spent in culture by the keratinocytes that were seeded into or cultured into DRT. In this study, the number of rete ridges synthesized by 20 d was 49 per centimeter cross section with cultured cells and only 14 with uncultured cells; furthermore, the epidermis synthesized was significantly thicker, when cultured, rather than uncultured, keratinocytes were used (Butler et al., 1999a). The dependence of rete ridge structure on the keratinocyte phenotype, which is presumably expressed in culture, provides direct evidence that keratinocytes significantly modify this structure that appears to require mesodermal elements for its synthesis.

Another phenomenon that cannot be explained by a hypothetical early independence between synthetic processes occurring in the epidermis and the dermis is the absence of skin appendages in skin that has been synthesized as described above. During development, appendages are synthesized as extensions of the epidermis that are projected into the dermis (Burkitt et al., 1993). As with the observed synthesis of rete ridges, an explanation of the failure to synthesize appendages also requires consideration of an epithelial-mesodermal interaction involving the two major tissues of skin.

10.3 Mechanism of Synthesis of the Dermis

The events that lead to partial synthesis of the dermis will be analyzed below in an effort to understand the mechanistic aspects of these processes. An outline of the mechanism for synthesis of an epidermis over an existing dermal surface has been presented in Chapter 2 and will not be repeated here; further details on epithelialization can be found in thorough reviews (Stenn and Malhotra, 1992; Woodley, 1996). The focus of the discussion of mechanism is on interpretation of certain critical observations involving the induction of stroma regeneration in skin. Reliance will be placed below on the mechanism of spontaneous healing discussed in Chapter 9; the latter will be treated as the negative control.

10.3.1 Depletion of Cells, Including Contractile Cells, in the Defect

The dermis-free defect grafted with keratinocyte-seeded DRT significantly differs from the ungrafted defect in certain features of its cell population. In a detailed study of synthesis of skin in the presence of the keratinocyte-seeded DRT it was observed that the proportion of dermal fibroblasts inside the defect that had expressed the contractile phenotype (myofibroblasts) was less than 10% at 14 d; in contrast, the proportion was more than 50% in the ungrafted control at the same day (Murphy et al., 1990). Although the onset in contraction of the grafted defect was delayed by 13.5 d compared with the ungrafted defect (Table 8.3), both defects were actively contracting at that time at near maximum levels of the contraction rate. In another study, it was observed that defects grafted with cell-free DRT were characterized by a much lower total density of cells relative to the ungrafted defect almost throughout the healing process (Troxel, 1994).

The observed myofibroblast depletion suggests a deficiency either in fibroblast proliferation or in fibroblast differentiation to the contractile cell phenotype. Furthermore, the observed depletion of the defect from cells of all types probably reflects lack of adequate upregulation either of migration or proliferation. Either one of the anticipated deficiencies that could account for these observations could result from lack of adequate signaling from soluble regulators. This reasoning leads to consideration of the effect of the keratinocyte-seeded DRT on the composition of the cytokine field present inside the defect.

Unlike their behavior with other collagen-containing matrices, platelets adhere to but are not aggregated following contact with the surface of DRT in vitro; as a result, they do not degranulate after adhering to the DRT surface (Yannas and Silver, 1975; Sylvester et al., 1989; Yannas, 1990). The platelet-collagen reaction requires the presence of the well-known banding periodicity of collagen (Sylvester et al., 1989). During DRT synthesis, the banding periodicity of collagen fibers is erased by lengthy incubation below the critical pH level, 4.25 ± 0.30, at which a reversible disorganization of banding takes place; banding is prevented from reforming when the copolymer is returned back to physiological pH by covalent crosslinking at the acidic pH level. The collagen triple helix is not affected by this treatment (Yannas, 1972a,b, 1990; Sylvester et al., 1989). Incorporation of a glycosaminoglycan in the graft copolymer also inhibits adhesion of platelets on collagen as well as serotonin release (Yannas and Silver, 1975; Silver et al., 1978, 1979). GAG-mediated suppression of platelet aggregation may also depend on manipulation of the banding periodicity of collagen during collagen precipitation in the presence of GAG.

In a DRT-free defect, platelets that are present inside the defect soon after injury bind on ECM that has become exposed due to the injury and degranulate, secreting several cytokines, including PDGF and TGF-β. In the presence of the very high specific surface of DRT, it would be expected that a substantial fraction of platelets in the defect would adhere on that surface and would, therefore, be prevented from degranulating. PDGF and TGF-β have been long recognized as potent upregulators of the inflammatory response that follows soon after injury. In particular, PDGF is recognized as a powerful mitogen for connective tissue cells and a stimulus for chemotaxis of fibroblasts (Heldin and Westermark, 1996), while TGF-β stimulates the migration of monocytes, lymphocytes, neutrophils, and fibroblasts, as well as upregulating collagen synthesis in the defect (Roberts et al., 1986; Roberts and Sporn, 1996). Quite importantly, there is strong evidence that TGF-β1 is the most effective upregulator for expression of α-SM actin, the recognized myofibroblast marker (Desmoulière and Gabbiani, 1996; Vaughan et al., 2000). The evidence suggests that grafting with DRT suppresses secretion of certain cytokines that are readily produced in the ungrafted defect; these cytokines are known to upregulate fibroblast proliferation as well as their differentiation to the contractile phenotype.

An additional pathway by which DRT hypothetically interferes with the cytokine field in the defect is suggested by the preliminary observation that cytokines, including TGF-β1, TGF-β2, and PDGF-BB, bind avidly, though apparently not specifically, on the extensive surface of DRT both in vivo and in vitro (Ellis et al., 1997). There have been many independent reports of significant binding of cytokines on several ECM components, including type IV collagen, fibronectin, and the proteoglycans betaglycan and decorin (Massagué and Like, 1985; Fava and McClure, 1987; Yamaguchi et al., 1990; Paralkar et al., 1991). However, it is not known whether the observed massive binding of PDGF and TGF-β on the DRT surface (Ellis et al., 1997) actually leads to depletion of unbound (free) cytokines; nor is it clear to what extent the activity of PDGF and TGF-β depends on their presence in an unbound form.

10.3.2 Delay in Onset of Contraction

It was observed that grafting with the cell-free DRT had a significant delaying effect on the onset of contraction, t_o, measured as the time after injury when the first inward movement of the dermal edges of the dermis-free defect was observed; t_o was measured following grafting the dermis-free defect in the guinea pig both with DRT and with another, less active ECM analog (analog B) that was used as a control. The two cell-free analogs structurally differed only in average pore diameter; analog B had a pore diameter of 400 μm while the pore diameter in DRT was 40 μm, with a resulting approximately 12-fold higher specific surface for DRT. All other structural features of DRT and analog B, including the chemical composi-

TABLE 10.1. Differences in contraction-delaying activity between two structurally very similar ECM analogs.[1]

	DRT	Less active ECM analog (analog B)
A. Characteristics of ECM analogs		
collagen/GAG, w/w	98/2	98/2
cross linking treatment	same in both	same in both
average pore diameter, μm	40	400
specific surface, mm²/cm³	ca. 25,000	ca. 2,000
B. Morphology of defect at onset of contraction		
contraction onset, d	8.5 ± 1.1 d	3.7 ± 1.1 d
thickness of granulation tissue at dermal edge, μm	ca. 100	ca. 100
cell density in defect	low	high
C. After onset; contraction delay and morphology		
delay in contraction half-life, d[2]	18.5 ± 2.5	1.5 ± 3
number of cells per graft pore cross section	2–5	30–50
% cells inside graft pores	90	60
alignment of cell axes inside graft	quasi-random	quasi-random
alignment of cell axes outside graft	axial	axial
cell density in defect	low	high

[1] Structural data on ECM analogs from Chang, 1988 and Troxel, 1994. Histological data from Murphy et al., 1990 and Troxel, 1994.
[2] Relative to ungrafted control.

tion and cross link density of the macromolecular network, were nearly identical (Table 10.1).

At the time of onset of contraction, as well as throughout the healing process, the total cell density was much lower in DRT-grafted defects than in those grafted with analog B. Grafting with the two ECM analogs had a significantly different effect on the onset of contraction; t_o occurred at 3.7 ± 1.1 d (numbers of days after injury and grafting) for analog B and at 8.5 ± 1.1 d for cell-free DRT (Troxel, 1994) (Figure 10.2). For comparison, t_o was 3 ± 1 d for the ungrafted defect (Chapter 9). Additional observations related to the thickness of the cell cluster that appears at the edge of the defect, δ, measured in a direction perpendicular to the surface of the defect (described in Chapter 9). Following injury, and prior to the start of contraction, δ remained negligibly thin in ungrafted defects and in those grafted with DRT or with analog B. At the onset of contraction, determined by the earliest sign of loss in area bounded by the dermal edges of the defect, δ exceeded a level, roughly approximated at 100 μm in all three defects. This finding was taken as an indication that contraction of the defect, whether grafted or not, did not start until δ reached this estimated minimal thickness. However, this level was reached several days later when DRT, rather than analog B, was grafted (Figure 10.3). Evidence that the onset of con-

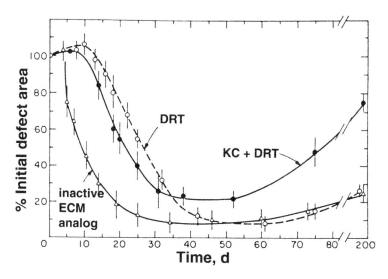

FIGURE 10.2. Contraction kinetics following grafting of the dermis-free defect in the guinea pig with cell-free and cell-seeded DRT, as well as with a relatively inactive (unseeded) analog of DRT (analog B). Analog B (inactive ECM analog) was identical to DRT in structure except having much higher average pore diameter than keratinocyte-seeded dermis regeneration template (KC + DRT) or cell-free DRT (Table 10.1). Cell-free DRT delayed contraction but did not arrest it; eventually, only a small mass of dermis was synthesized. KC-seeded DRT arrested contraction at 35 to 40 d and the defect perimeter continued increasing at a rate higher than predicted by animal growth to yield a partial skin regenerate (appendages missing) occupying 2/3 of initial defect area at 200 d. The inactive ECM analog did not delay contraction significantly; nor did it induce regeneration. (From Yannas et al., 1989.)

traction is controlled by formation of a cell cluster at the edge of the ungrafted dermis-free defect is presented in Chapter 9.

The significant delay in onset of contraction, as well as the delayed increase in thickness of the cell cluster, observed with DRT-grafted defects (Figure 10.3), appear to be directly related to the observation of a much lower total cell density inside the defect, relative to defects grafted with analog B. It is expected that, when other factors that describe the two grafted defects remained fixed, the rate of formation of the cell cluster at the edge should have been lower in the defect that was characterized by lower total cell density. Since DRT and analog B differed only in specific surface (Table 10.1), the lower cell density observed with DRT must be attributed to that single structural difference. In the discussion above, the observation that the DRT-grafted defect is severely depleted from myofibroblasts relative to the ungrafted defect was interpreted as the result of the observed lack of platelet-aggregating activity of DRT. The deficit in specific surface of analog B suggests that it binds (thereby preventing degran-

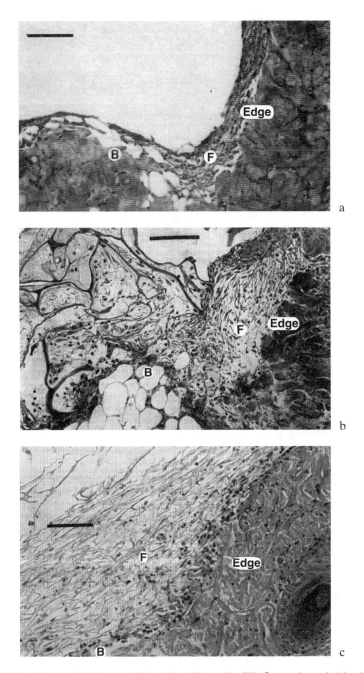

a

b

c

FIGURE 10.3. Cluster thickness of fibroblast-like cells (F), δ, at edge of skin defect 4 d after surgery following three treatments. δ was measured in a direction perpendicular to the point where the plane of the defect edge (Edge) intersected the defect base (B). *Top* (Figure 10.3a): Ungrafted; δ about 100 μm thick. *Middle* (Figure 10.3b): Grafted with cell-free analog B, a relatively inactive ECM analog (Table 10.1); δ somewhat larger than 100 μm thick. *Bottom* (Figure 10.3c): Grafted with cell-free dermis regeneration template; very few fibroblast-like cells were present at the point of observation for δ and the cluster thickness was much lower than 100 μm. Bar: 100 μm. (From Troxel, 1994.)

ulation) a smaller fraction of the platelet content of the defect relative to DRT.

10.3.3 Delay in Contraction Half-Life

The time of onset of contraction, t_o, and the contraction half-life, $t_{1/2}$, describe the rate of the process at distinctly different stages. In the ungrafted dermis-free defect in the guinea pig, t_o was observed at 3 ± 1 d whereas the half-life was 8 ± 1 d; in the DRT-grafted defect, t_o was observed at 8.5 ± 1 d whereas the half-life was 26.5 ± 2.5 d (Yannas et al., 1989; Troxel, 1994). The evidence, presented in Chapter 9, strongly suggested that two distinct mechanisms were necessary to account for defect closure by contraction: an early stage process dependent on cell activity at the defect edge and a later process that additionally recruited myofibroblasts and involved transfer of contractile forces across the entire defect. The data suggest the possibility that t_o describes the rate of the early-stage process whereas $t_{1/2}$ describes the later stage of contraction; however, there is need for additional data before such an assignment can be definitively made. The ensuing discussion focuses on the delay in $t_{1/2}$ observed when the defect was grafted with DRT or with one of several ECM analogs with related structure (Table 8.3) and will be limited to the later stage of contraction.

DRT, as well as several other ECM analogs, have been shown to significantly delay contraction. Contraction delay, Δt, is the difference between the contraction half-life of a treated and an untreated defect. As shown in Table 8.3, the delay reached a high point of about 20 d when DRT was studied. The magnitude of the delay depended very sensitively on structure, rapidly dropping when the following modifications were made to the structure of DRT: the average pore diameter was either higher or lower than the estimated range 20 to 120 μm; the crosslink density did not stay within limits consistent with a half-life of degradation in vivo of 8 to 15 d; the GAG component was deleted; the ECM analog was replaced with a silicone membrane (Flynn, 1983; Yannas et al., 1989). The value of Δt was either not affected or slightly increased when chondroitin 6-sulfate was exchanged for several other GAGs or proteoglycans (Shafritz et al., 1994).

A preliminary interpretation of the observed delay in contraction half-life will be based once more on a comparison between DRT and the less active ECM analog (analog B); the two analogs differed only in average pore diameter, a difference reflected in a 12-fold higher specific surface for DRT. The contraction delay Δt was 18.5 ± 2.5 d for DRT and 1.5 ± 3 d for analog B (Table 10.1).

In contrast to the experimental protocol reported in the preceding section, observations of cell distribution were made at the center of the defect rather than at the edges (Table 10.1). There is considerable evidence that a variety of cells inside the defect, including contractile cells, bind extensively on the surface of DRT (Murphy et al., 1990; Troxel, 1994; Compton et al., 1998). Large numbers of cells were observed in intimate contact with the collagen-GAG fibers of the ECM analogs at the center of the defect. The observations, made 7 d after grafting, described conditions both inside each graft as well as at the interface between graft and defect surface. The pore density of cells (number of cells per single pore cross section) was 30 to 50 cells inside the much larger pores of the less active analog but only 2 to 5 cells per pore cross section inside the DRT. Contractile cells were clearly distributed in two "phases" either inside the porous graft, or outside it (at the interface between the graft and the surface of the defect). Sixty percent of all cells in the defect cross section had migrated inside analog B whereas as many as 90% had migrated inside the DRT. The long axes of cells located inside either of the grafts did not have a preferred orientation; however, at the graft-defect interface (outside the graft), cell axes were aligned entirely in the plane of the defect (Figure 10.4). The highly planar cell orientation at the graft-defect interface appeared very similar to that observed with the vigorously contracting, ungrafted defect (Table 10.1).

A simple analysis of the contractile forces originating from cells inside a defect will be based on the hypotheses that a contractile cell exerts traction on the ECM to which it is bound only along the direction of the long cell axis and that a cell axis oriented in the plane of the defect contributes to contraction whereas one oriented out of the plane is inactive. Use is also made of the observation that, in each graft, only a fraction of the cell axes were oriented in the plane of the defect (Figure 10.4), thereby actively contributing to defect contraction, whereas the remainder were oriented out of the plane and were inactive. Application of these simple rules to the three defects (ungrafted, grafted with DRT, or analog B) leads to a characterization of the observed differences in contraction behavior among these. Almost all of the cells in the ungrafted defect were oriented in the plane of the defect and contributed to contraction. In contrast, cell axes inside each graft were organized in a quasi-random, almost isotropic, arrangement, in which most of the cell axes were oriented out of the plane of the defect, suggesting that only a fraction of cells inside each graft contributed to contraction.

The difference in contraction half-life between DRT and analog B can be attributed to two factors, each contributing its share in reducing the ability of the DRT-grafted defect to mount a vigorous contractile response. First, of the total number of cells present in each defect, a smaller fraction was located at the DRT-defect than at the analog B-defect interface; it follows that the fraction of total cells present in the defect that could have mounted a contractile response was smaller in the DRT-grafted defect.

Second, the total number of cells in the DRT-grafted defect was smaller than in the analog B-grafted defect; it follows that a smaller number of cells were potentially available, both inside and outside DRT, to function in a contractile mode than in the analog B-grafted defect. It follows that grafting with either ECM analog should suppress contraction relative to the

100 microns

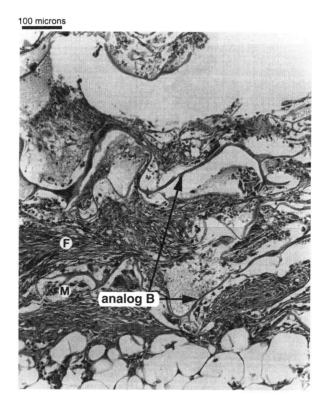

FIGURE 10.4. Fibroblast-like cells (F) inside two ECM analogs at center of defect at 7 d. *Top*: Inside the relatively inactive analog B. Notice high cell density and large numbers of cell inside pores. Arrows point at the fibers comprising analog B. *Bottom*: Inside DRT. Notice much lower cell density inside porous DRT and numerous cells outside it. M, macrophages. Bar: 100 μm. (From Troxel, 1994.)

ungrafted defect; furthermore, grafting with DRT should suppress contraction even more than with the less active analog. Both predictions agree with the data (Table 10.1).

Considering the effect of difference in specific surface between DRT and analog B on the fraction of cells that were observed inside each graft rather than at the graft-defect interface (outside the graft), we hypothesize that it reflects a difference in total capacity of each graft for binding cells on its surface. This suggestion is supported by recognition that the number of cell-binding domains (ligands) per unit volume of ECM analog is, to a good approximation, proportional to the specific surface of the porous solid (Yannas, 1997). According to the estimates of specific surface in each ECM analog (Table 10.1), the ligand density of DRT is about 12-fold higher than that of analog B. Since the mechanical stiffness of DRT and of the less active analog was not only extremely low but also identical for the two ECM analogs (Freyman et al., 2000), the possibility that either ECM analog delayed contraction by acting as a mechanical splint across the defect is ruled out. Instead, it is concluded that the high contraction-delaying activity of DRT compared with other ECM analogs with higher average pore diameter (Table 8.3) can be explained in terms of a maximal specific surface for the DRT, corresponding to a sufficiently high density of the appropriate ligands for capturing contractile cells in random orientations (Yannas, 1997).

The sharp decrease in contraction-delaying activity of ECM analogs when the average pore diameter was decreased much below about 10 μm (Table 8.3) is readily explained by using the observation that ECM analogs with pores much smaller than about 5 μm presented barriers to cell migration and remained practically free of cells following grafting. Presence of almost all cells outside the graft

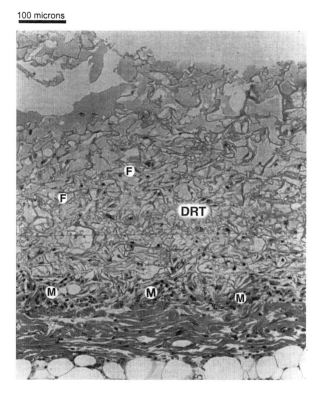

FIGURE 10.4. *Continued*

due to this barrier effect implies that these cells mounted a contractile response.

The nature of the DRT ligand(s) that binds with the fibroblast receptor and is responsible for the observed capture of contractile cells on the DRT scaffold (Figure 10.4) can be deduced from a variety of data. Deletion of the GAG component from the ECM analog reduced the contraction delay, Δt, assigned to DRT, an evidence of reduced activity. Substitution of aggrecan for chondroitin 6-sulfate in the copolymer had no significant effect whereas substitution with dermatan sulfate and decorin led to a small but significant increase in Δt, evidence of increased contraction-delaying activity (Table 8.3). The combined data suggest that the DRT ligand is probably not located in the GAG moiety; if it were, deletion of the GAG should have reduced Δt to near zero, rather than causing a modest reduction, as observed. This conclusion is consistent with the observed insensitivity of Δt to substitution of chondroitin 6-sulfate by other GAGs; however, the modest increase in activity observed following substitution of chondroitin 6-sulfate with each of the latter two GAGs is not readily explained by this mechanism.

Independent support to the conclusion that a GAG receptor in fibroblasts is not involved in contraction delay induced by DRT comes from the finding, discussed in Chapter 9, that integrin $\alpha_1\beta_1$, a known collagen receptor in fibroblasts (Xu and Clark, 2000), is the sole integrin utilized by contractile cells during contraction in spontaneously healing skin defects (Racine-Samson et al., 1997). If the latter evidence is directly applicable to the DRT-grafted skin defect, the binding of contractile cells on the DRT scaffold, responsible for disorientation of contractile cells (Figure 10.4) and for the hypothetical loss in their ability to contract the defect, can be assigned exclusively to the $\alpha_1\beta_1$ collagen receptor in fibroblasts.

Although the GAG component may not contribute directly to the contraction-delaying activity of DRT via a hypothetical GAG receptor in fibroblasts, it does contribute several days to the contraction-delaying activity of DRT, a significaint increment (Table 8.3). The contribution of GAG content to the value of Δt for DRT may reflect the confirmed increase in resistance to degradation of collagen implants following covalent attachment of GAG chains on it (Yannas et al., 1975a; Yannas, 1981, 1988). The observed requirement for a minimal resistance to degradation in contraction-delaying ECM analogs is discussed below in the context of the hypothetically required persistence of the active ECM analog in a nondiffucible state over a minimum period.

10.3.4 Persistence of the Regulator in a Nondiffusible State

When other structural parameters are maintained fixed, the contraction-delaying activity of ECM analogs depended relatively strongly on its degradation rate (Table 8.3). Resistance of collagen to degradation by collagenase has been shown to increase by crosslinking (Grillo and Gross, 1962; Kline and Hayes, 1964; Yannas et al., 1975b; Yannas, 1981) as well as by incorporation of a small mass of GAG into the ECM analog (Yannas et al., 1975a; Yannas, 1981, 1988). However, an unlimited increase in resistance to degradation led to synthesis of scar, rather than dermis, next to the implanted ECM analog (Yannas and Burke, 1980; Yannas, 1981). An analog that degraded too rapidly was not capable of effectively delaying contraction (Table 8.3). The hypothesis (partly based on observation) that upper and lower limits for degradation rate of DRT were both required for suppression of contraction was incorporated in the simple rule of "tissue isomorphous replacement"; the hypothetical rule requires that, during induced regeneration, tissue is synthesized at the same rate that the template is being degraded (Yannas and Burke, 1980; Yannas, 1997).

According to the hypothetical mechanism for the contraction-delaying activity of DRT discussed in the preceding section, the axes of contractile cells that have migrated inside the pores of DRT are maintained in a state of relatively random orientation. The ability of these cells to contribute to contraction of the defect is cancelled provided they remain inside DRT. Degradation of DRT should, therefore, lead to dismantling of the porous scaffold and to the hypothetical recovery of contractile cell activity. This reasoning explains qualitatively the existence of an upper limit of the degradation rate for retention of the contraction-delaying activity of ECM analogs. A lower limit of the degradation rate appeared hypothetically necessary in order to clear space for the ongoing tissue synthesis that would otherwise be physically blocked by the undegraded ECM analog (Yannas et al., 1979; Yannas and Burke, 1980).

In addition to the structure of the ECM analog itself, the presence of seeded keratinocytes also has an effect on the delay in half-life for contraction, Δt, as shown by comparing data in the presence of DRT alone ($\Delta t = 18.5 \pm 2.5$ d) and in the presence of DRT seeded with keratinocytes ($\Delta t = 13.5 \pm 1.5$ d) (Table 8.3). Since migratory keratinocytes produce collagenase (Woodley et al., 1986), it could be speculated, according to the hypothesis described above, that the keratinocyte-seeded defect provides for a higher concentration of collagenase than the unseeded one, presumably leading to faster DRT degradation and a corresponding drop to its contraction-delaying activity.

The hypothetical mechanism presented above suggests the existence of a simple relation between the persistence of the contraction process during spontaneous healing and the persistence of the DRT in a state that is consistent with inactivation of contractile cells. In the guinea pig, contraction of the dermal edges of the ungrafted defect was arrested at about 35 to 40 d; in a defect grafted with keratinocyte-free DRT it was 40 to 45 d (Yannas et al., 1989) whereas, in the keratinocyte-seeded DRT, arrest of contraction extended to 35 to 40 d (Yannas, 1981; Yannas et al., 1989).

Reports on the length of persistence of DRT particles inside the dermis-free defect have agreed only approximately. The keratinocyte-seeded DRT was observed to have completely disappeared by 21 d in the guinea pig model (Murphy et al., 1990). However, in a study with the swine model, there was evidence of multinucleated giant cells, the cell type that appears to digest DRT particles, by 35 d (Compton et al., 1998), an observation that indirectly suggested the persistence of DRT particles too small to directly detect at 35 d. Clearly, there is absence of data describing the relation between the size of DRT particles and their ability to support the hypothetical inactivation of contractile cells; for this reason, the sought-for hypothetical relation between the extent of duration of DRT in a nondegraded state and the time for arrest of contraction cannot be further pursued.

10.3.5 Mechanism for Contraction Arrest

We now consider the factors that determine the total length of the contraction process, specifically, the time of contraction arrest, observed to occur at 35 to 40 d in the ungrafted dermis-free defect in the guinea pig (Yannas, 1981). Reference is made to Figure 10.5, where the timing associated with synthesis of tissue components of skin and the onset, as well as arrest, of contraction are indicated based on data primarily from the guinea pig model (Yannas et al., 1989; Murphy et al., 1990) with some data from the swine model (Compton et al., 1998). The three curves in Figure 10.5 represent the contraction kinetics for an ungrafted dermis-free defect, the defect grafted with the cell-free dermis regeneration template (DRT), or the defect grafted with DRT that had been seeded with dissociated, uncultured keratinocytes.

We first consider a hypothetical relation between epidermal confluence and contraction arrest in defects grafted with KC-seeded DRT. We note that partial confluence was observed at 12 d and full confluence by 19 d, whereas contraction was arrested much later (35 to 40 d) (Figure 10.5). The significant difference in timing, at least 16 d, between full confluence and arrest of contraction makes it unlikely that they were directly associated with each other. A similar conclusion was reached with the ungrafted defect (Chapter 9). Furthermore, a continuous basement membrane was observed at 12 d, an event separated from the time of arrest of contraction by at least 23 d. However, in the ungrafted defect there was no evidence that remodeling processes involving hemidesmosomes and sub-basal plates were complete by 23 d (see Chapter 9). Likewise, the process of angiogenesis in the stroma started at about 10 d, far removed from the time of contraction arrest. As discussed in the preceding section, the likelihood that contraction arrest is related to the degradation of DRT cannot be evaluated on the basis of existing data.

Of the major synthetic events that took place inside the defect, the process of intensified synthesis of dermis was demonstrably taking place

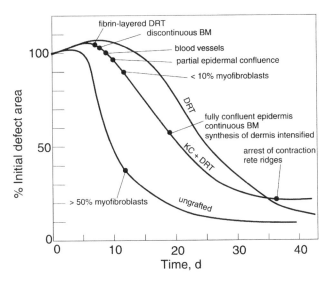

FIGURE 10.5. Kinetics of synthesis of skin tissues up to 40 d. Data shown for three treatments of the dermis-free defect in guinea pig: ungrafted; grafted with keratinocyte-seeded dermis regeneration template (KC + DRT); and KC-free DRT. An opaque, fully confluent epidermis and a continuous basement membrane were both synthesized by 19 d when grafted with the KC + DRT graft. Contraction arrest occurred at 35 to 40 d, roughly coinciding with the last stages of synthesis of dermis and rete ridges.

during the period when contraction was arrested. As reported above, synthesis of dermis started at about 14 to 19 d and became intensified at 19 d; the dermis appeared to have become homogeneous by about 35 d, approximately during the period that contraction was arrested (35 to 40 d).

The discussion of spontaneous healing of skin defects in the preceding chapter led to detailed consideration of two stromal mechanisms that could conceivably account for loss of traction between contractile cells and matrix, eventually leading to arrest of contraction. The first was based on the observed suppression of fibronectin synthesis, a process that hypothetically led to a change in the nature of cell-matrix interactions from "slip to grip." The second was based on the observed reduction in numbers of contractile cells, hypothetically due to loss of contractile phenotype resulting from the presence of newly synthesized collagen (Chapter 9). As with spontaneously healing skin defects, the available evidence cannot distinguish between these two hypothetical processes; nor can the evidence rule out the presence of an interaction between processes taking place in the epithelium and the stroma that hypothetically forces contraction to stop.

10.3.6 Blocking of Scar Synthesis.
Synthesis of the Dermis

The preceding discussion provides a mechanistic explanation for the strong contraction-delaying activity of DRT. In Chapter 8 the quantitative evidence from studies of induced regeneration in skin, peripheral nerves and the conjunctival stroma (Table 8.1) was marshaled to show that scar synthesis was abolished in all cases in which contraction was suppressed using specific ECM analogs and regeneration was induced instead. In spontaneously healing defects collagen fibers appear to be synthesized with their long axes oriented in the plane of the defect (Chapter 9). Suppression of contraction by DRT hypothetically cancelled the tensile field responsible for collagen fiber orientation and induced synthesis of fibers that lacked specific in-plane orientation, as observed in the physiological dermis. If we adhere to the mechanism proposed for the ungrafted defect (Chapter 9), it follows that the absence of scar in skin defects treated with DRT can be fully explained by the contraction-delaying activity of DRT.

Regeneration of the dermis by keratinocyte-free DRT appears, therefore, to depend strongly on a highly selective suppression of contraction. Once that specific inhibitory mechanism is in place, the hypothetical state of plane stress does not become established and the dermis is synthesized as a relatively random array of collagen fibers. Synthesis of an epidermis from migratory epithelia originating at the defect edge follows with delay depending on the size of the skin defect (sequential synthesis of dermis and epidermis; see Chapter 5). In contrast, following grafting of keratinocyte-seeded DRT, the dermis and epidermis are synthesized simultaneously. The synthetic processes that yield each of the two major tissues that comprise skin appear to proceed to some extent independently of each other in vivo, as described in detail above. However, the synthesis of rete ridges and associated transition tissues (e.g., anchoring fibrils) requires a specific interaction between epithelial and stromal cells that is not understood well.

10.3.7 Summary: Mechanism of Induced Regeneration of the Dermis

A variety of ECM analogs, differing in structure from dermis regeneration template (DRT) in well-defined respects, were used to obtain evidence that allowed construction of a mechanistic explanation for the regeneration of dermis by DRT in dermis-free skin defects of adults.

The observed reduction in total cell density, including myofibroblast density, in DRT-grafted defects was attributed to the observed blocking of platelet aggregation on the surface of DRT, and to the hypothetically ensuing deficiency in cytokine signaling that normally follows from platelet degranulation in spontaneously healing defects. The delay in onset of contraction observed in DRT-grafted defects was attributed to the observed delay in growth of the cell cluster at the edges of the defect that appears to control initiation of the inward movement of edges. Cluster growth at the edges was delayed following the hypothetical reduction in proliferative signals from cytokines that account for high total cell density in spontaneously healing defects. Myofibroblast depletion was attributed to the hypothetical depletion of signals from cytokines that appear to induce differentiation of fibroblasts in vigorously contracting defects.

The strong delay in contraction half-life that was observed in DRT-grafted defects was attributed to binding of a very large fraction of contractile cells on the surface of the collagen-GAG fibers comprising the DRT scaffold. Binding on DRT appeared to depend strongly on the $\alpha_1\beta_1$ collagen receptor in fibroblasts. The long axes of contractile cells bound on DRT fibers were oriented almost randomly in space, hypothetically preventing these cells from contributing to contraction of the defect. In contrast, a large fraction of contractile cells remained outside the graft and participated actively in contraction when the specific surface of a control ECM analog was not sufficiently high to bind these contractile cells.

DRT was required to persist in the defect as an insoluble (nondiffusible) scaffold over a minimal period (at least 10 d in guinea pig defects) in order to be effective in delaying contraction. It was hypothesized that the required duration of DRT as an insoluble network roughly matched the duration of the peak contractile activity in the defect. There was also an observed requirement for a maximum in the persistence period of DRT in an undegraded state, probably corresponding to the requirement for physical space to be occupied by newly synthesized tissues.

The abolition of scar synthesis observed in contraction-inhibited defects grafted with DRT was attributed to the effective suppression of the tensile field that is hypothetically generated in the plane of contracting defect and leads to the observed synthesis of collagen fibers with high planar orientation that characterizes scar. This hypothesis was consistent with the observation that scar synthesis in skin, peripheral nerve and conjunctival defects was abolished when contraction was suppressed in each case by an appropriate nondiffusible regulator.

The regenerative activity of DRT depends on its property of selectively blocking contraction by inhibiting the proliferation and contractile activity of fibroblasts without impairing other major processes that contribute to healing of a defect. Keratinocyte-free DRT induces synthesis of a dermis by blocking contractile forces; however, synthesis of an epidermis by migratory epithelia from the defect edges follows with delay. In contrast, keratinocyte-seeded DRT induces simultaneous synthesis of a dermis and an epidermis.

10.4 Kinetics of Synthesis of Peripheral Nerves

As with the discussion on skin, presented above, an account of the kinetics and mechanism of peripheral nerve synthesis will be based on an irreducible reaction diagram from Chapter 7. The simplest protocol used in the synthesis of a nerve trunk was reaction diagragm N19 (Table 7.2). In this widely used protocol, the two stumps of the transected nerve were inserted in a tube based on each of a variety of materials, including synthetic polymers and collagen. Use of fillings inside tubes was an alternative strategy that was employed (Dg. N20 in Table 7.2). Based on tabulated values of the length shift, ΔL, an objective measure of regenerative activity in the tubulated model (Chapter 6), tubes based either on a lactic acid homopolymer or one of the lactic acid copolymers, as well as tubes based on collagen tubes, clearly showed superior regenerative activity to that of the silicone tube that was used as a standard in this compilation (Tables 6.1, 6.2, and 6.3).

In spite of the typically superior regenerative activity of tubes made from certain materials other than silicone, especially those filled with oriented substrates, the published record of tubulation with silicone without an active filling is much more extensive than with any other single type of tubulated configuration. Only the silicone tube data obtained across a 10-mm gap provide the appropriate level of detail for a kinetic account. The discussion of the kinetics of induced peripheral nerve regeneration will therefore be based on several accounts, all focused on use of the unfilled silicone tube as a bridge across a gap of 10 mm in the transected rat sciatic nerve (Lundborg et al., 1982a; Longo et al., 1983a; Williams et al., 1983; Williams and Varon, 1985; Fields and Ellisman, 1986a,b; Williams, 1987; Le Beau et al., 1988; Fields et al., 1989; Danielsen, 1990; Azzam et al., 1991; Chamberlain et al., 1988b, 2000a; Chamberlain, 1998). Other studies, conducted under apparently identical conditions but at different gap lengths (Jenq and Coggeshall, 1984, 1985b; Scaravilli, 1984; Williams et al., 1987) or using a plastic film wrapping rather than a silicone tube (Scaravilli, 1984), have also been included in the ensuing discussion. A few remarks concerning the superior regenerative activity of tubes based on collagen and certain synthetic polymers over silicone appear at the end of this account.

10.4.1 Synthesis of Regenerative Tissues: Nerve Fibers

Prior to implantation, the silicone tubes, virtually impermeable to liquids, had an inside diameter of 1.2 to 1.5 mm and a wall thickness of about 0.25 mm. The stumps of the transected rat sciatic nerve were typically inserted about 5 mm each into each tube end and were sutured in place, leaving a gap of 10 ± 1 mm between the stumps that was occasionally filled with phosphate buffered saline (PBS). Relative to an initially unfilled tube, the regenerative activity of PBS is nearly insignificant. The gap distance employed in these studies, about 10 mm, is equal to the critical axon elongation for the silicone tube configuration (see Chapter 6).

In the discussion below, the gap was divided into 9 segments (S), each 1 mm long, and the spatial location of a morphological feature along the gap length was indicated by the numbers S1 to S9, S1 being the segment

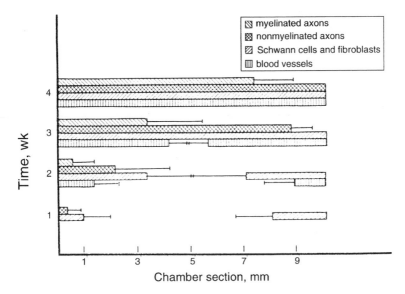

FIGURE 10.6. Kinetics of migration of axons and of nonneuronal cells of different types inside a 10-mm gap in the rat sciatic nerve bridged with a silicone tube. Schwann cells and fibroblasts led the way inside the gap, followed by nonmyelinated axons, blood vessels, and myelinated axons, in that order. (Copyright 1983. Wiley-Liss, Inc. From Williams et al., 1983. Spatial-temporal progress of peripheral nerve regeneration within a silicone chamber: Parameters for a bioassay. *Journal of Comparative Neurology* 218:460–470. Reprinted with permission of Wiley-Liss, Inc., a subsidiary of John Wiley & Sons, Inc.)

closest to the proximal stump (Williams et al., 1983). At given points in time, advancing cells of a given type, or elongating axons, comprised a "front" inside the gap, with the fastest cells of a given type located about two segments ahead of the slowest ones (Figure 10.6). Time points given below apply only to the 10-mm gap configuration. Tissues inside the chamber will be referred to as "cable," in order to distinguish them from relatively intact (uninjured) tissues in the regenerating stumps.

Connection of Stumps by a Fibrin Cable (7 d)

Following implantation, there was accumulation of a dark, yellow fluid, containing few red blood cells, at each end of the tubulated gap (chamber). The fluid fronts advanced toward each other, eventually filling the chamber by 9 to 12 h. The fluid was endoneurial in origin; it was hypertonic (Myers et al., 1983) and included the cytokines PDGF, aFGF, and NGF. At 7 d, the fluid had become yellowish brown; at 14 d, it became clear.

By 7 d, a cable had formed inside the chamber, immersed in the chamber fluid and connecting the two stumps. The cable diameter decreased toward the center of the gap, reaching a minimum about 7 mm away from the proximal stump; the diameter averaged about 0.4 mm, about one-third the internal diameter of the silicone tube. At 7 d, the cable was translucent; at 14 d, surface blood vessels were observed on its surface; eventually, it became opaque. The cable comprised primarily longitudinally oriented fibrin fibers; fibronectin was also present. Red blood cells were observed inside the cable; in addition, fibroblasts and Schwann cells were observed in the most proximal and most distal segments of the chamber (S1 and S9), indicating that both stumps were sources of these cells. Very few nonmyelinated axons were observed in S1.

Synthesis of Basement Membrane (14 d)

Schwann cells and fibroblasts, advancing from both stumps, were observed between S1 and S3 as well as between S7 and S9, but not in the center of the gap. Nonmyelinated axons were present only between S1 and S2, and were observed at different stages of the regenerative process, ranging from the presence of growth cones together with myelinated and nonmyelinated axons at S1 to growth cones with few nonmyelinated and no myelinated axons in S2. Nonmyelinated axons and growth cones were engulfed in Schwann cells. The latter were encased in an uninterrupted basement membrane that followed the irregularities of the axon-Schwann cell complexes and extended into deep indentations in the Schwann cell surface.

Myelinated axons were generally very thin, with a maximum diameter of 5 to 6 μm, and were surrounded by a thin myelin sheath. The axoplasm contained abundant filaments, 10 nm thick, aligned with their axes mostly parallel to the axon direction; particularly in larger axons, however, filament bundles that were oriented at an angle or even transversely were also observed.

Myelin Synthesis Across Entire Gap (32 to 34 d)

Comparison of the segments at both ends of the cable showed that myelination was well advanced in the proximal segments (S1–S2) before any axons had reached the distal side of the cable. This observation supported the conclusion that myelination is independent of contact of the axon with its target.

The gap length had been traversed by nonmyelinated axons elongating from the proximal stump by 23 to 25 d; myelinated axons had reached S5 at that time. Myelinated axons were observed at the distal end of the gap at an estimated 32 to 34 d, suggesting a delay of about 7 to 9 d for early observation of the myelin sheath on an elongating axon. The thickness of the myelin sheath was not uniform along the length of the gap; it was thicker near the proximal end, suggesting an ongoing axon maturation process.

Long-term data showed that regenerated axons did not achieve the morphological features of uninjured axons, even at 400 d. The total number of myelinated axons in the proximal nerve stump rapidly increased during the first 100 d, exceeding normal values, and remained approximately constant after that time. The thickness of the myelin sheath was slightly but significantly thinner compared with normal axons of the same diameter. Regenerated axons were clearly smaller and remained so (e.g., by 200 d, the average diameter of a regenerated axon was $2.6 \pm 0.2 \mu m$, compared with $8.5 \pm 0.2 \mu m$ for the uninjured control). Especially noticeable was the absence of axons greater than $7 \mu m$, even after a year of recovery; in contrast, uninjured nerves contain many axons as large as $9 \mu m$. Small axon diameters were reflected in low values of conduction velocity; values of 35 to 40 m/s, about 60% normal, were observed even after 300 d. The amplitude of the conducted signal was about 10% normal (Table 6.3).

10.4.2 Evidence for Synthesis of an Endoneurium and a Perineurium

We complete the kinetic description of synthesis of nerve trunk inside a silicone tube by focusing on nonneuronal cells and the synthesis of ECM.

Formation of Concentric Tissue Layers at the Perimeter
of the Trunk (14 d)

Several layers of elongated, concentrically arranged cells had formed at 14 d, at the perimeter of both stumps. These cells lacked a basement membrane and intercellular tight junctions at all times of observation and were not, therefore, candidates for classification as perineurial cells. Use of anti-α-smooth muscle actin showed that they were myofibroblasts. The thickness of the capsule, about $45 \mu m$, corresponding to 15 to 20 cell layers, remained unchanged at the three times it was observed, that is, 6, 30, and 60 wk (420 d). The morphology of the capsule was similar to that observed around capped stumps (neuromata) following untubulated healing.

Synthesis of Endoneurial Collagen Fibrils (14 to 18 d)

At 14 d, bundles of longitudinally oriented collagen fibrils were observed in the spaces between cells at the most distal part of the cable. Abundant collagen fibrils were observed in the space surrounding axon-Schwann cell complexes by 16 to 18 d at different segments of the cable. Collagen fibrils, with diameters of about 40 nm, were oriented with their axes approximately parallel to the growing axons. These diameters were similar to those observed in the absence of tubulation and were smaller than the diameters of collagen fibrils, averaging close to 50 nm, observed in normal endoneurium.

By 30 to 40 d, abundant collagen fibrils with highly variable diameters were present both inside and outside the perineurium (see below); fibrils outside the perineurium were observed to have higher diameters. (Data on fibril diameters were typically not reported by authors.)

Formation of Minifascicles (16 d)

By 16 d, numerous minifascicles with axons were observed between S1 and S6; fewer were observed in S8 and S9. Minifascicles, each containing 5 to 10 myelinated axons and several unmyelinated axons in a cross section, had diameters in the range 5 to 20 µm and were eventually surrounded by a perineurial sheath (see below). They were more numerous, and contained fewer axons, at the periphery of the nerve trunk than those located near the center.

Vascularization of Regenerated Nerve Trunk (21 d)

At 14 d, blood vessels were observed only at S1 and S9; however, by 21 d, vasculature was observed along the entire chamber length. Permeability data obtained at 182 d were consistent with presence of blood vessels between the perineurium (see below) and the trunk perimeter; however, blood vessels originating in this space were excluded from the immediate surroundings of the axons by the perineurial sheaths. No blood vessels were detected in the endoneurium.

Synthesis of a Perineurium (reported between 16 and 182 d)

By 20 d, each minifascicle was surrounded by cells that resembled perineurial cells. The cells were thin and had formed distinct layers while their cytoplasm contained very few pinocytotic vesicles. The thin processes of these cells were in contact with one another at their edges by means of tight junctions (zonulae occludentes). Very few collagen fibrils were present between cell layers; in contrast, the space on either side of the multilaminated structure was relatively richly appointed with fibrils. Although basement membrane covered wide areas of the cell surfaces, both on the endoneurial and perineurial side, encasement of perineurial cells in membrane was incomplete (see detailed description of perineurium in Chapter 6). A permeability study, conducted at 28 d, showed that the tissue lacked the barrier properties of a physiological perineurium.

Covering of perineurial cells by basement membrane was virtually complete by 30 d and abundant collagen fibrils were observed inside the cell layers. The cytoplasm of perineurial cells contained numerous pinocytotic vesicles.

By 182 d, the cells surrounding the minifacicles had all the features characteristic of mature perineurial cells; they were highly elongated, contained many vesicles, included collagen fibrils between cell layers, and were ensheathed on both sides with continuous basement membrane. Furthermore, the circular, multilaminated structure that they formed had the permeability barrier property of normal perineurium even when the sheaths were occasionally only one or two cell layers deep. In contrast, there was no endoneurial vasculature and, therefore, no endoneurial permeability barrier.

10.5 Mechanism of Peripheral Nerve Regeneration

In a review of the evidence for the mechanism of nerve regeneration across tubulated gaps we will emphasize the healing response of the transected organ that eventually leads to wound closure. Spontaneous (unaided) closure can be accomplished either by reconnection of the two stumps that have been kept close together after transection or, if the stumps have been separated by a sufficiently long gap, by individual closure of each stump.

Conclusions on the regenerative activity of several experimental configurations obtained with the rat sciatic nerve were generally in good agreement with conclusions reached based on the mouse model (Chapter 6). The discussion below will be limited largely to data from the rat sciatic nerve.

10.5.1 Length and Diameter of Regenerated Nerve Trunk

In studies of nerve regeneration across a tubulated gap it has been observed that a continuous nerve trunk has formed across the gap, reconnecting the two stumps, provided that the gap length was equal to or less than the critical axon elongation length, L_c, a characteristic of a specific experimental configuration. The definition of L_c is based on previously established findings of a "critical gap length" (Lundborg et al., 1982a) and emphasizes the fact that it is based on assays related to axons rather than on assays based on noregenerative tissues, such as the endoneurium. The procedure for estimating values of L_c standardizes the concept of the critical gap length, providing a self-consistent method for comparing the regenerative activity of a large variety of tubulated configurations. Values of L_c for various configurations have been tabulated in Chapter 6 (Table 6.1). Very low values of L_c, indicative of very poor regeneration, were observed when the distal stump had not been inserted inside the tube (Lundborg et al., 1982a; Williams et al., 1984), when the distal tube end had been ligated (Williams et al., 1984) or when use of the tube itself was entirely omitted (Chamberlain et al., 2000a).

Across a 10-mm gap in the silicone tube a cable formed in about 7 d inside the exudate that had filled the chamber (Williams et al., 1987). The cable resulted from polymerization of fibrinogen in the fluid, yielding fibrin fibers that were longitudinally oriented (Williams et al., 1983). Initially, the cable was acellular and comprised longitudinally oriented fibrin fibers, as well as fibronectin, the result of coagulation of exudate inside the tube (Williams and Varon, 1985). In the ensuing few weeks, the fibrin core was replaced by Schwann cells, fibroblasts, endothelial cells, and myelinated axons; the cable eventually became remodeled into a regenerated trunk that conducted electrical signals. Although a decrease in cable diameter was observed after 1 wk, the diameter remained approximately constant between 2 and 4 wk, as the acellular cable was being transformed into a nerve trunk (Williams et al., 1983; Williams and Varon, 1985).

Using a series of chambers with increasing volume, and allowing them to be filled up with exudate, it was shown that the diameter of the cable regularly increased with the total volume of exudate, suggesting that the polymerization process generated a mass of cable that increased with the total mass of fibrinogen available in the chamber (Williams and Varon, 1985). In a 10-mm chamber, large enough to be filled by exudate within 1 to 2 d, a dense and homogenous fibrin cable had formed inside (Williams and Varon, 1985; Williams, 1987); however, when the chamber length was increased to 15 mm, only a very thin cable connected the two stumps and, in several cases, no cable had formed across the gap (Williams et al., 1987). This and related results showed that the diameter of the cable was limited by the total volume of exudate flowing out of both stumps. Since the diameter of the cable determined the eventual diameter of the nerve trunk, the clear implication from the data is that a process that limits the total volume of exudate also limits the diameter of the nerve trunk that forms between the stumps.

The diameter of the regenerated trunk, measured at the center of the regenerated trunk (former gap center) at 8 wk following transection, was observed to decrease regularly as the initially established tubulated gap length increased from 0 mm (nerve transection followed by tubulation but without formation of a significant gap) to 4 and 8 mm (Jenq and Coggeshall, 1985a) (Figure 10.7). Tube composition had a strong effect on the diameter of the nerve trunk, measured at the center of the regenerated gap at 30 wk; it was observed to be 0.54 ± 0.15 mm for silicone tubes and 1.30 ± 0.05 mm for collagen tubes (Chamberlain et al., 2000a).

10.5.2 Contractile Cell Capsule Around Stumps and Regenerated Nerve Trunk

In a large number of studies of nerve regeneration across tubulated gaps it was observed microscopically that the regenerated nerve trunk was ensheathed at its periphery in a thick circumferential sheath of connective tissue comprising cells that resembled fibroblasts. The sheath was commonly observed in nerve trunks regenerated across a variety of gap lengths; however, most reports refer to a gap of 10 mm in silicone tubes with or without a filling (Lundborg et al., 1982a, Williams et al., 1983; Jenq and Coggeshall, 1985a,b; Williams and Varon, 1985; Hurtado et al., 1987; Yannas et al., 1987a; Madison et al., 1988; Fields et al., 1989; Azzam et al., 1991; Itoh et al., 1999; Chamberlain et al., 2000a). The sheath layer was almost absent when a porous collagen tube was used either with or without filling consisting of an oriented substrate (Chamberlain et al., 2000a).

The thickness of the sheath surrounding the nerve trunk inside the silicone tubes was observed to be $51 \pm 25\,\mu m$ and was continuous around the entire length of the regenerated cable; it comprised about 15 to 20 contractile cell layers. In contrast, the sheath surrounding the trunk regenerated inside the collagen tube comprised only a single cell layer, about 3 μm thick; this cell layer was not continuous around the entire length of the trunk (Chamberlain et al., 2000a). In several other studies, the sheath thickness was not directly reported but could be estimated from the published microphotographs; with silicone tubes, it was typically in the range 35 to 50 μm (Williams et al., 1983; Jenq and Coggeshall, 1985a,b; Fields et al., 1989).

Viewed in cross section, several circumferential tissue layers appeared to be indented or wrinkled at several locations around the circumferential sheath inside a silicone tube (Jenq and Coggeshall, 1985a; Madison et al., 1988; Hoppen et al., 1990; Azzam et al., 1991; Itoh et al., 1999; Chamberlain et al., 2000a); however, indentations were absent in the sheath present inside the collagen tube (Chamberlain, 1998). The cross-sectional area of the regenerated trunk bounded by the sheath was circular whereas the cross section of the uninjured rat sciatic nerve, used as internal control, was elliptical (Jenq and Coggeshall, 1985a) (Figure 10.7a). In one study, the silicone tube was removed after 4 wk of tubulation and the nerve trunks were reinserted in the appropriate anatomical site; when these nerve trunks were examined at 26 wk, the circumferential sheath was entirely absent (Azzam et al., 1991).

The nature of cells in the outer sheath was suggested from the observation that the cells stained positively for α-smooth muscle actin (Figures 4.5 and 4.6), as well as showing evidence of densely bundled microfilaments and specialized cell-matrix connections (Chamberlain et al., 1998a, 2000a). Cells with this type of immunohistochemical response and ultrastructural morphology have been referred to as myofibroblasts (i.e., fibroblasts that have expressed the contractile phenotype) (Desmoulière and Gabbiani, 1996; Masur et al., 1996; Gabbiani, 1998). Previously, filaments were reported in perineurial cells in the uninjured mouse sciatic nerve that were similar to those observed in smooth muscle (Ross and Reith, 1969). Also, myofibroblasts have been identified in human neuroma; they were observed to increase in number during the period from 2 to 6 months following injury and to decrease thereafter (Badalamente et al., 1985). The role of myofibroblasts in contractile closure (capping) of neuroma in untubulated transected nerves has been described in detail (see Chapter 9) (Chamberlain et al., 2000a). The myofibroblast layer was not limited around the regenerated nerve trunk; a particularly thick sheath of myofibroblasts was observed around both proximal and distal stumps of a transected nerve with a silicone tube (Figure 4.6). The concentric sheath of myofibroblasts was therefore observed to extend through the entire tubulated chamber, that is, it extended from the proximal stump (stump sheath) along the regenerated nerve trunk (trunk sheath) and also surrounded the distal stump.

The large difference in numbers of contractile cells observed in tissues that are in contact with tubes made of silicone and collagen has been frequently observed with various implants based on these biomaterials. Following implantation of a material that is not biodegradable or porous, the tissues in contact with the implant have synthesized a capsule of contrac-

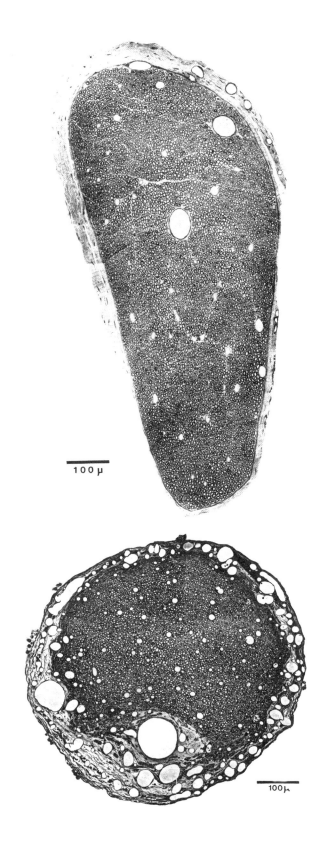

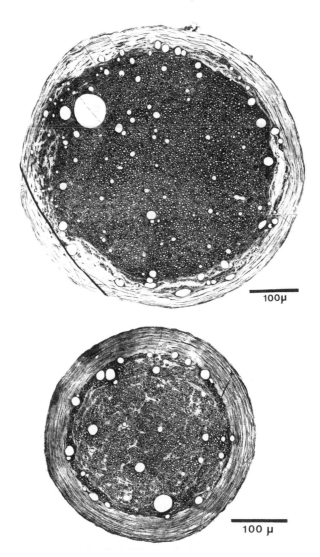

FIGURE 10.7. Cross sections of a normal nerve and of nerve trunks regenerated across gaps of different length 8 wk after transection and bridging with a silicone tube. Myelinated axons appear as very small open circles. Blood vessels appear as large open circles. *Top left*: Normal rat sciatic nerve. *Bottom left*: Nerve trunk regenerated across a 0-mm gap (stumps were opposed after transection). *Top right*: Regenerated across a 4-mm gap. *Bottom right*: Regenerated across an 8-mm gap. The trunk diameter significantly decreased as the gap length increased. Bar: 100 μm. (Reprinted from Jenq and Coggeshall, 1985a. Numbers of regenerating axons in parent and tributary peripheral nerves in the rat. *Brain Research* 326:29–33, Copyright 1985, with permission from Elsevier Science.)

tile cells and connective tissue that has chronically constrained the implant. Silicone implants (e.g., breast implants) are well-known examples of such a chronic response; it has been described in detail by several authors (Rudolph et al., 1978; Ginsbach et al., 1979; Brodsky and Ramshaw, 1994; Tarpila et al., 1997). Even a subcutaneous collagen implant that was non-degradable and nonporous has been shown to develop a capsule of con-tractile cells adjacent to it whereas the degradable and porous control did not (Yannas, 1981).

Not only inside the silicone tube bridging the nerve gap, but outside it as well, a thick capsule of contractile cells has been observed. The porous col-lagen tube developed no such sheath on its outside surface; instead, it was observed that contractile cells had migrated inside the pores in the colla-gen tube wall, where the axes of many cells had assumed an approximately circumferential orientation (Chamberlain, 1998; Chamberlain et al., 1998a, 2000a). Nevertheless, following removal of an implant from its capsule, tissue remodeling generally ensued and the residual contractile capsule gradually disappeared, as was observed when the silicone tube bridging the nerve stumps was removed after four weeks of implantation (Azzam et al., 1991).

Having reviewed the macroscopic experimental configurations (tubu-lated models) that led to induced regeneration as well as the evidence for the presence of contractile cells in the healing stumps, we wish to identify a mechanism that explains these data.

10.5.3 The Pressure Cuff Hypothesis

In Chapters 4 and 9 we reviewed the evidence that contractile cells stain-ing positively for α-smooth muscle actin (myofibroblasts) are present in the transected stump, arranged with their long axes aligned circumferen-tially around the stump perimeter, as well as in axial configuration inside the nerve trunk, aligned in parallel to the nerve axis. It was hypothesized that spontaneous closure of a stump results from a balance of three forces: the circumferential contractile force that restricts the stump perimeter at the transected face and leads to stump closure unless opposed; the axial contractile force that restricts the length of the stump along the nerve axis and also leads to stump closure; and lastly, the intrafascicular pressure that opposes the previous two forces and, if not adequately blocked, leads to outflow of exudate from the intrafascicular space (endoneurial fluid). A preliminary statement of this hypothesis has appeared (Chamberlain et al., 2000a).

It follows from the above that neuroma formation is the result of stump closure occurring when the circumferential and axial forces pulling tissues inside and away from the plane of transection at each stump overcome the force that causes outflow of endoneurial fluid. Neuroma can be hypotheti-cally prevented, therefore, if an experimental configuration can suppress formation of the two contractile forces. It has been shown that formation of a contractile capsule is partly suppressed by inserting the stumps inside a silicone tube, or even entirely blocked by use of a collagen tube; under these conditions, endoneurial fluid flows in spite of the continuing presence of the axial contractile force (Chamberlain et al., 2000a). This observation suggests that, in certain experimental configurations, the circumferential force plays a dominant role in spontaneous closure of a transected nerve.

Provided that the axial contractile force can be neglected during healing of a transected nerve, the extent of regeneration depends, according to the hypothesis presented above, entirely on the balance between the circumferential contractile force and the force of outflow of intrafascicular fluid. This simple "pressure cuff" hypothesis appears to explain certain features of the characteristic morphology of the regenerated nerve trunk as well as the existence of a critical gap length (critical axon elongation, L_c) that characterizes certain tubulated configurations, as described below.

10.5.4 Dependence of L_c on Macroscopic Experimental Configurations

In a preceding section the data showed that the cable diameter, and eventually the diameter of the resulting nerve trunk, were limited by the total volume of exudate flowing out of both stumps. It follows from these data that a restriction in the flow of exudate should lead to a nerve trunk with diminished diameter. Such a restriction could originate at the face of the transected stump, most probably at the opening in intrafascicular (endoneurial) space from which the exudate was presumably flowing out.

It follows from the pressure cuff hypothesis that a decrease in intrafascicular opening in an experimental series, resulting from an increase in hoop stress acting on the stumps, should restrict the flow of total exudate from the stumps, and should limit the nerve trunk diameter. If the restriction further increased, the cable diameter should become very thin; and, if the restriction led to a sufficiently low level of the flow, the flow of intrafascicular fluid should be arrested before the fluid extruded from each stump has had the opportunity to connect with its counterpart across the gap. In a related experimental series, in which the hoop stress acting on the stumps remained unchanged while the gap length was progressively being increased, one should eventually expect to observe the same loss in cable (or nerve trunk) continuity to occur when the gap became sufficiently long. Irrespective of whether the cable had become discontinuous because of increased flow restriction (increased hoop stress acting on stumps) or increased distance required for connection (increased gap length between stumps), the hypothesis predicts that, in either case, the length of the nerve trunk regenerated in the experiment, should reach a maximum. The maximum length regenerated by each stump is about one-half the critical axon elongation, L_c.

This qualitative hypothesis for the existence and magnitude of L_c can be tested by finding out whether it describes the observed differences in morphological features of the nerve trunk in a series of experimental configurations that are closely related. When only the composition of the tube is varied (e.g., change from silicone to collagen) without changing the gap length, the hypothesis predicts that the tube that restricts flow of exudate less should yield a trunk with a larger diameter. As described above, a thick concentric sheath of myofibroblasts was observed at each stump after the latter had been inserted in a silicone tube (Figure 4.6). In contrast, only a very thin concentric sheath of myofibroblasts was observed around stumps inserted inside collagen tubes (data not shown here) or around the nerve trunk regenerated inside collagen tubes. If we make the reasonable assumption that the hoop stress deforming the stump increases with the thickness of the stump sheath, it clearly follows that the hoop stress inside the silicone tube was higher, leading to a thinner trunk, as observed (Chamberlain et al., 2000a). Taking the L_c values for silicone tubes, 9.7 mm, and for collagen tubes, ≥ 13.4 mm (Table 6.1), we observe that the model accounts for the lower critical axon elongation observed with silicone tubes. The pressure cuff model interprets rather simply, although qualitatively, the substantial increase of a critical gap length (critical axon elongation, L_c) in this example.

In a different experimental series, the hypothesis predicts that, when all other experimental parameters are maintained constant, a gradual increase in gap length should lead to an increasingly smaller volume of exudate and, therefore, to an increasingly thinner cable, as observed with silicone tubes of increasing gap length (Figure 10.7) (Jenq and Coggeshall, 1985a). Furthermore, when the distal stump has not been inserted (Lundborg et al., 1982a; Williams et al., 1984), or when the tube end has been ligated (Williams et al., 1984), the value of L_c is expected to significantly decrease due to cancellation of distal stump contribution to the total flow of directed, although confined, exudate, as observed (Table 6.1). Omission of the tube totally prevents formation of a stream of confined exudate and is accordingly expected to lead to a very significant reduction in L_c, as is also observed (Table 6.2).

Further use of the pressure cuff model can provide a qualitative explanation of the observation of a circular cross section for trunks regenerated inside silicone tubes, compared with the elliptical cross section of the normal control (Figure 10.7). A symmetrical force field is generated around the circular cuff acting around the nerve trunk due to the presence of the circumferential sheath of contractile cells; these forces are absent in the normal nerve. Furthermore, this model accounts for the indentations frequently observed in the layers of trunk sheath inside silicone tubes; the indentations probably result from buckling, a mechanical instability observed when a slender beam (Euler column), corresponding to one of the thin connective tissue layers in the sheath, has been loaded above a limiting value (Crandall et al., 1972). In the nerve trunk, connective tissue fibers lying along a circular path are forced, due to compressive forces originating in the sheath, to occupy a circle of shorter diameter; as a result, buckling of fibers occurs around the circumference of the sheath.

The contractile sheath is present both around the entire regenerated nerve trunk (trunk sheath) as well as around the stumps (stump sheath); it follows that both stumps as well as the trunk are subjected to hoop stresses. The question arises whether the observed reduction in nerve trunk diameter inside the silicone tube results entirely from the restriction to flow of exudate by forces originating in the stump sheath or whether it results in part from compressive deformation resulting from hoop stresses directly applied on the previously regenerated nerve by the trunk sheath. The data show that the cable diameter had been established across the entire gap by about 7 d and did not significantly change through the next 4 wk (Williams et al., 1983; Williams and Varon, 1985) (see section 10.4.1). The first waves of fibroblasts migrating along the cable from both stumps were reported to have met near the center at about 14 d, a clear delay of several days from the time when the cable diameter had been established (Williams et al., 1983). These data suggest that myofibroblasts comprising the stump sheath, rather than those in the trunk sheath, are primarily responsible for shaping the cable diameter. One would, however, expect that the observed circular shape of the cross section, together with the hypothetical buckling of fibers inside the sheath, resulted from forces originating in the trunk sheath rather than the stump.

There is insufficient morphological or other information on the concentric cell sheath with which to attempt an explanation of several observations reported in Table 6.1. Prominent among these are the significant regenerative activity shown by tubes fabricated from two synthetic biodegradable polymers, plasticized poly(lactic acid) and a copolymer of lactic acid and ε-caprolactone, and the relative lack of activity observed with a tube based on an ethylene-vinyl acetate copolymer. Other sets of data that cannot be readily explained without additional morphological information include the very high regenerative activity observed when the impermeable silicone tube was replaced with a cell-permeable tube; the significantly higher activity of a cell-permeable compared with a protein-permeable tube wall; or the lack of regenerative activity of a protein-permeable tube compared with an impermeable tube (Table 6.1).

The pressure cuff hypothesis does not appear to be useful in explaining the very significant effect on L_c of several types of tube fillings (Chapter 6; Table 6.1). In one study, it was observed that one of the tube fillings used with the silicone tube, the nerve regeneration template, had a very significant effect on L_c, whereas it had no significant effect on the morphology of the contractile cell sheath (Chamberlain et al., 2000a). Although the data are very limited, they suggest that the pressure cuff hypothesis is generally not applicable to the effects of fillings on L_c.

10.5.5 *Hypothetical Synthesis of Basement Membrane Microtubes*

Although changes in dimensions of the nerve trunk and the relative magnitude of the critical axon elongation can be qualitatively explained in many cases by use of the pressure cuff hypothesis, other facts pertaining to nerve regeneration require use of a different hypothesis, closer to the scale of a cell. In particular, there is need for an additional hypothesis to explain the effects of various tube fillings on the value of L_c. Many of these fillings have shown very high regenerative activity (Table 6.1).

The synthetic events in the fibrin cable that forms inside the tubulated gap present an interesting pattern. It has been observed that the fibrin matrix in the nerve gap is loosely organized during the first week and that cell migration occurs both along its periphery as well as through its interior (Williams et al., 1983). Schwann cells and fibroblasts lead the procession; they are followed in order by nonmyelinated axons, endothelial cells, and myelinated axons (Williams et al., 1983). It has been shown that basement membrane was synthesized around "isolated" Schwann cells (i.e., Schwann cells isolated from axons) inside a silicone chamber that incorporated a collagen matrix bridging a 10-mm gap in the rat sciatic nerve. In this study, axons were excluded from the chamber interior by interposition of Millipore filters at the ends of the tube; use of the filters led to exclusion of axons but allowed entry of exudate from the stumps (Chapter 6) (Ikeda et al., 1989). In another study, the stumps were inserted in a Y-shaped silicone tube configuration in which regeneration could be studied inside a tubulated gap in the absence of axons. It was observed that, following formation of a fibrin cable, Schwann cells migrated into the regenerate and became arranged in longitudinally oriented columns that spanned the 4-mm gap. The experimental protocol did not include a study of the possible synthesis of basement membrane around the Schwann cell columns (Zhao et al., 1992) (Figure 10.8). It is known that Schwann cells can also synthesize basement membrane in the absence of neurons in culture (Chapter 7) (Obremski et al., 1993).

The combined data lead to the conclusion that Schwann cells migrating inside the fibrin cable are capable of assembling to form long columns, longitudinally oriented toward the nerve axis, as well as synthesizing basement membrane, even though nonmyelinated axons may not be present. The spontaneous synthesis of basement membrane by Schwann cells is analogous to that occurring during reepithelialization of a skin defect. The essential difference between these processes in the two organs is that keratinocytes synthesize an approximately two-dimensional sheet whereas Schwann cells synthesize cylindrical sheets of basement membrane.

Accordingly, it is hypothesized that a sequence of Schwann cells, migrating along the fibrin fibers inside the cable, spontaneously synthesize long segments of cylindrical tubes of basement membrane along the cable axis; and that nonmyelinated axons eventually enter these cylinders from the

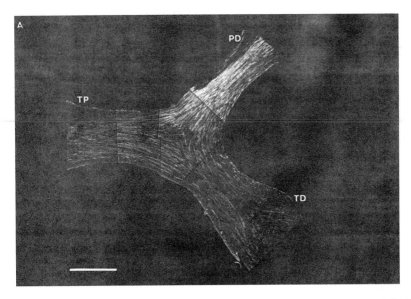

FIGURE 10.8. Longitudinally oriented columns of Schwann cells formed inside regenerated trunk in the absence of axons. An isolated segment of rat nerve was used as a proximal insert (TP, proximal tibial fascicle) into a Y-shaped silicone chamber; the distal tibial fascicle (TD) and the distal peroneal fascicle (PD) were used as distal inserts. A 4-mm gap was left between the proximal and distal inserts. In this preparation, columns of Schwann cells are visible as longitudinally oriented white lines. Bar: 1mm. (Reprinted from Zhao et al., 1992. The formation of a "pseudo-nerve" in silicone chambers in the absence of regenerating axons. *Brain Research* 592:109, Copyright 1992, with permission from Elsevier Science.)

proximal stump, elongate, and become myelinated inside them. There is insufficient information on which to base an estimate of the average length of these BM cylinders; data on formation of longitudinally oriented columns of Schwann cells along distances of a few mm (Zhao et al., 1992), however, suggest that they could reach lengths comparable to the gap length separating the stumps in some experimental configurations. Furthermore, to the extent, that the structure of a BM cylinder approximated that of endoneurial tubes (endoneurial sheaths) observed in the spontaneously healed distal stump (Chapter 9), their diameter would approach 10 to 20 μm and their structure would be very similar to that of a myelin-free basement membrane. In view of their anticipated diameter in the region of several microns, these hypothetical cylinders will be referred to below as "BM microtubes."

There is considerable evidence that empty endoneurial tubes, commonly present in the distal stump following spontaneous healing, support axon elongation and myelination (Fu and Gordon, 1997). Accordingly, it is suggested that the hypothetical BM microtubes described above somewhat resemble the endoneurial tubes observed in the distal stump in diameter and regenerative activity.

What are the substrate preferences of Schwann cells that migrate inside a cable spanning the distance between the stumps, especially those preferences that facilitate the synthesis of BM mictotubes lengthy enough to bridge a long gap? The collective data from the use of insoluble matrices (nondiffusible regulators) suggest strongly that certain structural features enhance significantly axon elongation and myelination across a gap (Table 6.1). These preferences can be summed up as the early availability of the substrate (24 h or less after tubulation), high specific surface, high orientation and a modest degradation rate (Chapter 6). The combined structural features of these highly regenerative surfaces suggest that they perform as a degradable surface for deposition of fibrin/fibrinogen fibers with high axial orientation; and that, eventually, Schwann cells migrate along these oriented channels and synthesize BM microtubes that are later occupied by elongating axons.

10.5.6 Substrate Preferences of Schwann Cells and Elongating Axons

The hypothesis stated above predicts that an experimental configuration that enhances synthesis of BM microtubes by Schwann cells, is capable of enhancing elongation of myelinated axons along the length of the cable, eventually leading to relatively large values of L_c. The hypothesis further suggests that an experimental configuration that promotes synthesis of BM microtubes by Schwann cells in a very large number (thousands) of independent locations inside the cable cross section, rather than in a few locations, should eventually lead to a nerve trunk characterized by relatively higher values of axon density (number of axons per cross-section area of nerve trunk). Predictions from this hypothesis will be compared below with relevant values of L_c and the shift length ΔL; the latter allows comparison of the critical axon elongation of a device with that for the standard silicone tube (Table 6.1). The discussion below will be largely limited to data from the rat sciatic nerve; the latter are in good general agreement with data from the mouse model for most tube fillings.

The requirements suggested by the hypothesis described above should be met by an experimental protocol involving supply of the chamber with exogenous Schwann cell suspensions, thereby adding a further source of migratory Schwann cells. The result of addition of Schwann cells is reflected in the high value of L_c or the shift length, ΔL, as shown in Table 6.1 (Ansselin et al., 1997). Supply of solutions of bFGF and aFGF, both known as very active mitogens and inducers of migratory behavior of Schwann cells in vitro (Krikorian et al., 1982; Burgess and Maciag, 1989), should induce an increase in density of Schwann cells migrating toward the gap center. The observed role of these added cytokines is reflected in significant to very significant values of the regenerative activity of such preparations in Table 6.1 (Aebischer et al., 1989; Walter et al., 1993). Schwann cells have been shown to start synthesizing NGF after losing axonal contact and to interrupt the synthesis once axonal contact has been reestablished (Taniuchi et al., 1986, 1988); however, the available data suggest that NGF shows much smaller regenerative activity than either aFGF or bFGF in the tubulated configuration (Table 6.1).

Gels based on fibronectin or laminin, prepared without allowance for orientation of macromolecular constituents prior to implantation, did not have significant regenerative activity (Table 6.1). It is speculated that gel formation in vivo traps either fibrinogen, the monomer of fibrin, or fibrin polymer in a relatively isotropic, semisolid medium, possibly erasing the orientation inside the fibrin cable. In contrast, a very high regenerative activity was observed when a highly oriented fibrin matrix, rather than an unoriented one, was established inside the gap; or when the oriented fibrin matrix was established in 24 h rather than in several days (Table 6.1) (Williams, 1987; Williams et al., 1987). Furthermore, use of six polyamide filaments, diameter 250 μm, also led to a very high value of the regenerative activity (Table 6.1) (Lundborg et al., 1997).

The contribution of specific surface and degradation rate on the regenerative activity of the insoluble substrate can be evaluated by analyzing the data obtained with homologous series of ECM analogs (Table 6.1). In each series, all relevant structural parameters, except one, were kept constant, thereby isolating effects due to the one parameter that was being systematically varied in the series. Filling the silicone tube with a porous collagen-GAG matrix in which the pore channel axes were highly oriented along the nerve axis (axial orientation) led to a very highly significant increase in regenerative activity compared with the same matrix in which the orientation was perpendicular to the nerve axis (radial orientation) (Chang et al., 1990; Chang and Yannas, 1992). A rapidly degrading matrix (nerve regeneration template, NRT; half-life about 6 wk) showed much higher regenerative activity than a matrix that degraded much more slowly (half-life much longer than 6 wk) (Yannas et al., 1988).

Even a collagen-GAG copolymer with randomly oriented pore channel axes, but very high specific surface due to its porosity, showed a much higher regenerative activity than the unfilled silicone tube (Yannas et al., 1985, 1987a). Deliberate modification of the average pore diameter in another series from 300 to 5 μm, corresponding to an approximately 50-fold increase in specific surface with decreasing average pore diameter for the series, led to a significantly closer approach of electrophysiological properties to normal (latency, conduction velocity, and amplitude of conducted signal) (Chang et al., 1990; Yannas et al., 1991; Chang and Yannas, 1992) (Figure 10.9).

The performance of insoluble substrates used as tube fillings generally supports a requirement for a nondiffusible regulator with appropriately high density of specific ligands that persists in an insoluble state for an optimal period.

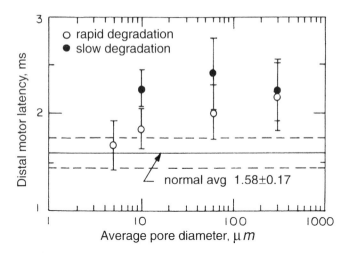

FIGURE 10.9. The fidelity of peripheral nerve regeneration strongly depends on the average pore diameter of the nondiffusible regulator. A 10-mm gap in the rat sciatic nerve was transected and bridged with silicone tubes filled with ECM analogs prepared at various levels of the average pore diameter. Two series of ECM analogs, each at a different level of the degradation rate (rapid degradation, open circles; slow degradation, closed circles), were studied. The latency (time delay for signal to reach the muscle) was measured along the x-axis from the stimulus to the peak (see Figure 6.6) and is an inverse measure of conduction velocity. An average pore diameter in the region 1 to 10 µm led to synthesis of a regenerated trunk with near normal latency. (From Chang and Yannas, 1992.)

10.5.7 Mechanistic Considerations for Synthesis of Nonregenerative Tissues in Nerves

Description of specific conditions for synthesis of an endoneurium, a perineurium, or an epineurium cannot proceed far due to paucity of morphological data available on induced regeneration of these structures. The axonocentric viewpoint that characterizes studies of peripheral nerve regeneration (Chapter 2) deemphasizes assays featuring recovery of nonregenerative tissues.

The persistent presence of a minifascicular structure in regenerated nerves somewhat speculatively suggests the hypothesis that the physically constrained endoneurial space that characterizes these "compartmented" structures (Morris et al., 1972d) prevented formation of an endoneurial vasculature. Suppression of formation of endoneurial vasculature was observed with nerve trunks, characterized by minifascicle morphology, that were regenerated inside silicone tubes (Azzam et al., 1991). The observed compartmentation may have been completed by synthesis of the multilayered perineurial structure around the small pockets of residual endoneurium that may have resulted from contraction of the stump. These hypotheses can be readily tested by observing changes in compartmentation resulting from release of contractile forces; such release can result from the appropriate choice of tube composition, as described above in detail.

10.5.8 Summary of Mechanisms for Nerve Regeneration

Certain tubes used to bridge the transected stumps of a peripheral nerve have regenerative activity and a number of tube fillings also add their own independent regenerative activity.

The regenerative activity of tubulation has been hypothetically explained in terms of its observed effect on the thickness of the sheath of contractile cells (myofibroblasts) that surrounds the nerve stump as well as the regenerated nerve trunk. It was hypothesized that the contractile cell layer exerts circumferential stresses that compress the stump and restrict the flow of exudate from the stumps, thereby interfering with a critical requirement for regeneration of a long nerve trunk. It was speculated that, of the processes required for promotion of axon elongation, the most sensitive to circumferential compression is vascularization of the endoneurial space. This pressure cuff hypothesis explains the existence of a critical axon elongation, L_c, and describes its dependence on tube composition and on other macroscopic experimental configurations.

The activity of tube fillings based on oriented substrates is hypothetically due to a specific interaction between Schwann cells and the surface of the temporarily insoluble regulator. Data on the regenerative activity of several substrates as well as of a family of ECM analogs have been used to investigate the mechanism of regeneration. It is hypothesized that Schwann cells synthesize highly oriented channels of basement membrane (BM microtubes) that, acting as if they were highly elongated endoneurial tubes, facilitate axon regeneration. BM microtube synthesis is facilitated in the presence of oriented substrates coated with fibrin.

Peripheral nerve regeneration along a tubulated gap is described above hypothetically as requiring a two-stage process. In the first, it is necessary to block formation of a capsule of contractile cells that applies circumferential stresses to the healing stumps and restricts the outflow of endoneurial fluid. The second process requires the presence inside the gap of oriented substrates, that become coated with endogenous fibrin and facilitate the synthesis of long, axially oriented basement membrane microtubes by migrating Schwann cells; the resulting dense array of BM microtubes eventually guides large numbers of elongating axons along lengthy gaps.

10.6 Similarities and Differences of Induced Regeneration in Skin and Nerves

Induced regeneration was treated in this volume as the synthesis of tissues and organs at the original anatomical site. Tissues in the adult organ were classified into those that are spontaneously synthesized during healing of wounds (regenerative tissues) and those that are not (nonregenerative). Epithelia (epidermis in skin, myelin sheath in nerve) are regenerative whereas stroma (dermis in skin, endoneurial stroma in nerve) is nonregenerative; a similar classification was applicable in several other organs. The central problem of induced organ regeneration is therefore the discovery of conditions for synthesis of physiological stroma.

A large number of experimental protocols that have induced synthesis of regenerative and nonregenerative tissues in various laboratories were analyzed. The protocols included in this analysis were limited to those that had been investigated in standardized wounds (anatomically well-defined defects) and could, therefore, be relied upon to lead to unambiguous conclusions about the incidence or absence of induced regeneration. Defects were considered subject to closure by one of three modes: contraction, scar synthesis or regeneration. Out of a large variety of independently used protocols, the simplest that led to the desired synthesis of each tissue or organ was selected for a detailed analysis of its mechanism.

The similarities in mechanistic hypotheses for inducing regeneration in skin and peripheral nerves originate in their common response to irreversible injury. Both organs spontaneously respond to injury by recruiting contractile cells that, if not selectively suppressed, drive closure of the defect by contraction and scar synthesis rather than by regeneration. Contraction of skin defects started from a cell cluster at the edge of the defect and later extended across the entire defect area. In peripheral nerves, contraction primarily resulted from the activity of a circumferential sheath of contractile cells. In each organ, the mechanism of defect closure was adapted to the peculiarities of its unique topography.

Synthesis of individual tissues (epithelia or stroma) in an organ required strikingly different approaches. Cells separated from the epithelia of the organ sufficed to synthesize both the epithelia and the associated basement membrane, provided that they were placed in an appropriate culture medium or were implanted in the defect. However, synthesis of the stroma, an essentially nonregenerative tissue, required the presence of one or more nondiffusible (insoluble) regulators with highly specific structure. Partial synthesis of the organ, either skin and peripheral nerve, was accomplished using a pathway that required implantation only of cells that had been dissociated from the epithelia of the organ together with a nondiffusible regulator that possessed a minimal density of specific ligands for contractile cells and an optimal persistence time in the insoluble state.

A major conceptual difference between the two organs derives from the topology of epithelia in each organ: planar in skin and cylindrical in peripheral nerve. During simultaneous synthesis of an epidermis and a dermis, keratinocytes have been observed to condense into islands and cords that are often deeply embedded into the immature, yet emerging, stroma. Eventually, there is a sorting-out process, reminiscent of the spontaneous phase separation of two immiscible liquids, and each tissue finds its physiological anatomical location. In synthesis of a peripheral nerves along a gap, it has been hypothesized that Schwann cells organize themselves into long cylinders that eventually accommodate elongating axons and guide the newly synthesized nerve fibers along the gap. Here, the process of sorting out the epithelia (nerve fibers) from the stroma (endoneurial stroma and perineurium) during regeneration of the nerve trunk has not been studied as extensively as with skin.

It is this spontaneous grasp by epithelial cells of the appropriate topology, planar in skin, cylindrical in nerve, that almost eludes detailed description. Even in the often artificial surroundings of the typical experimental configuration that leads to induced regeneration, migratory epithelia appear to know where to go and what to do once they get there. In often-quoted words (Trinkaus, 1969), "an epithelium will not tolerate a free edge. Accompanying the advance of the free edge and thoroughly integrated with it is a similar advance of the (epithelial) sheet behind it." Is it possible that the newly synthesized stroma (the "free edge") determines the local topology of the new organ? If so, the cells synthesizing the stroma (fibroblasts) must surely receive spatial directions from an appropriate environment; that clearly includes the nondiffusible regulatory required in the synthesis. Examples of such temporarily insoluble regulators that are suitable for coaxing cells to express their "regenerative" phenotype were described in this volume. These thoughts lead me to anticipate that extension of this simple synthetic approach to other organs may soon be possible.

APPENDIX
Method of Estimation of Critical Axon Elongation of an Arbitrary Tubulated Device Bridging Two Nerve Stumps

A.1 Shift in Critical Elongation Relative to the Standard Device

The following discussion is an extension of the treatment in Chapter 6.

If sufficient data were available to construct a complete characteristic curve for every device configuration of interest, a value for the critical axon elongation for each such device, L_c, could be immediately estimated. With the exception of the silicone tube, however, extensive data of the type shown in Figure 6.1 are not available in the literature for different types of devices used in bridging the rat or mouse sciatic nerve. There are, instead, numerous reports in which a group of investigators has reported a single value of % N (frequency of reinnervation) obtained at a given gap length bridged by an arbitrary tubulation device. How can such isolated data points be compared with the standard?

Data from the literature obtained with devices other than the silicone tube can be referred (reduced) to the standard conditions of the silicone tube by making a simple hypothesis: Every tubulated device exhibits a drop in frequency of reinnervation with increase in gap length that is just as sharp as it is for the silicone tube standard; in other words, the characteristic curve of any tubulated device is identical in shape to that for the silicone standard (Figures 6.1 and 6.2). We will refer to it as the hypothesis of "universal shape." If the hypothesis is supported by data, it would follow that a curve with the general shape shown in Figures 6.1 and 6.2 is not an exclusive characteristic of silicone tubes but also characterizes tubes constructed from other materials, as well as tubes filled with solutions of regulators or with insoluble regulators. Comparison of one device with another could then be made with only a minimal amount of information.

There is currently little direct experimental evidence that can be used to test this hypothesis that all characteristic curves of different experimental configurations conform to a universal shape. We recall, however, that data from rat and mouse studies can be fitted to the same S-shaped curve provided that the difference in scale is taken into account (Figure 6.2), suggesting that the basic phenomenon responsible for the drop in % N with gap length may be persistent enough to remain unchanged even by a change in species. Although the evidence is insufficient, in the following we will assume the existence of a universal shape as a working hypothesis.

This hypothesis has a useful consequence. If we accept that all characteristic curves have the same shape, it follows that the length that separates the curves for any two devices is a constant at all values of % N. The distance between the characteristic curves of the nonstandard (test) configuration and the internal control used by the investigator will be referred to as the shift in critical axon elongation, ΔL (length shift). Under this hypothesis, the shape of the characteristic curve for each of these configurations is identical to that for the silicone tube standard, which is known (Figure 6.1). It follows that the length shift between test and control can be deduced by reference to the standard at all values of % N. Let us assume that the gap lengths corresponding to (say) % $N = 30$ for the test configuration, control, and silicone standard are L^t, L^c, and L^s, respectively. The length shift between test and standard is $L^t - L^s$, while that between control and standard is $L^c - L^s$. Accordingly, the length shift between test and control is $L^t - L^s - (L^c - L^s) = L^t - L^c$, clearly independent of the standard. However, if no internal control has been provided in a study, the length shift for the test configuration can be deduced simply by comparison with the standard curve; in this case, it should be made clear that the "control" used is the silicone tube. The shift ΔL will be positive if the test device encourages higher levels of reinnervation frequency than does the internal control (or standard) and negative if it inhibits reinnervation relative to the control.

We now have the basic procedure to generate the entire characteristic curve of a test device from a single data point: We simply draw an S-shaped curve, which includes the data point for the test device and is identical in shape to the standard curve (Figure 6.1). The available reports in the literature are usually in the form of a single observation of % N each for the test device and for an internal control selected by the investigator. By use of the simple construct described above, it is possible to estimate the desired value of critical axon elongation for the nonstandard device, as well as for the internal control by referring both to the standard curve.

Three examples of such a graphical construction are shown below based on data points from the literature of studies on the rat sciatic nerve. In the first example, an isolated observation, located at point A in Figure A.1, corresponded to a value of % N equal to 57.0 (4 successful reinnervations out of 7 trials) at a gap length of 15.0 mm, using a silicone tube filled with dialyzed plasma to bridge the transected nerve. The control, a PBS solution, showed % $N = 14.0$ at the same gap length; it is located at point C in Figure A.1. These observations have been reported in the literature (Williams et al., 1987). The observation represented by point A has coordinates [% N = 57.0, L = 15.0 mm], or briefly represented as [57%, 15.0 mm], and is located clearly to the right of corresponding point B [57%, 9.2 mm] on the standard

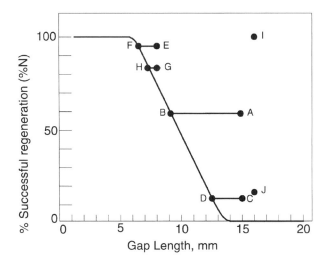

FIGURE A.1. Graphical construction used to describe the procedure for estimating the length shift, ΔL, of an experimental tubulated configuration for nerve regeneration relative to the silicone tube standard. The solid curve passes through data points reported for the silicone tube (Figure 6.1). The significance of the horizontal segments is explained in the text of the Appendix in detail.

curve that is located along the same ordinate, % $N = 57.0$. According to the hypothesis of universal shape, described above, Point A is located on a curve, identical in shape to the standard curve but shifted to the right by the distance AB, equal to the difference between the gap length on the non-standard curve (15.0 mm) and that on the standard curve (9.2 mm). This difference, $15.0 - 9.2 = 5.8$ mm, is the horizontal shift (length shift) between the two curves. It leads to a L_c value for the test device equal to (L_c for standard + length shift between the test and standard curve) = $9.7 + 5.8 = 15.5$ mm. The data point for the investigator's control is represented by point C with coordinates [14.0%, 15.0 mm]; the difference between C and corresponding point D [14.0%, 12.2 mm] on the standard curve (measured along the ordinate % $N = 14.0$) is $15.0 - 12.2 = 2.8$ mm, leading to a L_c value of $9.7 + 2.8 = 12.5$ mm for the control. The length shift that characterizes the difference between the test device and the investigator's control is, therefore, $\Delta L = (L_c$ for test device) $- (L_c$ for internal control) $= 15.5 - 12.5 = 3.0$ mm, a shift toward a longer gap length than the standard. In view of the magnitude of the estimated standard error in measuring L_c, about ± 2 mm, this result suggests significant upregulation of innervation frequency when the silicone tube is prefilled with dialyzed plasma rather than with PBS. This analysis is in agreement with the conclusion reached by the investigators (Williams et al., 1987).

In another example, it has been reported that % N was equal to 95.0 (18/19) at a gap length of 8.0 mm in the rat sciatic nerve bridged by a silicone tube filled with a 1 mg/ml solution of nerve growth factor (NGF); the control, a solution of cytochrome C filling the silicone tube, gave a value of % $N = 84.0$ at the same gap length (Hollowell et al., 1990). Point E [95.0%, 8.0 mm] for the test configuration is located at a distance $8.0 - 6.6 = 1.4$ mm to the right of point F [95.0%, 6.6 mm] on the standard curve, leading to the L_c value of $9.7 + 1.4 = 11.1$ mm while point G [84.0%, 8.0 mm] for the control is located $8.0 - 7.3 = 0.7$ mm to the right, leading to an L_c value of $9.7 + 0.7 = 10.4$ mm. It follows that $\Delta L = 11.1 - 10.4 = 0.7$ mm, a value too small to be considered significant in view of the experimental error of the L_c for the standard (± 1.8 mm). This result is in agreement with the investigators' conclusion that there was no significant difference between the NGF-treated group and the untreated control (Hollowell et al., 1990).

In a third example, % N was equal to 100.0% (6/6) for a silicone tube that had four holes, each 0.6 by 2 mm, cut into the wall and was used to bridge a 16.0-mm gap in the rat sciatic nerve; the control was an impermeable silicone tube that led to % $N = 17.0$ (1/6) (Jenq and Coggeshall, 1987). The first experimental point, point I [100.0%, 16.0], is located "off scale," that is, on the flat (zero-slope) segment of the characteristic curve for the test device. The off-scale location of point I most probably resulted from choice of a gap length in the experimental protocol that was apparently too small to test the regenerative capacity of the device adequately. The observation for the test device lies, therefore, at a distance at least equal ($\geq$) to $16.0 - 6.3 = 9.7$ from the standard along the % $N = 100$ ordinate; accordingly, L_c for the test device takes a value that is estimated at $\geq 9.7 + 9.7 \geq 19.4$ mm. The observation for the control is "on scale," represented by point J [17.0%, 16.0 mm], leading to an L_c value of $9.7 + (16.0 - 12.0) = 13.7$ mm. The length shift in this case is $\Delta L \geq 19.4 - 13.7 \geq 5.7$ mm, clearly a lower limit for a very significant advantage in innervation frequency. In direct contrast, if an observation is % $N = 0$, falling off scale on the zero-slope segment to the left of the inflection point of the standard curve, the device has a critical axon elongation that is at most equal ($\leq$) to that of the standard; here, the gap length employed was most probably too long to provide for a useful comparison of the device with the standard. In general, % N values equal to 100 lead to ΔL values that are expressed as being larger than or equal ($\geq$) to the standard; the reverse is true for % N values equal to 0. Data expressed as inequalities are not useless; they provide valuable information about the upper and lower performance limits for a device.

A.2 Limitations and Uses of Critical Axon Elongation Data

The choice of % N as an assay for the extent of regeneration is obviously arbitrary and based on the need to analyze, by use of a common benchmark, the largest possible body of data in the literature in a self-consistent manner. This procedure is limited by the nature of % N as a frequency of reinnervation that is not directly related to the information contained in other commonly used morphological or functional assays. Thus, there is no way in which % N data can be used to reconstruct, by themselves, either the structure or function of the regenerate.

The use of data from the literature to construct the characteristic curve for the standard configuration, Figure 6.1, is subject to criticism since not all of these data have been obtained under identical experimental conditions. For example, some of the data included in Figure 6.1 were obtained before completion of a period long enough (about 6 weeks) to ensure that maximum values of % N had been reached; also, most but not all of the data were obtained using the same surgical procedure for transecting the sciatic nerve. Furthermore, the precision of most data on the frequency of reinnervation, % N, is rather low due to a relatively small size of samples generally studied.

A further limitation derives from the abruptness with which % N drops off with gap length. Such abruptness suggests that values of % N between 0 and 100 can be recorded only inside a relatively short interval of the gap length; if an observation of % N falls outside of this interval in gap length, only an upper or lower bound (limit) of % N can be recorded, as explained above. In Table 6.1 it is clear that a large number of data from the literature are, in fact, available only in the form of upper and lower limits of % N. Although such bounds are still useful, they are less informative than absolute values of % N.

Finally, we recall the use of the hypothesis of universal shape for the characteristic curves of all configurations. This hypothesis is supported by very limited data.

In spite of these important limitations, data relating % N to gap length for a test configuration form the basis of an approximate but self-consistent method that has been used (Table 6.1) to characterize regeneration across widely different tubulated devices.

A.3 Evaluation of Short-Term Data Using the Length Shift

ΔL provides a measure of comparison between the test device and the investigator's control; the magnitude of ΔL is a measure of the regenerative activity of a test configuration compared with the silicone tube standard. Listed in Table 6.1 are values for L_c and ΔL for representative structural characteristics of a tubulated configuration and for the internal control used by the investigator. In the absence of an internal control, ΔL for a device has been obtained by direct comparison with the standard (silicone tube). The tabulated data form the basis of a discussion of the structural features that are associated with very high, modest, or negligible regeneration in the peripheral nervous system. The implications of the entries in Table 6.1 have been discussed in Chapter 6.

Considering that the uncertainty in values of L_c calculated by this method has been estimated at about ± 1.8 mm (see above), it becomes clear that L_c values that lie closer to the standard than this value are not significantly different from it. We recall that ΔL for the 10-mm gap bridged by the silicone tube is, by definition, zero. Positive and negative values of ΔL signify upregulation and downregulation, respectively, of regenerative activity over that for the internal control employed in the study. In Chapter 6, ΔL values in the range +2 to +4 mm for the rat sciatic nerve model and +1 to +2 mm for the mouse sciatic nerve model are being referred to as "significant" (corresponding to a high value of the regenerative activity); values above +4 mm (rat) and +2 mm (mouse) are "very significant" (corresponding to a very high value of the regenerative activity). Negative values obviously reflect downregulation of regenerative processes relative to the silicone tube standard. The quality of available data does not merit a more detailed statistical analysis.

References

Abercrombie, M., D.W. James, and J.F. Newcombe. 1960. Wound contraction in rabbit skin, studied by splinting the wound margins. *J. Anat.* 94:170–182.

Abraham, J.A. and M. Klagsbrun. 1996. Modulation of wound repair by members of the fibroblast growth factor family. In *The Molecular and Cellular Biology of Wound Repair*, edited by Clark, R.A.F. New York: Plenum Press.

Adzick, N.S. and H.P. Lorenz. 1994. Cells, matrix, growth factors, and the surgeon. The biology of scarless fetal wound repair. *Ann. Surg.* 220:10–18.

Aebischer, P., V. Guénard, S.R. Winn, R.F. Valentini, and P.M. Galletti. 1988. Blind-ended semipermeable guidance channels support peripheral nerve regeneration in the absence of a distal nerve stump. *Brain Res.* 454:179–187.

Aebischer, P., A.N. Salessiotis, and S.R. Winn. 1989. Basic fibroblast growth factor released from synthetic guidance channels facilitates regeneration across long nerve gaps. *J. Neurosci. Res.* 23:282–289.

Aguayo, A.J., J.M. Peyronnard, and G.M. Bray. 1973. A qualitative ultrastructural study of regeneration from isolated proximal stumps of transected umyelinated nerves. *J. Neuropath. Exp. Neurol.* 32:256–270.

Aihara, M. 1989. Ultrastructural study of grafted autologous cultured human epithelium. *Br. J. Plast. Surg.* 42:35–42.

Albertson, S., R.P. Hummel, M. Breeden, and D.S. Greenhalgh. 1993. PDGF and FGF reverse the healing impairment in protein-malnourished diabetic mice. *Surgery* 114:368–373.

Aldini, N.N., G. Perego, G.D. Cella, M.C. Maltarello, M. Fini, M. Rocca, and R. Giardino. 1996. Effectiveness of a bioresorbable conduit in the repair of peripheral nerves. *Biomater.* 17:959–962.

Allbrook, D. 1962. An electron microscopic study of regenerating skeletal muscle. *J. Anat.* 96:137–152.

Alvarez, O.M., J.B. Goslen, W.H. Eaglestein, H.G. Welgus, and G.P. Stricklin. 1987. Wound Healing. In *Dermatology in General Medicine*, edited by Fitzpatrick, T.B., A.Z. Eisen, K. Wolff, I.M. Freedberg, and K.F. Austen. 3rd ed. New York: McGraw-Hill.

Amadio, P.C. 1992. Tendon and Ligament. In *Wound Healing*, edited by Cohen, I.K., R.F. Diegelmann, and W.J. Lindblad. Philadelphia: W. B. Saunders.

Ansselin, A.D., T. Fink, and D.F. Davey. 1997. Peripheral nerve regeneration through nerve guides seeded with adult Schwann cells. *Neuropathol. Appl. Neurobiol.* 23:387–398.

Arbuthnot, R., I.A. Boyd, and K.U. Kalu. 1980. Ultrastructural dimensions of myelinated peripheral nerve fibers in the cat and their relation to conduction velocity. *J. Physiol.* 308:125–157.

Archibald, S.J. and T.R. Fisher. 1987. Micro-surgical fascicular nerve repair: A morphological study of the endoneurial bulge. *J. Hand Surg.* 12-B:5–10.

Archibald, S.J., C. Krarup, J. Sheffner, S.-T. Li, and R.D. Madison. 1991. A collagen-based nerve guide conduit for peripheral nerve repair: An electrophysiological study of nerve regeneration in rodents and nonhuman primates. *J. Comp. Neurol.* 306:685–696.

Archibald, S.J., J. Sheffner, C. Krarup, and R.D. Madison. 1995. Monkey median nerve repaired by nerve graft or collagen nerve guide tube. *J. Neurosci.* 15: 4109–4123.

Arora, P.D., N. Narani, and C.A. McCulloch. 1999. The compliance of collagen gels regulates transforming growth factor-beta induction of alpha-smooth muscle actin in fibroblasts. *Am. J. Pathol.* 154:871–882.

Asmussen, P.D. and B. Sollner. 1993. *Wound Care*. Stuttgart: Hippokrates.

Avgoustiniatos, E.S. and C.K. Colton. 1997. Design considerations for immuno-isolation. In *Principles of Tissue Engineering*, edited by Lanza, R.P., R. Langer, and W.L. Chick. San Diego: Academic Press.

Azzam, N.A., A.A. Zalewski, L.R. Williams, and R.N. Azzam. 1991. Nerve cables formed in silicone chambers reconstitute a perineurial but not a vascular endoneurial permeability barrier. *J. Comp. Neurol.* 314:807–819.

Bach, F.H., S.C. Robson, H. Winkler, C. Ferran, K.M. Stuhlmeier, C.J. Wrighton, and W.W. Hancock. 1995. Barriers to xenotransplantation. *Nature Med.* 1:869–873.

Badalamente, M.A., L.C. Hurst, J. Eilstein, and C.A. McDevitt. 1985. The pathobiology of human neuromas: An electron microscopic and biochemical study. *J. Hand Surg.* 10:49–53.

Bailey, A.J., S. Bazin, T.J. Sims, M. LeLous, C. Nicoletis, and A. Delaunay. 1975. Characterization of the collagen of human hypertrophic and normal scars. *Biochim. Biophys. Acta* 405:412–421.

Bailey, S.B., M.E. Eichler, A. Villadiego, and K.M. Rich. 1993. The influence of fibronectin and laminin during Schwann cell migration and peripheral nerve regeneration through silicone chambers. *J. Neurocytol.* 22:176–184.

Balazs, E. and N.E. Larsen. 2000. The role of hyaluronan-receptor interactions in wound repair. In *Scarless Wound Healing*, edited by Garg, H.G. and M.T. Longaker. New York: Marcel Dekker.

Banks-Schlegel, S. and H. Green. 1980. Formation of epidermis by serially cultivated human epidermal cells transplanted as an epithelium to athymic mice. *Transplant.* 29:308–313.

Baron-Van Ebercooren, A., A. Gansmuller, M. Gumpel, N. Baumann, and H.K. Kleinman. 1986. Schwann cell differentition *in vitro*: Extracellular matrix deposition and interaction. *Dev. Neurosci.* 8:182–196.

Barrandon, Y., V. Li, and H. Green. 1988. New techniques for the grafting of cultured human epidermal cells onto athymic animals. *J. Invest. Dermatol.* 91:315–318.

Barsa, J., M. Batra, R. Fink, and S.M. Sumi. 1982. A comparative in vivo study of local neurotoxicityof lidocaine, bupivacaine, 2-chloroprocaine, and a mixture of 2-chloroprocaine and bupivacaine. *Anesth. Analg.* 61:961–967.

Bauer, E.A., J.M. Gordon, M.E. Reddick, and A.Z. Eisen. 1977. Quantitative and immunohistochemical localization of human skin collagenase in basal cell carcinoma. *J. Invest. Dermatol.* 69:363–367.

Beck, L.S., T.L. Chen, P. Mikalauski, and A.J. Ammann. 1990a. Recombinant human transforming growth factor-beta 1(rhTGF-β1) enhances healing and strength of granulation skin wounds. *Growth Factors* 3:267–275.

Beck, L.S., T.L. Chen, S.E. Hirabayashi, L. Deguzman, W.P. Lee, L.L. McFatridge, Y. Xu, R.L. Bates, and A.J. Ammann. 1990b. Accelerated healing of ulcer wounds in the rabbit ear by recombinant human transforming growth factor-b1. *Growth Factors* 2:273–282.

Beerens, E., J. Slot, and J. VanDerLeun. 1975. Rapid regeneration of the dermal-epidermal junction after partial separation by vacuum: An electron microscopic study. *J. Invest. Dermatol.* 65:513–521.

Behrman, J.E. and R.D. Acland. 1981. Experimental study of the regenerative potential of perineurium at a site of nerve transection. *J. Neurosurg.* 54:79–83.

Bell, E., B. Ivarsson, and C. Merrill. 1979. Production of a tissue-like structure by contraction of collagen lattices by human fibroblasts of different proliferative potential in vitro. *Proc. Natl. Acad. Sci. USA* 76:1274–1278.

Bell, E., H.P. Ehrlich, D.J. Buttle, and T. Nakatsuji. 1981a. Living skin formed in vitro and accepted as skin-equivalent tissue of full thickness. *Science* 211:1052–1054.

Bell, E., H.P. Ehrlich, S. Sher, C. Merrill, R. Sarber, B. Hull, T. Nakatsuji, D. Church, and D.J. Buttle. 1981b. Development and use of a living skin equivalent. *Plast. Reconstr. Surg.* 67:386–392.

Bell, E., S. Sher, B. Hull, C. Merrill, S. Rosen, A. Chamson, D. Asselineau, L. Dubertret, B. Coulomb, C. Lapiere, et al. 1983. The reconstitution of living skin. *J. Invest. Dermatol.* 81:2s–10s.

Bell, E., S. Sher, and B. Hull. 1984. The living skin-equivalent as a structural and immunological model in skin grafting. *Scan. Electr. Micr.* 4:1957–1962.

Bently, J.P. 1967. Rate of chondroitin sulfate formation in wound healing. *Ann. Surg.* 165:186–191.

Bertolami, C. and R.B. Donoff. 1982. Identification, caracterization and partial purification of mammlian skin wound hyaluronidase. *J. Invest. Dermatol.* 79:417–421.

Besner, G.E. and J.E. Klamar. 1998. Integra Artificial Skin as a useful adjunct in the treatment of purpura fulminans. *J. Burn Care Rehabil.* 19:324–329.

Billingham, R.E. and P.B. Medawar. 1950. Pigment spread in mammalian skin: Serial propagation and immunity reactions. *Heredity* 4:141–164.

Billingham, R.E. and P.B. Medawar. 1951. The technique of free skin grafting in mammals. *J. Exp. Biol.* 28:385–402.

Billingham, R.E. and J. Reynolds. 1952. Transplantation studies on sheets of pure epidermal epithelium and epidermal cell suspensions. *Brit. J. Plast. Surg.* 5:25–36.

Billingham, R.E. and P.B. Medawar. 1955. Contracture and intussusceptive growth in the healing of extensive wounds in mammalian skin. *J. Anat.* 89:114–123.

Billingham, R.E. and P.S. Russell. 1956. Studies on wound healing, with special reference to the phenomenon of contracture in experimental wounds in rabbits' skin. *Ann. Surg.* 144:961–981.

Birk, D.E. and R.L. Trelstad. 1985. Fibroblasts compartmentalize the extracellular space to regulate and facilitate collagen fibril, bundle, amd macro-aggregate formation. In *Extracellular Matrix: Structure and Function*, edited by Reddi, A.H. New York: Alan R. Liss.

Bjorklund, A. and U. Stenevi. 1984. Intracerebral neural implants: Neuronal replacement and reconstruction of damaged circuitries. *Annu. Rev. Neurosci.* 7:279–308.

Borkenhagen, M., R.C. Stoll, P. Neuenschwander, U.W. Suter, and P. Aebischer. 1998. In vivo performance of anew bioegradable polyester urethane system used as a nerve guidance channel. *Biomaterials.* 19:2155–2165.

Bosca, A.R., E. Tinois, M. Faure, J. Kanitakis, P. Roche, and J. Thivolet. 1988. Epithelial differentiation of human skin equivalents after grafting onto nude mice. *J. Invest. Dermatol.* 91:136–141.

Boyce, S.T. and R.G. Ham. 1983. Calcium-regulated differentiation of normal human epidermal keratinocytes in chemically defined clonal culture and serum-free serial culture. *J. Invest. Dematol.* 81(Suppl.):33s–40s.

Boyce, S.T. and R.G. Ham. 1985. Cultivation, frozen storage, and clonal growth of normal human epidermal keratinocytes in serum-free medium. *J. Tissue Culture Meth.* 9:83–93.

Boyce, S.T. and J.F. Hansbrough. 1988. Biologic attachment and growth of cultured human keratinocytes onto a graftable collagen and chondroitin 6-sulfate substrate. *Surg.* 103:421–431.

Boyce, S.T., D. Christianson, and J.F. Hansbrough. 1988. Structure of a collagen-GAG substitute optimized for cultured human epidermal keratinocytes. *J. Biomed. Mater. Res.* 22:939–957.

Boyce, S.T., D.G. Greenhalgh, R.J. Kagan, T. Housinger, J.M. Sorrell, C.P. Childress, M. Rieman, and G.D. Warden. 1993. Skin anatomy and antigen expression after burn wound closure with composite grafts of cultured skin cells and biopolymers. *Plast. Resconstr. Surg.* 91:632–641.

Boykin, J.V. and J.A. Molnar. 1992. Burn scar and skin equivalents. In *Wound Healing*, edited by Cohen, I.K., R.F. Diegelmann, and W.J. Lindblad. Philadelphia: W. B. Saunders.

Bradley, J.L., D.A. Abernethy, R.H. King, J.R. Muddle, and P.K. Thomas. 1998. Neural architecture in transected rabbit sciatic nerve after prolonged nonreinnervation. *J. Anat.* 192:529–538.

Breuing, K., E. Eriksson, P.Y. Liu, and D.R. Miller. 1992. Healing of partial thickness porcine skin wounds in a liquid environment. *J. Surg. Res.* 52:50–58.

Briggaman, R.A. and C.E. Wheeler. 1975. The epidermal-dermal junction. *J. Invest. Dermatol.* 65:71–84.

Briggaman, R.A., F.G. Dalldorf, and J.C.E. Wheeler. 1971. Formation and origin of basal lamina and anchoring fibrils in adult human skin. *J. Cell Biol.* 51:384–395.

Brockes, J.P. 1997. Amphibian limb regeneration: Rebuilding a complex structure. *Science* 275:81–87.

Brodsky, B. and J.A.M. Ramshaw. 1994. Collagen organization in an oriented fibrous capsule. *Int. J. Biol. Macromol.* 16:27–30.

Brown, G.L., L.C. III, J.R. Brightwell, D.M. Ackerman, G.R. Tobin, J.H.C. Polk, C. George-Nacimento, P. Valenzuela, and G.S. Schultz. 1986. Enhancement of epidermal regeneration by biosynthetic epidermal growth factor. *J. Exp. Med.* 163:1319–1324.

Brown, H. 1992. Wound healing research through the ages. In *Wound Healing*, edited by Cohen, I.K., R.F. Diegelmann, and W.J. Lindblad. Philadelphia: W. B. Saunders.

Brown, I.A. 1972. Scanning electron microscopy of human dermal fibrous tissue. *J. Anat.* 113:159–168.

Brown, R.E., D. Erdmann, S.F. Lyons, and H. Suchy. 1996. The use of cultured Schwann cells in nerve repair in a rabit hind-limb model. *J. Reconstr. Microsurg.* 12:149–152.

Bucher, N.L.R. 1963. Regeneration of mammalian liver. *Intern. Rev. Cytol.* 15: 245–300.

Bunge, M.B., A.K. Willams, P.M. Wood, J. Uitto, and J.J. Jeffrey. 1980. Comparison of nerve cell and nerve cell plus Schwann cell cultures, with particular emphasis on basal lamina and collagen formation. *J. Cell Biol.* 84:184–202.

Bunge, M.B., A.K. Williams, and P.M. Wood. 1982. Neuron-Schwann cell interaction in basal lamina formation. *Dev. Biol.* 92:449–460.

Bunge, M.B., P.M. Wood, L.B. Tynan, M.L. Bates, and J.B. Sanes. 1989. Perineurium originates from fibroblasts: Demonstration in vitro with a retroviral marker. *Science* 243:229–231.

Bunge, R.P. and M.B. Bunge. 1978. Evidence that contact with connective tissue matrix is required for normal interaction between Schwann cells and nerve fibers. *J. Cell Biol.* 78:943–950.

Bunge, R.P. and M.B. Bunge. 1983. Interrelationship between Schwann cell function and extracellular matrix production. *Trends Neurosci.* 6:499–505.

Burgess, W.H. and T. Maciag. 1989. The heparin-binding (fibroblast) growth factor family of proteins. *Annu. Rev. Biochem.* 58:575–606.

Burke, J.F. 1987. Observations on the development and clinical use of artificial skin: An attempt to employ regeneration rather than scar formation in wound healing. *Jpn. J. Surg.* 17:431–438.

Burke, J.F., C.C. Bondoc, and W.C. Quinby. 1974. Primary burn excision and immediate grafting: A method of shortening illness. *J. Trauma* 14:389–395.

Burke, J.F., I.V. Yannas, W.C.Q. Jr., C.C. Bondoc, and W.K. Jung. 1981. Successful use of a physiologically acceptable artificial skin in the treatment of extensive burn injury. *Ann. Surg.* 194:413–428.

Burkitt, H.G., B. Young, and J.W. Heath. 1993. *Wheater's Functional Histology*. 3rd ed. Edinburgh: Churchill Livingstone.

Burrington, J.D. 1971. Wound healing in the fetal lamb. *J. Pediatr. Surg.* 6:523–528.

Butí, M., E. Verdú, R.O. Labrador, J.J. Vilches, J. Forés, and X. Navarro. 1996. Influence of physical parameters of nerve chambers on peripheral nerve regeneration and reinnervation. *Exp. Neurol.* 137:26–33.

Butler, C.E., D.P. Orgill, I.V. Yannas, and C.C. Compton. 1998. Effect of keratinocyte seeding of collagen-glycosaminoglycan membranes on the regeneration of skin in a porcine model. *Plast. Reconstr. Surg.* 101:1572–1579.

Butler, C.E., I.V. Yannas, C.C. Compton, C.A. Correia, and D.P. Orgill. 1999a. Comparison of cultured and uncultured keratinocytes seeded into a collagen-GAG matrix for skin replacements. *Br. J. Plast. Surg.* 52:127–132.

Butler, P.E., C.D. Sims, M.A. Randolph, D. Menkes, J. Onorato, and W.P. Lee. 1999b. A comparative study of nerve healing in adult, neonatal, and fetal rabbits. *Plast. Reconstr. Surg.* 104:1386–1392.

Caballos, D., X. Navarro, N. Dubey, G. Wendelschafer-Crabb, W.R. Kennedy and R.T. Tranquillo. 1999. Magnetically aligned collagen gel filling a collagen nerve guide improves peripheral nerve regenertion. *Exp. Neurol.* 158:290–300.

Cajal, R.Y. 1928. *Degeneration and Regeneration of the Nervous System* (volume reissued in 1982). London: Oxford University Press.

Campbell, C.J. 1969. The healing of cartilage defects. *Clin. Orthop.* 64:45–63.

Carbonetto, S. 1991. Facilitatory and inhibitory effects of glial cells and extracellular matrix in axonal regeneration. *Curr. Opin. Neurobiol.* 1:407–413.

Carbonetto, S., M.M. Gruver, and D.C. Turner. 1983. Nerve fiber growth in culture on fibronectin, collagen, and glycosaminoglycan substrates. *J. Neurosci.* 3:2324–2335.

Carey, D.J. and M.S. Todd. 1987. Schwann cell myelination in a chemiclly defined medium: Demonstration of a requirement for additives that promote Schwann cell extracellular matrix formation. *Brain Res.* 429:95–102.

Carey, D.J., C.F. Eldridge, C.J. Cornbrooks, R. Timpl, and R.P. Bunge. 1983. Biosynthesis of type IV collagen by cultured rat Schwann cells. *J. Cell Biol.* 97:473–479.

Carey, D.J., M.S. Todd, and C.M. Rafferty. 1986. Schwann cell myelination: Induction by exogenous basement membrane-like extracellular matrix. *J. Cell Biol.* 102:2254–2263.

Carman, L.S., G.E. Schneider, and I.V. Yannas. 1988. Extension of critical age for retinal axon regeneration by polymer bridges conditioned in neonatal cortex. *Soc. Neurosci. Abs.* 14:498.

Carrel, A. and A. Hartmann. 1916. Cicatrization of wounds I: The relation between the size of a wound and the rate of its cicatrization. *J. Exp. Med.* 24:429–450.

Carver, N., H.A. Navsaria, C.J. Green, and I.M. Leigh. 1993a. The effect of backing materials on keratinocyte autograft take. *Br. J. Plast. Surg.* 46:228–234.

Carver, N., H.A. Navsaria, P. Fryer, C.J. Green, and I.M. Leigh. 1993b. Restoration of basement membrane structure in pigs following keratinocyte autografting. *J. Plast. Surg.* 46:384–392.

Cass, D.L., K.G. Sylvester, E.Y. Yang, T.M. Crombleholme, and N.S. Adzick. 1997. Myofibroblast persistence in fetal sheep wounds is associated with scar formation. *J. Pediatr. Surg.* 32:1017–1021.

Ceballos, D., X. Navarro, N. Dubey, G. Wendelschafer-Crabb, W.R. Kennedy, and R.T. Tranquillo. 1999. Magnetically aligned collegen gel filling a collagen nerve guide improves peripheral nerve regeneration. *Exp. Neurol.* 158:290–300.

Chamberlain, L.J. 1998. Influence of implant parameters on the mechanisms of peripheral nerve regeneration. Ph. D. thesis, Massachussetts Institute of Technology, Cambridge, MA.

Chamberlain, L.J. and I.V. Yannas. 1998. Preparation of collagen-glycosaminoglycan copolymers for tissue regeneration. In *Methods of Molecular Medicine*, edited by Morgan, J.R. and M.L. Yarmush. Tolowa, NJ: Humana Press.

Chamberlain, L.J., I.V. Yannas, A. Arrizabalaga, H.-P. Hsu, T.V. Norregaard, and M. Spector. 1998a. Early peripheral nerve healing in collagen and silicone tube implants: Myofibroblasts and the cellular response. *Biomaterials* 19:1393–1403.

Chamberlain, L.J., I.V. Yannas, H.-P. Hsu, G. Strichartz, and M. Spector. 1998b. Collagen-GAG substrate enhances the quality of nerve regeneration through collagen tubes up to level of autograft. *Exp. Neurol.* 154:315–329.

Chamberlain, L.J., I.V. Yannas, H.-P. Hsu, and M. Spector. 2000a. Connective tissue response to tubular implants for peripheral nerve regeneration: The role of myofibroblasts. *J. Comp. Neurol.* 417:415–430.

Chamberlain, L.J., I.V. Yannas, H.-P. Hsu, G.R. Strichartz, and M. Spector. 2000b. Near terminus axonal structure and function following rat sciatic nerve regeneration through a collagen-GAG matrix in a 10-mm gap. *J. Neurosci. Res.* 60:666–677.

Chamson, A., N. Germain, A. Clad, C. Perier, and J. Frey. 1989. Study of basement membrane formation in dermal-epidermal recombinants in vitro. *Arch. Dermatol. Res.* 281:267–272.

Chang, A.S. 1988. Electrophysiological recovery of peripheral nerves regenerated by biodegradable polymer matrix. M. S. thesis, Massachusetts Institute of Technology.

Chang, A.S. and I.V. Yannas. 1992. Peripheral nerve regeneration. In *Neuroscience Year,* edited by Smith, B. and G. Adelman. Boston: Birkhauser.

Chang, A.S., I.V. Yannas, S. Perutz, H. Loree, R.R. Sethi, C. Krarup, T.V. Norregaard, N.T. Zervas, and J. Silver. 1990. Electrophysiological study of recovery of peripheral nerves regenerated by a collagen-glycosaminoglycan copolymer matrix. In *Progress in Biomedical Polymers,* edited by Gebelein, C.G. New York: Plenum.

Chen, E.H.-Y. 1982. The effects of porosity and crosslinking of a collagen based artificial skin on wound healing. M. S. thesis, Massachusetts Institute of Technology, Cambridge, MA.

Chen, Y.S.H., L.T. Wang-Bennet, and N.J. Coker. 1989. Facial nerve regeneration in the silicone chamber: The influence of nerve growth factor. *Exp. Neurol.* 103:52–60.

Chin, G.S., E.J. Stelnicki, G.K. Gittes, and M.T. Longaker. 2000. Characteristics of fetal wound repair. In *Scarless Wound Healing,* edited by Garg, H.G. and M.T. Longaker. New York: Marcel Dekker.

Chvapil, M. and R. Holusa. 1968. Experimental experiences with the collagen sponge as hemostaticum and tampon. *J. Biomed. Mater. Res.* 2:245–264.

Chvapil, M., R. Holusa, K. Kliment, and M. Stoll. 1969. Some chemical and biological characteristics of a new collagen-polymer compound material. *J. Biomed. Mater. Res.* 3:315–332.

Clark, A.H. 1919. The effect of diet on the healing of wounds. *Bull. Johns Hopk. Hosp.* 30:117–120.

Clark, M.B. and M.B. Bunge. 1989. Cultured Schann cells assemble normal-appearing basal lamina only when they ensheathe axons. *Dev. Biol.* 133:393–404.

Clark, R.A.F. 1993. Regulation of fibroplasia in cutaneous wound repair. *Am. J. Med. Sci.* 306:42–48.

Clark, R.A.F., ed. 1996a. *The Molecular and Cellular Biology of Wound Repair.* 2nd ed. New York: Plenum Press.

Clark, R.A.F. 1996b. Wound repair. Overview and general considerations. In *The Molecular and Cellular Biology of Wound Repair,* edited by Clark, R.A.F. New York: Plenum Press.

Clark, R.A.F. 1997. Wound repair: Lessons for tissue engineering. In *Principles of Tissue Engineering,* edited by Lanza, R., R. Langer, and W. Chick. Austin, TX: R.G. Landes Company.

Clark, R.A.F. and P.M. Henson, eds. 1988. *The Molecular and Cellular Biology of Wound Repair.* 1st ed. New York: Plenum Press.

Clark, R.A.F., J. Lanigan, P. Dellapelle, E. Manseau, H. Dvorak, and R. Colvin. 1982. Fibronectin and fibrin provide a provisional matrix for epidermal-dermal cell migration during wound re-epithelialization. *J. Invest. Dermatol.* 79:264–269.

Clark, R.A.F., H.J. Quinn, H.J. Winn, and R.B. Colvin. 1983. Fibronectin beneath reepithelializing epidermis *in vivo*: Sources and significance. *J. Invest. Derm.* 80 (Suppl.):26S–30S.

Clark, R.A.F., L.D. Nielsen, M.P. Welch, and J.M. McPherson. 1995. Collagen matrices attenuate the collagen synthetic response of cultured fibroblasts to TGF-b. *J. Cell Sci.* 108:1251–1261.

Cohen, I.K. 1991. Wound healing models to study connective tissue metabolism: Normal and chronic wounds. In *Clinical and Experimental Approaches to Dermal and Epidermal Repair*, edited by Barbul, A., M. Caldwell, W. Eaglstein, T. Hunt, D. Marshall, E. Pines, and G. Skover. New York: Alan R. Liss.

Cohen, J., J.F. Burne, J. Winter, and P.F. Bartlett. 1986. Retinal ganglion cells lose response to laminin with maturation. *Nature* 322:465–467.

Cohen, S. 1959. Purification and metabolic effects of a nerve growth-promoting protein from snake venom. *J. Biol. Chem.* 234:1129–1137.

Coleman, C., T.L. Tuan, S. Buckley, K.D. Anderson, and D. Warburton. 1998. Contractility, transforming growth factor-beta, and plasmin in fetal skin fibroblasts: Role in scarless wound healing. *Pediatr. Res.* 43:403–409.

Compton, C.C. 1994. Keratinocyte grafting models. In *The Keratinocycte Handbook*, edited by Lane, E.B., I. Leigh, and F. Watt. London: Cambridge University Press.

Compton, C.C., J.M. Gill, D.A. Bradford, S. Regauer, G.G. Gallico, and N.E. O'Connor. 1989. Skin regenerated from cultured epithelial autografts on full-thickness burn wounds from 6 days to 5 years after grafting. *Lab. Invest.* 60:600–612.

Compton, C.C., C.E. Butler, I.V. Yannas, G. Warland, and D.P. Orgill. 1998. Organized skin structure is regenerated in vivo from collagen-GAG matrices seeded with autologous keratinocytes. *J. Invest. Dermatol.* 110:908–916.

Contard, P., R.L. Bartel, L. Jacobs 2d, J.S. Perlish, E.D. MacDonald 2d, L. Handler, D. Cone, and R. Fleischmajer. 1993. Culturing keratinocytes and fibroblasts in a three-dimensional mesh results in epidermal differentiation and formation of a basal lamina-anchoring zone. *J. Invest. Dermatol.* 100:35–39.

Cook, J.R. and R.G. Van Buskirk. 1995. The matrix form of collagen and basal microporosity influence basal lamina deposition and laminin synthesis/secretion by stratified human keratinocytes in vitro. *In Vitro Cell Dev. Biol. Anim.* 31:132–139.

Cooper, D.K.C., E. Kemp, J.L. Platt, and D.J.G. White, eds. 1997. *Xenotransplantation*. New York: Springer-Verlag.

Cooper, M.L. and J.F. Hansbrough. 1991. Use of a composite skin graft composed of cultured human keratinocytes and fibroblasts and a collagen-GAG matrix to cover full-thickness wounds on athymic mice. *Surg.* 109:198–207.

Cooper, M.L., J.F. Hansbrough, R.L. Spielvogel, R. Cohen, R.L. Bartel, and G. Naughton. 1991. In vivo optimization of a living dermal substitute employing cultured human fibroblasts on a biodegradable polyglycolic acid or polyglactin mesh. *Biomaterials* 12:243–248.

Cooper, M.L., C. Andree, J.F. Hansbrough, R.L. Zapata-Sirvent, and R.L. Spielvogel. 1993. Direct comparison of a cultured composite skin substitute containing human keratinocytes and fibroblasts to an epidermal sheet graft containing human keratinocytes on athymic mice. *J. Invest. Dermatol.* 101:811–819.

Cordeiro, P.G., B.R. Seckel, S.A. Lipton, P.A. D'Amore, J. Wagner, and R. Madison. 1989. Acidic fibroblast growth factor enhances peripheral nerve regeneration in vivo. *Plast. Reconstr. Surg.* 83:1013–1019.

Cornbrooks, C.J., D.J. Carey, J.A. McDonald, R. Timpl, and R.P. Bunge. 1983. In vivo and in vitro observations on laminin production by Schwann cells. *Proc. Natl. Acad. Sci. USA* 80:3850–3854.

Cowin, A.J., M.P. Brosnan, T.M. Holmes, and M.W. Ferguson. 1998. Endogenous inflammatory response to dermal wound healing in the fetal and adult mouse. *Dev. Dyn.* 212:385–393.

Crandall, S.H., N.C. Dahl, and T.J. Lardner. 1972. *An Introduction to the Mechanics of Solids.* New York: McGraw-Hill.

Cruickshank, C.N.D., J.R. Cooper, and C. Hooper. 1960. The cultivation of cells from adult epidermis. *J. Invest. Dematol.* 34:339–342.

Cumpstone, M.B., A.H. Kennedy, C.S. Harmon, and R.O. Potts. 1989. The water permeability of primary mouse keartinocyte cultures grown at the air-liquid interface. *J. Invest. Dermatol.* 92:598–600.

Cuppage, F.E., D.R. Neagoy, and A. Tate. 1967. Repair of the nephron following temporary occlusion of the renal pedicle. *Lab. Invest.* 17:660–674.

Cuthbertson, A.M. 1959. Contraction of full thickness skin wounds in the rat. *Surg. Gynec. Obstet.* 108:421–432.

Dagalakis, N., J. Flink, P. Stasikelis, J.F. Burke, and I.V. Yannas. 1980. Design of an artificial skin. Part III. Control of pore structure. *J. Biomed. Mater. Res.* 14:511–528.

Dahners, L.E., A.J. Banes, and K.W.T. Burridge. 1986. The relationship of actin to ligament contraction. *Clin. Orthop.* 210:246–251.

Danielsen, N. 1990. Regeneration of the rat sciatic nerve within the silicone chamber model. *Restorative Neurol. Neurosci.* 1:253–259.

Danielsen, N., B. Pettman, H.L. Vahlsing, M. Manthorpe, and S. Varon. 1988. Fibroblast growth factor effects on peripheral nerve regeneration in a silicone chamber model. *J. Neurosci. Res.* 20:320–330.

Darden, D.L., F.Z. Hu, M.D. Ehrlich, M.C. Gorry, D. Dressman, H.S. Li, D.C. Whitcomb, P.A. Hebda, J.E. Dohar, and G.D. Ehrlich. 2000. RNA differential display of scarless wound healing in fetal rabbit indicates downregulation of a CCT chaperonin subunit and upregulation of a glycophorin-like gene transcript. *J. Pediatr. Surg.* 35:406–419.

Darwin, C. 1872. *On the Origin of Species* (republished 1991). Norwalk, CT: Easton Press.

DaSilva, C.F. and F. Langone. 1989. Addition of nerve growth factor to the interior of a tubular prosthesis increases sensory neuron regeneration in vivo. *Braz. J. M Biol. Res.* 22:691–694.

DaSilva, C.F., R. Madison, P. Dikkes, T.-H. Chiu, and R.L. Sidman. 1985. An in vivo model to quantify motor and sensory peripheral nerve regeneration using bioresorbable nerve guide tubes. *Brain Res.* 342:307–315.

David, G., B.V.d. Schueren, and M. Bernfield. 1981. Basal lamina formation by normal and transformed mouse mammary epithelial cells duplicated in vitro. *Nat. Cancer Inst.* 67:719–728.

Davidson, J.M., M. Klagsbrun, K.E. Hill, A. Buckley, R. Sullivan, P.S. Brewer, and S.C. Woodward. 1985. Accelereated wound repair, cell proliferation, and collagen accumulation are produced by a cartilage-derived growth factor. *J. Cell Biol.* 100:1219–1227.

Davidson, J.M., G. Giro, and D. Quaglino. 1992. Elastin Repair. In *Wound Healing,* edited by Cohen, I.K., R.F. Diegelmann, and W.J. Lindblad. Philadelphia: W. B. Saunders.

Davison, S.P., T.V. McCaffrey, M.N. Porter, and E. Manders. 1999. Improved nerve regeneration with neutralization of transforming growth factor-$\beta 1$. *Laryngoscope* 109:631–635.

Dawber, R. and S. Shuster. 1971. Scanning electron microscopy of dermal fibrous tissue. *Br. J. Dermatol.* 84:130–134.

Dawson, J.A. 1997. Personal communication with the author.

Delecluse, C., M. Regnier, and M. Prunieras. 1974. Studies on guinea pig skin cell cultures II: Effect of a pif skin extract on DNA synthesis. *Acta Dermatovener (Stockholm)* 54:1–6.

Dellon, A.L. and S.E. MacKinnon. 1988. Basic scientific and clinical applications of peripheral nerve regeneration. *Surg. Ann.* 20:59–100.

de Medinacelli, L., R.J. Wyatt, and W.J. Freed. 1983. Peripheral nerve reconnection: Mechanical, thermal, and ionic conditions that promote the return of function. *Exp. Neurol.* 81:469–487.

den Dunnen, W.F.A., J.M. Schakenraad, G.Z. Zondervan, A.J. Pennings, B. van der Lei, and P.H. Robinson. 1993a. A new PLLA/PCL copolymer for nerve regeneration. *J. Mater. Sci. Mater. Med.* 4:521–525.

den Dunnen, W.F.A., B. van der Lei, J.M. Schakenraad, E.H. Blaauw, I. Stokroos, A.J. Pennings, and P.H. Robinson. 1993b. Long-term evaluation of nerve regeneration in a biodegradable nerve guide. *Microsurg.* 14:508–515.

den Dunnen, W.F.A., I. Stickroos, E.H. Blaauw, A. Holwerda, A.J. Pennings, P.H. Robinson, and J.M. Schakenraad. 1996. Light-microscopic and electron-microscopic evaluation of short-term nerve regeneration using a biodegradable poly(DL-lactide-ε–caprolacton) nerve guide. *J. Biomed. Mater. Res.* 31:105–115.

Denny-Brown, D. 1946. Importance of neural fibroblasts in the regeneration of nerve. *Arch. Neurol. Psychiat.* 55:171–215.

Derby, A., V.W. Engleman, G.E. Frierdich, G. Neises, S.R. Rapp, and D.G. Roufa. 1993. Nerve growth factor facilitates regeneration across nerve gaps: Morphological and behavioral studies in rat sciatic nerve. *Exp. Neurol.* 119:176–191.

Desmoulière, A. and G. Gabbiani. 1996. The role of the myofibroblast in wound healing and fibrocontractive diseases. In *The Molecular and Cellular Biology of Wound Repair*, edited by Clark, R.A.F. New York: Plenum Press.

Desmoulière, A., A. Genioz, F. Gabbiani, and G. Gabbiani. 1993. Transforming growth factor-β1 induces α-smooth muscle actin expression in granulation tissue, myofibroblasts and in quiescent and growing cultured fibroblasts. *J. Cell Biol.* 122:103–111.

Desmoulière, A., M. Redard, I. Darby, and G. Gabbiani. 1995. Apoptosis mediates the decrease in cellularity during the transition between granulation tissue and scar. *Am. J. Pathol.* 146:56–66.

Desmoulière, A., C. Badid, M.-L. Bochaton-Piallat, and G. Gabbiani. 1997. Apoptosis during wound healing, fibrocontractive diseases and vascular wall injury. *Int. J. Biochem. Cell Biol.* 29:19–30.

Diegelmann, R.F., W.J. Lindblad, and I.K. Cohen. 1988. Fibrogenic processes during tissue repair. In *Collagen*, edited by Nimni, M.E. Boca Raton: CRC Press.

Dore, C., J. Noordenbos, and J.F. Hansbrough. 1998. Management of partial thickness burns with Dermagraft-TC. *J. Burn Care Rehabil.* 19:S172.

Drumheller, P.D. and J.A. Hubbell. 1997. Surface immobilization of adhesion ligands for investigations of cell-substrate interactions. In *The Biomedical Engineering Handbook*, edited by Bronzino, J.D. Boca Raton: CRC Press.

Ducker, T.B. and G.J. Hayes. 1967. A comparative study of the technique of nerve repair. *Surg. Forum* 28:443–445.

Ducker, T.B. and G.J. Hayes. 1968a. Experimetal improvements in the use of silastic cuff for peripheral nerve repair. *J. Neurosurg.* 28:52–587.

Ducker, T.B. and G.J. Hayes. 1968b. Peripheral nerve injuries: A comparative study of the anatomical and functional results following primary nerve repair in chimpanzees. *Milit. Med.* 133:298–302.

Dunn, M.G. and F.H. Silver. 1983. Viscoelastic behavior of human connective tissues: Relative contribution of viscous and elastic components. *Connect. Tissue Res.* 12:59–70.

Dunn, M.G., F.H. Silver, and D.A. Swann. 1985. Mechanical analysis of hypertrophic scar tissue: Structural basis for apparent increased rigidity. *J. Invest. Dermatol.* 84:9–13.

Dunphy, J.E. and W. Van Winkle. 1968. *Repair and Regeneration: The Scientific Basis for Surgical Practice.* New York: McGraw-Hill.

Eaglstein, W.H., M. Iriondo, and K. Laszlo. 1995. A composite skin substitute (Graftskin) for surgical wounds. *Dermatol. Surg.* 21:839–843.

Eather, T.F., M. Pollock, and D.B. Myers. 1986. Proximal and distal changes in collagen content of peripheral nerve that follow transection and crush lesions. *Exp. Neurol.* 92:299–310.

Eckes, B., M. Aumailley, and T. Krieg. 1996. Collagens and the reestablishment of dermal integrity. In *The Molecular and Cellular Biology of Wound Repair*, edited by Clark, R.A.F., 2nd ed, Chap. 16. New York: Plenum Press, pp. 493–512.

Ehrlich, H.P. 1988. Wound closure: Evidence of cooperation between fibrobasts and collagen matrix. *Eye* 2:149–157.

Ehrlich, H.P. 2000. Collagen considerations in scarring and regenerative repair. In *Scarless Wound Healing*, edited by Garg, H.G. and M.T. Longaker. New York: Marcel Dekker, pp. 99–113.

Ehrlich, H.P. and J.B.M. Rajaratnam. 1990. Cell locomotion forces versus cell contraction forces for collagen lattice contraction: An in vitro model of wound contraction. *Tiss. Cell* 22:407–417.

Eisinger, M., J.S. Lee, J.M. Hefton, Z. Darzynkiewicz, J.W. Chiao, and E. DeHarven. 1979. Human epidermal cell cultures: Growth and differentiation in the absence of dermal components or medium supplements. *Proc. Natl. Acad. Sci. USA* 76: 5340–5344.

Eisinger, M., M. Monden, J.H. Raaf, and J.G. Fortner. 1980. Wound coverage by a sheet of epidermal cells grown in vitro from dispersed single cell preparations. *Surg.* 88:287–293.

Eisinger, M., E.R. Kraft, and J.G. Fortner. 1984. Wound coverage by epidermal cells grown in vitro. In *Soft and Hard Tissue Repair: Biological and Clinical Aspects*, edited by Hunt, T.K., R.B. Heppenstall, E. Pines, and D. Rovee. New York: Praeger.

Eldad, A., A. Burt, J.A. Clarke, and B. Gusterson. 1987. Cultured epithelium as a skin substitute. *Burns* 13:173–180.

Eldridge, C.F., M.B. Bunge, R.P. Bunge, and P.M. Wood. 1987. Differentiation of axon-related Schwann cells in vitro I: Ascorbic acid regulates basal lamina assembly and myelin formation. *J. Cell Biol.* 105:1023–1034.

Eldridge, C.F., M.B. Bunge, and R.P. Bunge. 1989. Differentiation of axon-related Schwann cells in vitro II: Control of myelin formation by basal lamina. *J. Neurosci.* 9:625–638.

Ellis, D., S. Tholpady, S. Thies, and I.V. Yannas. 1997. Unpublished observations.

Eng, L.F., P.J. Reier, and J.D. Houle. 1987. Astrocyte activation and fibrous gliosis: Glial fibrillary acidic protein immunostaining of astrocytes following intraspinal cord grafting of fetal CNS tissue. *Prog. Brain Res.* 71:439–455.

English, K.B., N. Stayner, G.G. Krueger, and R.P. Tuckett. 1992. Functional innervation of cultured skin grafts. *J. Invest. Dermatol.* 99:120–128.

Eriksson, E., K. Breuing, L.B. Johansen, and D.R. Miller. 1989. Growth factor solutions for wound treatment in pigs. *Surg. Forum* 40:618–620.

Estes, J.M., J.S. Vande Berg, N.S. Adzick, T.E. MacGillivray, A. Desmoulière, and G. Gabbiani. 1994. Phenotype and functional features of myofibroblasts in sheep fetal wounds. *Differentiation (Berl.)* 56:173–181.

Eyden, B. 2001. The fibronexus in reactive and tumoral myofibroblasts: further characterisation by electron microscopy. *Histol. Histopathol.* 16:57–70.

Falanga, V., D. Margolis, O. Alvarez, M. Auletta, F. Maggiacomo, M. Altman, J. Jensen, M. Sabolinski, and J. Hardin-Young. 1998. Rapid healing of venous ulcers and lack of clinical rejection with an allogeneic cultured human skin equivalent. *Arch. Dermatol.* 134:293–300.

Farquhar, M.G. 1981. The glomerular basement membrane: A selective macromolecular filter. In *Cell Biology of Extracellular Matrix*, edited by Hay, E.D. New York: Plenum Press, pp. 335–378.

Faure, M., G. Mauduit, D. Schmitt, J. Kanitakis, A. Demidem, and J. Thivolet. 1987. Growth and differentiation of human epidermal cultures used as auto- and allografts in humans. *Br. J. Dermatol.* 116:161–170.

Fava, R.A. and D.B. McClure. 1987. Fibronectin-associated transforming growth factor. *J. Cell Physiol.* 131:184–191.

Ferdman, A. 1987. The measurement of collagen fiber orientation in tissue by small-angle light scattering. Ph.D. thesis, Massachusetts Institute of Technology.

Ferdman, A. and I.V. Yannas. 1986. Small-angle light scattering from dermal tissues. MIT Laser Research Center, Massachusetts Institute of Technology.

Ferdman, A. and I.V. Yannas. 1987. Small angle light scattering from histological sections of connective tissue. *Trans. Soc. Biomaterials* 10:207.

Ferdman, A.G. and I.V. Yannas. 1993. Scattering of light from histologic sections: A new method for the analysis of connective tissue. *J. Invest. Dermatol.* 100:710–716.

Fernandez-Valle, C., D. Gorman, A.M. Gomez, and M.B. Bunge. 1997. Actin plays a role in both changes in cell shape and gene-expression associated with Schwann cell myelination. *J. Neurosci.* 17:241–250.

Fessler, J.H., G. Lunstrum, K.G. Duncan, A.G. Campbell, R. Sterne, H.P. Bächinger, and L.I. Fessler. 1984. Evolutionary constancy of basement membrane components. In *The Role of Extracellular Matrix in Development*, edited by Trelstad, R.L. New York: Alan R. Liss, pp. 207–219.

ffrench-Constant, C., L. Van de Water, H.F. Dvorak, and R.O. Hynes. 1989. Reappearance of an embryonic pattern of fibronectin splicing during wound healing in the adult rat. *J. Cell Biol.* 109:903–914.

Fiddes, J.C., P.A. Hebda, P. Hayward, M.C. Robson, J.A. Abraham, and C.K. Klingbeil. 1991. Preclinical wound-healing studies with recombinant human basic fibroblast growth factor. *Ann. NY Acad. Sci.* 638:316–328.

Fields, R.D. and M.H. Ellisman. 1986a. Axons regenerated through silicone tube splices I: Conduction properties. *Exp. Neurol.* 92:48–60.

Fields, R.D. and M.H. Ellisman. 1986b. Axons regenerated through silicone tube splices II: Functional morphology. *Exp. Neurol.* 92:61–74.

Fields, R.D., J.M. Le Beau, F.M. Longo, and M.H. Ellisman. 1989. Nerve regeneration through artificial tubular implants. *Progr. Neurobiol.* 33:8–134.

Fischer, D.W., J.L. Beggs, A.G. Shetter, and J.D. Waggener. 1983. Comparative study of neuroma formation in the rat sciatic nerve after CO_2 laser and scalpel neurectomy. *Neurosurgery* 13:287–294.

Fitzgerald, P.J., L. Herman, B. Carol, A. Roque, W.H. Marsh, L. Rosenstock, C. Richards, and D. Perl. 1968. Pancreatic acinal cell regeneration I: Cytologic, cytochemical and pancreatic weight changes. *Am. J. Pathol.* 52:983–1011.

Fleischmajer, R., A. Schechter, M. Bruns, J.S. Perlish, E.D. Macdonald, T.C. Pan, and R. Timpl. 1995. Skin fibroblasts are the only source of nidogen during early basal lamina formtion in vitro. *J. Invest. Dermatol.* 105:597–601.

Flory, P.J. 1953. *Principles of Polymer Chemistry*. Ithaca, NY: Cornell University Press.

Flynn, S. 1983. Effects of glutaraldehyde crosslinking and chondroitin 6-sulfate upon the mechanical properties and in vivo healing response of an artificial skin. B. S. thesis, Massachusetts Institute of Technology, Cambridge, MA.

Freed, L.E. and G. Vunjak-Novakovic. 1995. Cultivation of cell-polymer tissue consructs in simulated microgravity. *Biotechnol. Bioeng.* 46:306–313.

Freed, L.E., G. Vunjak-Novakovic, R.J. Biton, D.B. Eagles, D.C. Lesnoy, S.K. Barlow, and R. Langer. 1994. Biodegradable polymer scaffolds for tissue engineering. *Biotechnol.* 12:689–693.

Freeman, A.E., H.J. Igel, B.J. Herrman, and K.L. Kleinfeld. 1976. Growth and characterization of human skin epithelial cultures. *In Vitro* 12:352–362.

Freyman, T., I.V. Yannas, and L. Gibson. 2000. Unpublished observations.

Frykman, G.K., J. Adams, and W.W. Bowen. 1981. Neurolysis. *Orthop. Clin. North Am.* 12:325–342.

Fu, S.Y. and T. Gordon. 1997. The cellular and molecular basis of peripheral nerve regeneration. *Molec. Neurobiol.* 14:67–116.

Furthmayr, H. 1988. Basement Membranes. In *The Molecular and Cellular Biology of Wound Repair*, edited by Clark, R.A.F. and P.M. Henson. New York: Plenum Press.

Gabbiani, G. 1998. Evolution and clinical implications of the myofibroblast concept. *Cardiov. Res.* 38:545–548.

Gabbiani, G., G.B. Ryan, and G. Majno. 1971. Presence of modified fibroblasts in granulation tissue and possible role in wound contraction. *Experientia* 27:549-550.

Gabbiani, G., B.J. Hirschel, G.B. Ryan, P.R. Stakov, and G. Majno. 1972. Granulation tissue as a contractile organ. *J. Exp. Med.* 135:719–734.

Gage, F.H. 2000. Mammalian neural stem cells. *Science* 287:1433–1438.

Gallico, G.G., N.E. O'Connor, C.C. Compton, O. Kehinde, and H. Green. 1984. Permanent coverage of large burn wounds with autologous cultured human epithelium. *N. Engl. J. Med.* 311:448–451.

Garbay, B., A.M. Heape, F. Sargueil, and C. Cassagne. 2000. Myelin synthesis in the peripheral nervous system. *Prog. Neurobiol.* 61:267–304.

Garg, H.G., D.A.R. Burd, and D.A. Swann. 1989. Small dermatan sulfate proteoglycans in human epidermis and dermis. *Biomed. Res.* 10:197–207.

Garg, H.G., E.W. Lippay, and D.A.R. Burd. 1990. Purification and characterization of iduronic acid-rich and glucuronic acid-rich proteoglycans implicated in human post-burn keloid scar. *Carbohydr. Res.* 207:295–305.

Garg, H.G., C.D. Warren, and J.W. Siebert. 2000. Chemistry of scarring. In *Scarless Wound Healing*, edited by Garg, H.G. and M.T. Longaker. New York: Marcel Dekker.

Gerwins, P., E. Skoldenberg, and L. Claesson-Welsh. 2000. Function of fibroblast growth factors and vascular endothelial growth factors and their receptors in angiogenesis. *Crit. Rev. Oncol. Hematol.* 34:185–194.

Giannini, C. and P.J. Dyck. 1990. The fate of Schwann cell basement membranes in permanently transected nerves. *J. Neuropathol. Exp. Neurol.* 49:550–563.

Gibson, K.L., L. Remson, A. Smith, N. Satterlee, G.M. Strain, and J.K. Daniloff. 1991. Comparison of nerve regeneration through different types of neural prostheses. *Microsurg.* 12:80–85.

Gibson, T., R.M. Kenedi, and J.E. Craik. 1965. The mobile microarchitecture of dermal collagen: A bioengineering study. *Br. J. Surg.* 52:764–770.

Ginsbach, G., L.C. Busch, and W. Kühnel. 1979. The nature of the collagenous capsules around breast implants. *Plast. Reconst. Surg.* 64:456–464.

Goodrum, J.F., J.E. Weaver, N.D. Goines, and T.W. Bouldin. 1995. Fatty acids from degenerating myelin lipids are conserved and reutilized for myelin synthesis during regeneration in peripheral nerve. *J. Neurochem.* 65:1752–1759.

Goodrum, J.F., K.A. Fowler, J.D. Hostetter. 2000. Peripheral nerve regeneration and cholesterol reutilization are normal in the low-density lipoprotein receptor knockout mouse. *J. Neurosci. Res.* 15:581–586.

Gordon, P.L., C. Huang, R.C. Lord, and I.V. Yannas. 1974. The far infrared spectrum of collagen. *Macromol.* 7:954–956.

Goss, R.J. 1964. *Adaptive growth.* New York: Academic Press.

Goss, R.J. 1969. *Principles of Regeneration.* New York: Academic Press.

Goss, R.J. 1980. Prospects for regeneration in man. *Clin. Orth.* 151:270–282.

Goss, R.J. 1987. Why mammals don't regenerate—or do they? *News Physiol. Sci.* 2:112–115.

Goss, R.J. 1992. Regeneration versus repair. In *Wound Healing,* edited by Cohen, I.K., R.F. Diegelmann, and W.J. Lindblad. Philadelphia: W. B. Saunders.

Goss, R.J. and L.N. Grimes. 1972. Tissue interactions in the regeneration of rabbit ear holes. *Am. Zool.* 12:151–157.

Goss, R.J. and L.N. Grimes. 1975. Epidermal downgrowths in regenerating rabbit ear holes. *J. Morphol.* 146:533–542.

Graham, M.F., P. Blomquist, and B. Zederfeldt. 1992. The alimentary canal. In *Wound Healing,* edited by Cohen, I.K., R.F. Diegelmann, and W.J. Lindblad. Philadelphia: W. B. Saunders.

Green, H. and J.G. Rheinwald. 1977. Process for serially culturing keratinocytes. US Patent No. 4,016,036. Washington, DC: United States Patent Office.

Green, H., O. Kehinde, and J. Thomas. 1979. Growth of cultured human epidermal cells into multiple epithelia suitable for grafting. *Proc. Natl. Acad. Sci. USA* 76:5665–5668.

Green, H.A., E. Burd, N.S. Nishioka, U. Brüggermann, and C.C. Compton. 1992. Mid-dermal wound healing. *Arch. Dermatol.* 128:639–645.

Greenhalgh, D.G., K.H. Sprugel, M.J. Murray, and R. Ross. 1990. PDGF and FGF stimulate wound healing in the genetically diabetic mouse. *Am. J. Pathol.* 136: 1235–1246.

Griffith, L. 2000. Polymeric biomaterials. *Acta mater.* 48:263–277.

Griffith Cima, L. 1994. Polymer substrates for controlled biological interactions. *J. Cell Biochem.* 56:155–161.

Grillo, H.C. and J. Gross. 1962. Thermal reconstitution of collagen from solution, and the response to its heterologous implantation. *J. Surg. Res.* 2:69–82.

Grillo, H.C., G.T. Watts, and J. Gross. 1958. Studies in wound healing. I. Contraction and the wound contents. *Ann. Surg.* 148:145–152.

Grinnell, F. 1992. Cell adhesion. In *Wound Healing*, edited by Cohen, I.K., R.F. Diegelmann, and W.J. Lindblad. Philadelphia: W. B. Saunders.

Grinnell, F. 1994. Fibroblasts, myofibroblasts, and wound contraction. *J. Cell Biol.* 124:401–404.

Grondin, C.M., I. Campeau, J.C. Thornton, J.C. Engle, F.S. Cross, and H. Schreiber. 1989. Coronary artery bypass grafting with saphenous vein. *Circ.* 79(I):24–29.

Gross, J., W. Farinelli, P. Sadow, R. Anderson, and R. Burns. 1995. On the mechanism of skin wound "contraction": A granulation tissue "knockout" with a normal phenotype. *Proc. Natl. Acad. Sci. USA* 92:5982–5986.

Guénard, V., N. Kleitman, T.K. Morrissey, R.P. Bunge, and P. Aebischer. 1992. Syngeneic Schwann cells derived from adult nerves seeded in semipermeable guidance channels enhance peripheral nerve regeneration. *J. Neurosci.* 12:3310–3320.

Guo, M. and F. Grinnell. 1989. Basement membrane formation and human epidermal differentiation in vitro. *J. Invest. Dermatol.* 93:372–378.

Haber, R.M., W. Hanna, C.A. Ramsay, and L.B. Boxall. 1985. Cicatricial junctional epidermolysis bullosa. *J. Am. Acad. Dermatol.* 12:836–844.

Haftek, J. and P.K. Thomas. 1968. Electron-microscope observations on the effects of localized crush injuries on the connective tissues of peripheral nerves. *J. Anat.* 103:233–243.

Hall, S.M. 1986a. Regeneration in cellular and acellular autografts in the peripheral nervous system. *J. Neuropathol. Appl. Neurobiol.* 12:27–46.

Hall, S.M. 1986b. The effect of inhibiting Schwann cell mitosis on the reinnervation of acellular autografts in the peripheral nervous system of the mouse. *J. Neuropathol. Appl. Neurobiol.* 12:402–414.

Ham, A.W. 1965. *Histology.* Philadelphia: J. B. Lippincott.

Hansbrough, J.F., S.T. Boyce, M.L. Cooper, and T.J. Foreman. 1989. Burn wound closure with cultured autologous keratinocytes atached to a collagen-glycosaminoglycan substrate. *JAMA* 262:2125–2130.

Hansbrough, J.F., M.L. Cooper, R. Cohen, R. Spielvogel, G. Greenleaf, R.L. Bartel, and G. Naughton. 1992a. Evaluation of a biodegradable matrix containing cultured human fibroblasts as a dermal replacement beneath meshed skin grafts on athymic mice. *Surgery* 111:438–446.

Hansbrough, J.F., C. Dore, and W.B. Hansbrough. 1992b. Clinical trials of a living dermal tissue replacement placed beneath meshed, split-thickness skin grafts on excised burn wounds. *J. Burn Care Rehab.* 13:519–529.

Hansbrough, J.F., J.L. Morgan, G.E. Greenleaf, and R. Bartel. 1993. Composite grafts of human keratinocytes grown on a polyglactin mesh-cultured fibroblast dermal substitute function as a bilayer skin replacement in full-thickness wounds on athymic mice. *J. Burn Care Rehab.* 14:485–494.

Hansbrough, J.F., J. Morgan, G. Greenleaf, M. Parikh, C. Nolte, and L. Wilkins. 1994. Evaluation of Graftskin composite grafts on full-thickness wounds on athymic mice. *J. Burn Care Rehab.* 15:346–353.

Harriger, M.D. and B.E. Hull. 1992. Cornification and basement membrane formation in a bilayered human skin equivalent maintained at an air-liquid interface. *J. Burn Care Rehabil.* 13:187–193.

Harris, A.K., P. Wild, and D. Stopak. 1980. Silicone rubber substrate: A new wrinkle in the study of cell locomotion. *Science* 280:177–179.

Harris, A.K., D. Stopak, and P. Wild. 1981. Fibroblast traction as a mechanism for collagen morphogenesis. *Nature* 290:249–251.

Hartwell, S.W. 1955. *The Mechanisms of Healing in Human Wounds*. Springfield, IL: Charles C. Thomas.

Hay, E.D. 1966. *Regeneration*. New York: Holt, Rinehart & Winston.

Hay, E.D. 1981. Collagen and embryonic development. In *Cell Biology of the Extracellular Matrix*, edited by Hay, E.D. New York: Plenum.

Hayward, P. and M.C. Robson. 1991. Animal models of wound contraction. In *Clinical and Experimental Approaches to Dermal and Epidermal Repair: Normal and Chronic Wounds*, edited by Barbul, A., M. Caldwell, W. Eaglstein, T. Hunt, D. Marshall, E. Pines, and G. Skover. New York: Alan R. Liss.

Hayward, P., J. Hokanson, J. Heggers, J. Fiddes, and C. Klingbeil. 1992. Fibroblast growth factor reverses the bacterial retardation of wound contraction. *Am. J. Surg.* 163:288–293.

Hefton, J.M., M.R. Madden, J.L. Finkelstein, and G.T. Shires. 1983. Grafting of burn patients with allografts of cultured epidermal cells. *Lancet* 2:428–430.

Heimbach, D., A. Luterman, J. Burke, A. Cram, D. Herndon, J. Hunt, M. Jordan, W. McManus, L. Solem, G. Warden, et al. 1988. Artificial dermis for major burns. *Ann. Surg.* 208:313–320.

Heldin, C.-H. and B. Westermark. 1996. Role of Platelet-derived growth factor in vivo. In *The Molecular and Cellular Biology of Wound Repair*, edited by Clark, R.A.F. New York: Plenum Press.

Henry, E.W., T.-H. Chiu, E. Nyilas, T.M. Brushart, P. Dikkes, and R.L. Sidman. 1985. Nerve regeneration through biodegradable polyester tubes. *Exp. Neurol.* 90:652–676.

Hertz, M.I., L. Snyder, K.R. Harmon, and P.B. Bitterman. 1992. Acute lung injury. In *Wound Healing*, edited by Cohen, I.K., R.F. Diegelmann, and W.J. Lindblad. Philadelphia: W. B. Saunders.

Higgins, G.M. and R.M. Anderson. 1931. Experimental pathology of the liver I: Restoration of the liver of the white rat following partial surgical removal. *Arch. Pathol.* 12:186–202.

Hirone, T. and S. Taniguchi. 1980. Basal lamina formation by epidermal cells in cell culture. *Curr. Probl. Dermatol.* 10:159–169.

Holbrook, K.A., P.H. Byers, and S.R. Pinnell. 1982. The structure and function of dermal connective tissue in normal individuals and patients with inherited connective tissue disorder. *Scan. Electron Micros.* 4:1731–1744.

Hollowell, J.P., A. Villadiego, and K.M. Rich. 1990. Sciatic nerve regeneration across gaps within silicone chambers: Long-term effects of NGF and consideration of axonal branching. *Exp. Neurol.* 110:45–51.

Holmes, W. and J.Z. Young. 1942. Nerve regeneration after immediate and delayed suture. *J. Anat. (London)* 77:63–96.

Hoppen, H.J., J.W. Leenslag, A.J. Pennings, B. van der Lei, and P.H. Robinson. 1990. Two-ply biodegradable nerve guide: Basic aspects of design, construction and biological performance. *Biomater.* 11:286–290.

Horne, R.S.C., J.V. Hurley, D.M. Crowe, M. Ritz, B.M. O'Brien, and L.I. Arnold. 1992. Wound healing in foetal sheep: A histological and electron microscopic study. *Br. J. Plast. Surg.* 45:333–344.

Hsu, W.-C., M.H. Spilker, I.V. Yannas, and P.A.D. Rubin. 2000. Inhibition of conjunctival scarring and contraction by a porous collagen-GAG implant. *Invest. Ophthalmol. Vis. Sci.* 41:2404–2411.

Huang, C. 1974. Physicochemical studies of collagen and collagen-mucopolysaccharide composite materials. D. Sc. thesis, Massachussetts Institute of Technology, Cambridge, MA.

Huang, C. and I.V. Yannas. 1977. Mechanochemical studies of enzymatic degradation of insoluble collagen fibers. *J. Biomed. Mater. Res.* 11:137–154.

Hubbell, J.A. 2000. Matrix effects. In *Principles of Tissue Engineering*, edited by Lanza, R.P., R. Langer, and J. Vacanti. San Diego: Academic Press.

Hull, B.E., S.E. Sher, S. Rosen, D. Church, and E. Bell. 1983a. Fibroblasts in isogeneic skin equivalents persist for long periods after grafting. *J. Invest. Dermatol.* 81: 436–438.

Hull, B.E., S.E. Sher, S. Rosen, D. Church, and E. Bell. 1983b. Structural integration of skin equivalents grafted to Lewis and Sprague-Dawley rats. *J. Invest. Dermatol.* 81:429–436.

Hunter, J.A.A. and J.B. Finlay. 1976. Scanning electron microscopy of normal scar tissue and keloids. *Br. J. Plasto. Surg.* 63:826–830.

Hurtado, H., B. Knoops, and P. Van den Bousch de Aguilar. 1987. Rat sciatic nerve regeneration in semipermeable artificial tubes. *Exp. Neurol.* 97:751–757.

Hynes, R.O. 1990. *Fibronectins*. New York: Springer-Verlag.

Igel, H.J., A.E. Freeman, C.R. Boeckman, and K.L. Kleinfeld. 1974. A new method for covering large surface area wounds with autografts II: Surgical application of tissue culture expanded rabbit-skin autografts. *Arch. Surg.* 108:724–729.

Ignotz, R.A. and J. Massague. 1986. Transforming growth factor-β stimulates the expression of fibronectin and collagen and their incorporation into extracellular matrix. *J. Biol. Chem.* 261:4337–4340.

Ikeda, K., Y. Oda, K. Tomita, S. Nomura, and I. Nakanishi. 1989. Isolated Schwann cells can synthesize the basement membrane in vitro. *J. Electron Miscrosc. (Tokyo)* 38:230–234.

Illingworth, C.M. 1974. Trapped fingers and amputated finger tips in children. *J. Pediatr. Surg.* 9:853–858.

Inoue, M., G. Kratz, A. Haegerstrand, and M. Stahle-Backdahl. 1995. Collagenase expression is rapidly induced in wound-edge keratinocytes after acute injury in human skin, persists during healing, and stops at re-epithelialization. *J. Invest. Dermatol.* 104:479–483.

Ippolito, E., P.G. Natali, F. Postacchini, L. Acccinni, and C. DeMartino. 1980. Morphological, immunochemical and biochemical study of rabbit Achilles tendon at various ages. *J. Bone Joint Surg.* 62A:583–598.

Itoh, S., K. Takakuda, H. Samejima, T. Ohta, K. Shinomiya, and S. Ichinose. 1999. Synthetic collagen fibers coated with a synthetic peptide containing the YISGR sequence of laminin to promote peripheral nerve regeneration in vivo. *J. Mater. Sci. Mat. Med.* 10:129–134.

Jenq, C.-B. and R.E. Coggeshall. 1984. Effects of sciatic nerve regeneration and axonal populations in tributary nerves. *Brain Res.* 295:91–100.

Jenq, C.-B. and R.E. Coggeshall. 1985a. Numbers of regenerating axons in parent and tributary peripheral nerves in the rat. *Brain Res.* 326:27–40.

Jenq, C.-B. and R.E. Coggeshall. 1985b. Long-term patterns of axon regeneration in the sciatic nerve and its tributaries. *Brain Res.* 345:34–44.

Jenq, C.-B. and R.E. Coggeshall. 1985c. Nerve regeneration through holey silicone tubes. *Brain Res.* 361:233–241.

Jenq, C.-B. and R.E. Coggeshall. 1987. Permeable tubes increase the length of the gap that regenerating axons can span. *Brain Res.* 408:239–242.

Jenq, C.-B., L.L. Jenq, and R.E. Coggeshall. 1987. Nerve regeneration changes with filters of different pore size. *Exp. Neurol.* 97:662–671.

Joseph, J. and M. Dyson. 1966. Tissue replacement in the rabbit's ear. *Brit. J. Surg.* 53:372–380.

Kaiser, J. 1996. IOM backs cautious experimentation. *Science* 273:305–306.

Kangesu, T., H.A. Navsaria, S. Manek, C.B. Shurey, C.R. Jones, P.R. Fryer, I.M. Leigh, and C.J. Green. 1993a. A porcine model using skin graft chambers for studies on cultured keratinocytes. *Br. J. Plast. Surg.* 46:393–400.

Kangesu, T., H.A. Navsaria, S. Manek, P.R. Fryer, I.M. Leigh, and C.J. Green. 1993b. Kerato-dermal grafts: The importance of dermis for the in vivo growth of cultured keratinocytes. *Br. J. Plast. Surg.* 46:401–409.

Karasek, M.A. 1966. In vitro culture of human skin epithelial cells. *J. Invest. Dermatol.* 47:533–540.

Karasek, M.A. 1968. Growth and differentiation of transplanted epithelial cell cultures. *J. Invest. Dermatol.* 51:247–252.

Kauppila, T., E. Jyväsjärvi, T. Huopaniemi, E. Hujanen, and P. Liesi. 1993. A laminin graft replaces neurorrhaphy in the restorative surgery of the rat sciatic nerve. *Exp. Neurol.* 123:181–191.

Keeley, R.D., K.D. Nguyen, M. Stephanides, J. Padilla, and J.M. Rosen. 1991. The artificial nerve graft: A comparison of blended elastomer hydrogel with polyglycolic acid conduits. *J. Reconstr. Microsurg.* 7:93–100.

Kefalides, N.A. and R. Alper. 1988. Structure and organization of macromolecules in basement membranes. In *Collagen*, edited by Nimni, M.E. Boca Raton: CRC Press.

Kennedy, D.F. and W.J. Cliff. 1979. A systematic study of wound contraction in mammalian skin. *Pathol.* 11:207–222.

Kiernan, J.A. 1979. Hypotheses concerned with axonal regeneration in the mammalian nervous system. *Biol. Revs.* 54:155–197.

Kiistala, U. 1972. Dermal-epidermal separation. *Ann. Clin. Res.* 4:10–22.

Kim, D.H., S.E. Connolly, S. Zhao, R.W. Beuerman, R.M. Voorhies, and D.G. Kline. 1993. Comparison of macropore, semipermeable, and nonpermeable collagen conduits in nerve repair. *J. Reconstr. Microsurg.* 9:415–420.

Kim, D.H., S.E. Connoly, D.G. Kline, R.M. Voorhies, A. Smith, M. Powell, T. Yoes, and J.K. Daniloff. 1994. Labeled Schwann cell transplants versus sural nerve grafts in nerve repair. *J. Neurosurg.* 80:254–260.

Kim, J.P., K. Zhang, R.H. Kramer, T.J. Schall, and D.T. Woodley. 1992. Integrin receptors and RGD sequences in human keratinocyte migration: Unique anitmigratory function of $\alpha 3\beta 1$. *J. Clin. Invest.* 98:764–770.

Kiviat, M.D., R. Ross, and J.S. Ansell. 1973. Smooth muscle regeneration in the ureter. *Am. J. Pathol.* 72:403–416.

Kivirikko, K.I. and R. Myllylä. 1984. Biosynthesis of the collagens. In *Extracellular Matrix Biochemistry*, edited by Piez, K.A. and A.H. Reddi. New York: Elsevier.

Kiyotani, T., M. Teramachi, Y. Takimoto, T. Nakamura, Y. Shimizu, and K. Endo. 1996. Nerve regeneration across a 25-mm gap bridged by a polyglycolic acid-collagen tube: A histological and electrophysiological evaluation of regenerated nerves. *Brain Res.* 740:66–74.

Klagsbrun, M. 1989. The fibroblast growth factor family: Structure and biological properties. *Prog. Growth Factor Res.* 1:207–235.

Kline, D.G. and G.J. Hayes. 1964. The use of resorbable wrapper for peripheral nerve repair. *J. Neurosurg.* 21:737–750.

Klingbeil, C.K., L.B. Cesar, and J.C. Fiddes. 1991. Basic fibroblast growth factor accelerated tissue repair in models of impaired wound healing. In *Clinical and Experimental Approaches to Dermal and Epidermal Repair: Normal and Chronic Wounds*, edited by Barbul, A., M. Caldwell, W. Eaglstein, T. Hunt, D. Marshall, E. Pines, and G. Skover. New York: Alan R. Liss.

Kljavin, I.J. and R.D. Madison. 1991. Peripheral nerve regeneration within tubular prostheses: Effects of laminin and collagen matrices on cellular ingrowth. *Cells & Mater.* 1:17–28s.

Knapp, T.R., J.R. Daniels, and E.N. Kaplan. 1977. Pathologic scar formation. *Am. J. Pathol.* 80:47–63.

Knoops, B., H. Hurtado, and P.B. Aguilar. 1990. Rat sciatic nerve regeneration within an acrylic semipermeable tube and comparison with a silicone impermeable material. *J. Neuropath. Exp. Neurol.* 49:438–448.

Kohn, D.H. and P. Ducheyne. 1992. Materials for bone and joint replacement. In *Materials Science and Technology*, edited by Williams, D.F. New York: VCH Publishers.

Konig, A. and L. Bruckner-Tuderman. 1991. Epithelial-mesenchymal interactions enhance expression of collagen VII in vitro. *J. Invest. Dermatol.* 96:803–808.

Krawczyk, W.S. and G. Wilgram. 1973. Hemidesmosome and desmosome morphogenesis during epidermal wound healing. *J. Ultrastruct. Res.* 45:93–101.

Krikorian, D., M. Manthorpe, and S. Varon. 1982. Purified mouse Schwann cells: Mitogenic effects of fetal calf serum and fibrobalst growth factor. *Dev. Neurosci.* 5:77–91.

Kronick, P.L. and P.R. Buechler. 1986. Fiber orientation in calfskin by laser light scattering or x-ray diffraction and quantitative relation to mechanical properties. *J. Amer. Leather Chem. Assoc.* 81:221–230.

Krummel, T.M., J.M. Nelson, R.F. Diegelmann, W.J. Lindblad, A.M. Salzberg, L.J. Greenfield, and I.K. Cohen. 1987. Fetal response to injury in the rabbit. *J. Pediatr. Surg.* 22:640–644.

Krummel, T.M., B.A. Michna, B.L. Thomas, M.B. Sporn, J.M. Nelson, A.M. Salzberg, I.K. Cohen, and R.F. Diegelmann. 1988. Transforming growth factor beta (TGF-beta) induced fibrosis in a fetal wound model. *J. Pediatr. Surg.* 23:647–652.

Krummel, T.M., H.P. Ehrlich, J.M. Nelson, B.A. Michna, B.L. Thomas, J.M. Haynes, I.K. Cohen, and R.F. Diegelmann. 1989. Fetal wounds do not contract in utero. *Surg. Forum* 40:613–614.

Krummel, T.M., H.P. Ehrlich, J.M. Nelson, B.A. Michna, B.L. Thomas, J.H. Haynes, L.K. Cohen, and R.F. Diegelmann. 1993. In vitro and in vivo analysis of the inability of fetal rabbit wounds to contract. *Wound Rep. Reg.* 1:15–21.

Ksander, G.A., G.H. Chu, H. McMullin, Y. Ogawa, B.M. Pratt, J.S. Rosenblatt, and J.M. McPherson. 1990. Transforming growth factors-beta1 and beta2 enhance connective tissue formation in animal models of dermal wound healing by secondary intent. *Ann. NY Acad. Sci.* 593:135–147.

Labrador, R.O., M. Butí, and X. Navarro. 1995. Peripheral nerve repar: Role of agarose matrix density on functional recovery. *NeuroReport* 6:2022–2026.

Labrador, R.O., M. Butí, and X. Navarro. 1998. Influence of collagen and laminin gels concentration on nerve regeneration after resection and tube repair. *Exp. Neurol.* 149:243–252.

Langer, R. and J.P. Vacanti. 1993. Tissue engineering. *Science* 260:920–928.

Lanning, D.A., B.C. Nwomeh, S.J. Montante, D.R. Yager, R.F. Diegelmann, and J.H. Haynes. 1999. TGF-beta1 alters the healing of cutaneous fetal excisional wounds. *J. Pediatr. Surg.* 34:695–700.

Lanning, D.A., R.F. Diegelmann, D.R. Yager, M.L. Wallace, C.E. Bagwell, and J.H. Haynes. 2000. Myofibroblast induction with transforming growth factor beta1 and beta3 in cutaneous fetal excisional wounds. *J. Pediatr. Surg.* 35:183–187.

Lanza, R.P. and W.L. Chick. 1997. Endocrinology: Pancreas. In *Principles of Tissue Engineering*, edited by Lanza, R.P., R. Langer, and W.L. Chick. San Diego: Academic Press.

Lanza, R.P., D.K.C. Cooper, and W.L. Chick. 1997a. Xenotransplantation. *Sci. Am.* (July):54–59.

Lanza, R.P., R. Langer, and W.L. Chick, eds. 1997b. *Principles of Tissue Engineering.* 1st ed. San Diego: Academic Press.

Lanza, R.P., R. Langer, and J. Vacanti, eds. 2000. *Principles of Tissue Engineering.* 2nd ed. San Diego: Academic Press.

Latarjet, J., M. Gangolphe, G. Hezez, C. Masson, P.Y. Chomel, J.B. Cognet, J.P. Galoisy, R. Joly, A. Robert, J.L. Foyatier, et al. 1987. The grafting of burns with cultured epidermis as autografts in man. *Scand. J. Plast. Reconstr. Surg.* 21:241–244.

Lau, H.T., A. Fontana, and C.J. Stoeckert. 1996. Prevention of islet allograft rejection wih engineered myoblasts expressing FasL in mice. *Science* 273:109–112.

Lavker, R.M. 1979. Structural alterations in exposed and unexposed aged skin. *J. Invest. Dermatol.* 73:59–66.

Le Beau, J.M., M.H. Ellisman, and H.C. Powell. 1988. Ultrastructural and morphometric analysis of long-term peripheral nerve regeneration through silicone tubes. *J. Neurocytol.* 17:161–172.

Lehv, M. and P.J. Fitzgerald. 1968. Pancreatic acinar cell regeneration IV: Regeneration after surgical resection. *Am. J. Pathol.* 53:513–535.

Leigh, I.M., P.E. Purkis, H.A. Navsaria, and T.J. Phillips. 1987. Treatment of chronic venous ulcers with sheets of cultured allogenic keratinocytes. *Br. J. Dermatol.* 117:591–597.

Leipziger, L.S., V. Glushko, B. DiBernardo, F. Shafaie, J. Noble, J. Nichols, and O.M. Alvarez. 1985. Dermal wound repair: Role of collagen matrix implants and synthetic polymer dressings. *J. Am. Acad. Dermatol.* 12:409–419.

Lever, W.F. and G. Schaumburg-Lever. 1990. *Histopathology of the Skin.* 7th ed. Philadelphia: J.B. Lippincott.

Levi-Montalcini, R. and V. Hamburger. 1951. Selective growth stimulating effects of mouse sarcoma on sensory and sympathetic nervous system of the chick embryo. *J. Exp. Zool.* 116:321–362.

Levine, J.H., H.J. Moses, L.I. Gold, and L.B. Nanney. 1993. Spatial and temporal patterns of immunoreactive transforming growth factor beta1, beta2, and beta3 during excisional wound repair. *Am. J. Pathol.* 143:368–380.

Lillie, J.H., D.K. MacCallum, and A. Jepsen. 1988. Growth of stratified squamous epithelium on reconstituted extracellular matrices: Long-term culture. *J. Invest. Dermatol.* 90:100–109.

Lim, F. and A.M. Sun. 1980. Microencapsulated islets as bioartificial endocrine pancreas. *Science* 210:908–910.

Lin, K.Y., J.C. Posnick, M.M. al-Qattan, J. Vajsar, and L.E. Becker. 1994. Fetal nerve healing: An experimental study. *Plast. Reconstr. Surg.* 93:1323–1333.

Lindquist, G. 1946. The healing of skin defects: An experimental study on the white rat. *Acta Chir. Scand.* 94 (suppl. 107):1–163.

Liuzzi, F.J. and R.J. Lasek. 1987. Astrocytes block axonal regeneration in mammals by activating the physiological stop pathway. *Science* 237:642–645.

Longaker, M.T. and N.S. Adzick. 1991. The biology of fetal wound healing: A review. *Plast. Reconstr. Surg.* 87:788–798.

Longaker, M.T., D.A.R. Burd, A.M. Gown, T.S.B. Yen, R.W. Jennings, B.W. Duncan, M.R. Harrison, and N.S. Adzick. 1991a. Midgestation fetal lamb wounds contract in utero. *J. Pediatr. Surg.* 26:942–948.

Longaker, M.T., D.J. Whitby, R.W. Jennings, B.W. Duncan, M.W.J. Ferguson, M.R. Harrison, and N.S. Adzick. 1991b. Fetal diaphragmatic wounds heal with scar formation. *J. Surg. Res.* 50:375–385.

Longaker, M.T., E.S. Chiu, N.S. Adzick, M. Stern, M.R. Harrison, and R. Stern. 1991c. Studies on fetal wound healing V: A prolonged presence of hyaluronic acid characterizes fetal wound fluid. *Ann. Surg.* 213:292–296.

Longaker, M.T., B.R.W. Moelleken, J.C. Cheng, R.W. Jennings, N.S. Adzick, J. Mintorovich, D.G. Levinsohn, L. Gordon, M.R. Harrison, and D.J. Simmons. 1992. Fetal fracture healing in a lamb model. *Plast. Reconstr. Surg.* 90:161–171.

Longaker, M.T., K.S. Bouhana, and M.R. Harrison. 1994. Wound healing in the fetus. Possible role for macrophages and transforming growth factor-beta isoforms. *Wound Rep. Reg.* 2:104–112.

Longo, F.M., S.D. Skaper, M. Manthorpe, L.R. Williams, G. Lundborg, and S. Varon. 1983a. Temporal changes of neuronotrophic activities accumulating in vivo within nerve regeneration chambers. *Exp. Neurol.* 81:756–769.

Longo, F.M., M. Manthorpe, S.D. Skaper, G. Lundborg, and S. Varon. 1983b. Neuronotrophic activities accumulate in vivo within silicone nerve regeneration chambers. *Brain Res.* 261:109–117.

Lorenz, C., A. Petracic, H.-P. Hohl, L. Wessel, and K.-L. Waag. 1997. Early wound closure and early reconstruction: Experience with a dermal substitute in a child with 60 per cent surface area burn. *Burns* 23:505–508.

Lorenz, H.P. and N.S. Adzick. 1993. Scarless skin wound repair in the fetus. *West. J. Med.* 159:350–355.

Lorenz, H.P., M.T. Longaker, L.A. Perkocha, R.W. Jennings, M.R. Harrison, and N.S. Adzick. 1992. Scarless wound repair: A human fetal skin model. *Development* 114:253–259.

Lovvorn, H.N., D.L. Cass, K.G. Sylvester, E.Y. Yang, T.M. Crombleholme, N.S. Adzick, and R.C. Savani. 1998. Hyaluronan receptor expression increases in fetal excisional skin wounds and correlates with fibroplasia. *J. Pediatr. Surg.* 33:1062–1069.

Luccioli, G.M., D.S. Kahn, and H.R. Robertson. 1964. Histologic study of wound contraction in the rabbit. *Ann. Surg.* 160:1030–1040.

Lui, S.C. and M. Karasek. 1978. Isolation and serial cultivation of rabbit skin epithelial cells. *J. Invest. Dermatol.* 70:288–293.

Lundborg, G. 1987. Nerve regeneration and repair. *Acta Orthop. Scand.* 58:145–169.

Lundborg, G. 1988. The nerve chamber as an experimental tool. In *In Nerve Injury and Repair*, edited by Lundborg, G. New York: Churchill Livingstone.

Lundborg, G. 2000. A 25-year perspective of peripheral nerve surgery: evolving neuroscientific concepts and clinical significance. *J. Hand Surg.* 25:391–414.

Lundborg, G., L.B. Fahlin, N. Danielsen, R.H. Gelberman, F.M. Longo, H.C. Powell, and S. Varon. 1982a. Nerve regeneration in silicone model chambers: Influence of gap length and of distal stump components. *Exp. Neurol.* 76:361–375.

Lundborg, G., L.B. Dahlin, N. Danielsen, A. Johannesson, H.A. Hansson, F. Longo, and S. Varon. 1982b. Nerve regeneration across an extended gap: A neuronobiological view of nerve repair and the possible involvement of neuronotrophic factors. *J. Hand Surg.* 7:580–587.

Lundborg, G., R.H. Gelberman, F.M. Longo, H.C. Powell, and S. Varon. 1982c. In vivo regeneration of cut nerves encased in silicone tubes: Growth across a six-millimeter gap. *J. Neuropathol. Exp. Neurol.* 41:412–422.

Lundborg, G., F.M. Longo, and S. Varon. 1982d. Nerve regeneration model and trophic factors in vivo. *Brain Res.* 232:157–161.

Lundborg, G., L.B. Dahlin, and N. Danielsen. 1991. Ulnar nerve repair by the silicone chamber technique. *Scand. J. Plast. Reconstr. Hand Surg.* 25:79–82.

Lundborg, G., B. Rosén, S.O. Abrahamson, L. Dahlin, and N. Danielsen. 1994. Tubular repair of the median nerve in the human forearm. *J. Hand Surg. (Br. Eur.)* 19B:273–276.

Lundborg, G., L. Dahlin, D. Dohi, M. Kanje, and N.Terada. 1997. A new type of "bioartificial" nerve graft for bridging extended defects in nerves. *J. Hand Surg. (Br. Eur.)* 22B:299–303.

Mackinnon, S.E. and A.L. Dellon. 1990. A study of nerve regeneration across synthetic (Maxon) and biologic (collagen) nerve conduits for nerve gaps up to 5 cm in the primate. *J. Reconstr. Microsurg.* 6:117–121.

Mackinnon, S.E., A.L. Dellon, A.R. Hudson, and D.A. Hunter. 1986. Chronic human nerve compresion: A histological assessment. *Neuropathol. Appl. Neurobiol.* 12:547–565.

Madden, J.W. 1972. Wound healing: Biologic and clinical features. In *Textbook of Surgery*, edited by Sabison, D. Philadelphia: W.B. Saunders.

Madison, R.D. and S.J. Archibald. 1994. Point sources of Schwann cells result in growth into a nerve entubulation repair site in the absence of axons: Effects of freeze thawing. *Exp. Neurol.* 128:266–275.

Madison, R.D., C.F.D. Silva, P. Dikkes, T.-H. Chiu, and R.L. Sidman. 1985. Increased rate of peripheral nerve regeneration using bioresorbable nerve guides and a laminin-containing gel. *Exp. Neurol.* 88:767–772.

Madison, R.D., C.F.D. Silva, and P. Dikkes. 1988. Entubulation repair with protein additives increases the maximum nerve gap distance successfully bridged with tubular prostheses. *Brain Res.* 447:325–334.

Madison, R.D., S.J. Archibald, and C. Krarup. 1992. Peripheral nerve injury. In *Wound Healing*, edited by Cohen, I.K., R.F. Diegelmann, and W.J. Lindblad. Philadelphia: W.B. Saunders.

Madrazo, A., Y. Suzuki, and J. Churg. 1970. Radiation nephritis II: Radiation changes after high doses of radiation. *Am J. Pathol.* 61:37–56.

Madri, J.A., S. Sankar, and A.M. Romanic. 1996. Angiogenesis. In *The Molecular and Cellular Biology of Wound Repair*, edited by Clark, R.A.F. New York: Plenum Press.

Majno, G. 1982. *The Healing Hand. Man and Wound in the Ancient World.* Cambridge, MA: Harvard University Press.

Majno, G., G. Gabbiani, B.J. Hirschel, G. Ryan, and P.R. Statkov. 1971. Contraction of granulation tissue in vitro: Similarity to smooth muscle. *Science* 173:548–550.

Mak, V.H.W., M.B. Cumpstone, A.H. Kennedy, C.S. Harmon, R.H. Guy, and R.O. Potts. 1991. Barrier function of human keratinocyte cultures grown at the air-liquid interface. *J. Invest. Dermatol.* 96:323–327.

Mann, P. and H. Constable. 1977. Induction of basal lamina formation in epidermal cell cultures in vitro. *Br. J. Dermatol.* 96:421–426.

Marinkovich, M.P., D.R. Keene, C.S. Rimberg, and R.E. Burgeson. 1993. Cellular origin of the dermal-epidermal basement membrane. *Dev. Dyn.* 197:255–267.

Marinkovich, M.P., C.L. Peavey, R.E. Burgeson, and D.T. Woodley. 1994. Kalinin inhibits collagen-driven human keratinocyte migration. *J. Clin. Invest.* 102:157.

Marks, R., E. Abell, and T. Nishikawa. 1975. The junctional zone beneath migrating epidermis. *Br. J. Dermatol.* 92:311–319.

Martin, P. 1996. Mechanisms of wound healing in the embryo and fetus. *Curr. Top. Dev. Biol.* 32:175–203.

Martin, P. 1997. Wound healing: Aiming for perfect skin regeneration. *Science* 276:75–81.

Martinez-Hernandez, A. 1988. Repair, regeneration and fibrosis. In *Pathology*, edited by Rubin, E. and J.L. Farber. Philadelphia: J.B. Lippincott.

Massagué, J. and B. Like. 1985. Cellular receptors for type-b transforming growth factor. *J. Biol. Chem.* 260:2636–2645.

Mast, B.A. 1992. The skin. In *Wound Healing*, edited by Cohen, I.K., R.F. Diegelmann, and W.J. Lindblad. Philadelphia: W.B. Saunders.

Mast, B.A., R.F. Diegelmann, T.M. Krummel, and I.K. Cohen. 1992a. Scarless wound healing in the mammalian fetus. *Surg. Gynecol. Obstet.* 174:441–451.

Mast, B.A., J.M. Neslon, and T.M. Krummel. 1992b. Tissue repair in the mammalian fetus. In *Wound Healing*, edited by Cohen, I.K., R.F. Diegelmann, and W.J. Lindblad. Philadelphia: W.B. Saunders.

Masur, S.K., H.S. Dewal, T.T. Dinh, I. Erenburg, and S. Petridou. 1996. Myofibroblasts differentiate from fibroblasts when plated at low density. *Proc. Natl. Acad. Sci. USA* 93:4219–4223.

Mayr, E. 1996. *This Is Biology*. Cambridge, MA: Bellknap/Harvard University Press.

McCallion, R.L. and M.W.J. Ferguson. 1996. Fetal wound healing and the development of antiscarring therapies for adult wound healing. In *The Molecular and Cellular Biology of Wound Repair*, edited by Clark, R.A.F. New York: Plenum Press.

McGarvey, M.L., A.G.V. Evercooren, H.K. Kleinman, and M. Dubois-Dalcq. 1984. Synthesis and effects of basement membrane components in cultured rat Schwann cells. *Dev. Biol.* 105:18–28.

McGrath, M.H. 1982. The effect of prostaglandin inhibitors on wound contraction and the myofibroblast. *Plast. Reconstr. Surg.* 69:71–83.

McMinn, R.M.H. 1969. *Tissue Repair*. New York: Academic Press.

McNeil, P.L. and S. Ito. 1990. Molecular traffic through plasma membrane disruptions of cells in vivo. *J. Cell Sci.* 96:549–556.

McNeil, P.L., L. Muthukrishnan, E. Warder, and P.A. D'Amore. 1989. Growth factors are released by mechanically wounded endothelial cells. *J. Cell Biol.* 109:811–822.

McNeil, P.L., S.S. Vogel, K. Miyake, and M. Terasaki. 2000. Patching plasma membrane disruptions with cytoplasmic membrane. *J. Cell Sci.* 113:1891–1902.

McPherson, J.M. and K.A. Piez, eds. 1988. *Collagen in Dermal Wound Repair.* Edited by Clark, R.A.F. 2nd ed. New York: Plenum Press.

Medawar, P.B. 1944. The behavior and fate of skin autografts and skin homografts in rabbits. *J. Anat.* 78:176–199.

Medawar, P.B. 1954. The storage of living skin. *Proc. Roy. Soc. Med.* 47:62–64.

Mellin, T.N., R.J. Mennie, D.E. Cashen, J.J. Ronan, J. Capparella, M.L. James, J. Disalvo, J. Frank, D. Linemeyer, G. Gimenez-Gallego, and K.A. Thomas. 1992. Acid fibroblast growht factor accelerates dermal wound healing. *Growth Factors* 7:1–14.

Merle, M., A.L. Dellon, J.N. Campbell, and P.S. Chang. 1989. Complications from silicon polymer intubulation of nerves. *Microsurg.* 10:130–133.

Meuli-Simmen, C., M. Meuli, C.D. Yingling, T. Eiman, G.B. Timmel, H.J. Buncke, W. Lineaweaver, and M.R. Harrison. 1997. Midgestational sciatic nerve transection in fetal sheep results in absent nerve regeneration and neurogenic muscle atrophy. *Plast. Reconstr. Surg.* 99:486–492.

Michaeli, D. and M. McPherson. 1990. Immunologic study of artificial skin used in the treatment of thermal injuries. *J. Burn Care & Rehab.* 11:21–26.

Michalopoulos, G.K. 1990. Liver regeneration: Molecular mechanisms and growth control. *FASEB J.* 4:176–187.

Michalopoulos, G.K. and M.C. DeFrances. 1997. Liver regeneration. *Science* 276:60–66.

Mikuz, G., G. Hoinkes, A. Propst, and P. Wilflingseder. 1984. Tissue reactions with silicone rubber implants (morphological, microchemical, and clinical investigations in humans and laboratory animals). In *Macromolecular Biomaterials,* edited by Hastings, G.W., and P. Ducheyne. Boca Raton: CRC Press.

Miller, E.J. 1984. Chemistry of the collagens and their distribution. In *Extracellular Matrix Biochemistry,* edited by Piez, K.A., and A.H. Reddi. New York: Elsevier.

Millesi, H. 1967. Erfahrungen mit der Mikrochirurgie peripherer Nerven. *Chir. Plast. Reconstr.* 3:47–55.

Millesi, H., G. Meissl, and G. Berger. 1972. The interfascicular nerve grafting of the median and ulnar nerves. *J. Bone Joint Surg.* 54-A:727–750.

Millesi, H., G. Meissl, and G. Berger. 1976. Further experience with interfascicular grafting of the median, ulnar and radial nerves. *J. Bone Joint Surg.* 58-A:209–216.

Molander, H., O. Engkvist, J. Hagglund, Y. Olsson, and E. Torebjork. 1983. Nerve repair using a polyglactin tube and nerve graft: An experimnetal study in the rabbit. *Biomaterials* 4:276–280.

Morris, J.A., A.F. Hudson, and G. Weddell. 1972a. A study of degeneration and regeneration in the divided rat sciatic nerve based on electron microscopy I: The traumatic degeneration of myelin in the proximal stump of the divided nerve. *Z. Zellforsch.* 124:76–102.

Morris, J.A., A.F. Hudson, and G. Weddell. 1972b. A study of degeneration and regeneration in the divided rat sciatic nerve based on electron microscopy II: The development of the "regenerating unit." *Z. Zellforsch.* 124:103–130.

Morris, J.A., A.F. Hudson, and G. Weddell. 1972c. A study of degeneration and regeneration in the divided rat sciatic nerve based on electron microscopy III: Changes in the axons of the proximal stump. *Z. Zellforsch.* 124:131–164.

Morris, J.A., A.F. Hudson, and G. Weddell. 1972d. A study of degeneration and regeneration in the divided rat sciatic nerve based on electron microscopy IV: Changes in fascicular microtopography, perineurium and endoneurial fibroblasts. *Z. Zellforsch.* 124:165–203.

Moss, T.H. and S.J. Lewkowicz. 1981. A comparative scanning electron-microscopical study of endoneurial collagen around normal mouse nerve fibres, nerve fibres following crush injury and nerve fires of the dystonic mouse mutant (dt/dt). *Cell Tissue Res.* 220:881–887.

Moya, F., M.B. Bunge, and R.P. Bunge. 1980. Schwann cells proliferate but fail to differentiate in defined medium. *Proc. Natl. Acad. Sci. USA* 77:6902–6906.

Müller, H., K. Shibib, H. Friedrich, and M. Modrack. 1987a. Evoked muscle action potentials from regenerated rat tibial and peroneal nerves: Synthetic versus autologous interfascicular grafts. *Exp. Neurol.* 95:21–33.

Munster, A.M. 1992. Use of cultured epidermal autograft in ten patients. *J. Burn Care Rehabil.* 13:124–126.

Munster, A.M. 1996. Cultured skin for massive burns. *Ann. Surg.* 224:372–377.

Murphy, G.F., D.P. Orgill, and I.V. Yannas. 1990. Partial dermal regeneration is induced by biodegradable collagen-glycosaminoglycan grafts. *Lab. Invest.* 62:305–313.

Murray, J.E., J.P. Merrill, and J.H. Harrison. 1955. Renal homotransplantation in identical twins. *Surg. For.* 6:432–436.

Mustoe, T.A., G.F. Pierce, C. Morishima, and T.F. Deuel. 1991. Growth-factor induced acceleration of tissue repair through direct and inductive activities in a rabbit dermal ulcer model. *J. Clin. Invest.* 87:694–703.

Myers, R.R., H.M. Heckman, and H.C. Powell. 1983. Endoneurial fluid is hypertonic. *J. Neuropath. Exp. Neurol.* 42:217–224.

Nanney, L.B. 1990. Epidermal and dermal effects of epidermal growth factor during wound repair. *J. Invest. Dermatol.* 94:624–629.

Nanney, L.B. and L.E. King, Jr. 1996. Epidermal growth and transforming growth factor–α. In *The Molecular and Cellular Biology of Wound Repair*, edited by Clark, R.A.F. New York: Plenum Press.

Nanney, L.B., C.M. Stoschek, L.E. King, Jr., R.A. Underwood, and K.A. Holbrook. 1990. Immunolocalization of epidermal growth factor receptors in normal developing human skin. *J. Invest. Dermatol.* 94:742–748.

Nath, R.K., B. Kwon, S.E. McKinnon, J.N. Jensen, S. Reznik, and S. Boutros. 1998. Antibody to transforming growth factor beta reduces collagen production in injured peripheral nerve. *Plast. Reconstr. Surg.* 102:1100–1106.

Nathaniel, E.L. and D.C. Pease. 1963. Degenerative changes in rat dorsal roots following Wallerian degeneration. *J. Ultrastruct. Res.* 9:511–532.

Naughton, G., J. Mansbridge, and G. Gentzkow. 1997. A metabolically active human dermal replacement for the treatment of diabetic foot ulcers. *Artif. Org.* 21:1–7.

Navarro, X., F.J. Rodríguez, R.O. Labrador, M. Butí, D. Ceballos, N. Gómez, J. Cuadra, and G. Perego. 1996. Peripheral nerve regeneration through bioresorbable and durable nerve guides. *J. Peripheral Nerv. Syst.* 1:53–64.

Nesbitt, J.A. and R.D. Acland. 1980. Histopathological changes following removal of the perineurium. *J. Neurosurg.* 53:233–238.

Neuman, M.R. 1998. Therapeutic and prosthetic devices. In *Medican Instrumentation*, edited by Webster, J.G. New York: Wiley.

Nimni, M.E. 1983. Collagen: Structure, function, and metabolism in normal and fibrotic tissues. *Sem. Arthr. Rheum.* 13:1–86.

Nimni, M.E., ed. 1988. *Biochemistry*. Vol. 1, *Collagen*. Boca Raton: CRC Press.

Noback, C.R., J. Husby, J.M. Girado, C. Andrew, L. Bassett, and J.B. Campbell. 1958. Neural regeneration across long gaps in mammalian peripheral nerves: Early morphological findings. *Anat. Rec.* 131:633–647.

Nolte, C.J.M., M.A. Oleson, P.R. Bilbo, and N.L. Parenteau. 1993. Development of a stratum corneum and barrier function in an organotypic skin culure. *Arch. Dermatol. Res.* 285:466–474.

Nolte, C.J.M., M.A. Oleson, J.F. Hansbrough, J. Morgan, G. Greenleaf, and L. Wilkins. 1994. Ultrastructural features of composite skin culutres grafted onto athymic mice. *J. Anat.* 185:325–333.

Obremski, V.J. and M.B. Bunge. 1995. Addition of purified basal lamina molecules enables Schwann cell ensheathment of sympathetic neurites in culture. *Dev. Biol.* 168:124–137.

Obremski, V.J., P.M. Wood, and M.B. Bunge. 1993. Fibroblasts promote Schwann cell basal lamina deposition and elongation in the absence of neurons in culture. *Dev. Biol.* 160:119–134.

O'Connor, N.E., J.B. Mulliken, S. Banks-Schlegel, O. Kehinde, and H. Green. 1981. Grafting of burns with cultured epithelium prepared from autologous epidermal cells. *Lancet.* 1:75–78.

Ogawa, M.M., T. Hashimoto, T. Suzuki, and T. Nishikawa. 1990. The establishment of optimum conditions for keratinocytes from human adult skin, and an attempt to graft cultured epidermal sheets onto athymic mice. *Keio J. Med.* 39:14–20.

Ohbayashi, K., H.K. Inoue, A. Awaya, S. Kobayashi, H. Kohga, M. Nakamura, and C. Ohye. 1996. Peripheral nerve regeneration in a silicone tube: Effect of collagen sponge prosthesis, laminin, and pyrimidine compound administration. *Neurol. Med. Chir. (Tokyo)* 36:428–433.

Okamoto, E. and Y. Kitano. 1993. Expression of basement membrane components in skin equivalents: Influence of dermal fibroblasts. *J. Dermatol. Sci.* 5:81–88.

Oliver, J. 1953. Correlations of structure and function and mechanisms of recovery in acute tubular necrosis. *Am. J. Med.* 15:535–557.

Olsson, Y. 1990. Microenvironment of the peripheral nervous system under normal and pathological conditions. *Crit. Revs. Neurobiol.* 5:285–311.

Oppenheimer, R. and F. Hinman. Jr. 1955. Ureteral regeneration: Contracture vs. hyperplasia of smooth muscle. *J. Urol.* 74:476–484.

Orgill, D.P. 1983. The effects of an artificial skin on scarring and contraction in open wounds. Ph.D. thesis, Massachusetts Institute of Technology, Cambridge, MA.

Orgill, D.P. and I.V. Yannas. 1998. Design of an artificial skin IV: Use of island graft to isolate organ regeneration from scar synthesis and other processes leading to skin wound closure. *J. Biomed. Mater. Res.* 36:531–535.

Orgill, D.P., C.E. Butler, and J.F. Regan. 1996. Behavior of collagen-GAG matrices as dermal replacements in rodent and porcine models. *Wounds* 8:151–157.

Orgill, D.P., C. Butler, J.F. Regan, M.S. Barlow, I.V. Yannas, and C.C. Compton. 1998. Vascularized collagen-glycosaminoglycan marix provides a dermal substrate and improves take of cultured epithelial autografts. *Plast. Reconstr. Surg.* 102:423–429.

Pandya, A.N., B. Woodward, and N. Parkhouse. 1998. The use of cultured autologous keratinocytes with Integra in the resurfacing of acute burns. *Plast. Reconstr. Surg.* 102:825–828.

Paralkar, V.M., S. Vukicevic, and A.H. Reddi. 1991. Transforming growth factor type-b1 binds to collagen IV basement membrane matrix: Implications for development. *Dev. Biol.* 143:303–308.

Parenteau, N.L., C.M. Nolte, P. Bilbo, M. Rosenberg, L.M. Wilkins, E.W. Johnson, S. Watson, V.S. Mason, and E. Bell. 1991. Epidermis generated in vitro: Practical considerations and applications. *J. Cell. Biochem.* 45:245–251.

Parenteau, N.L., P. Bilbo, C.J.M. Nolte, V.S. Mason, and M. Rosenberg. 1992. The organotypic culture of human skin keratinocytes and fibroblasts to achieve form and function. *Cytotechnol.* 9:163–171.

Parenteau, N., M. Sabolinski, S. Prosky, C. Nolte, M. Oleson, K. Kriwet, and P. Bilbo. 1996. Biological and physical factors influencing the successful engraftment of a cultured human skin substitute. *Biotechnol. Bioeng.* 52:3–14.

Patience, C., Y. Takeuchi, and R.A. Weiss. 1997. Infection of human cells by an endogenous retrovirus of pigs. *Nature Med.* 3:282–286.

Peacock, Jr., E.E. 1971. Wound healing and care of the wound. In *Manual of Pre-operative and Postoperative Care*. Philadelphia: A.C.S., W.B. Saunders.

Peacock Jr, E.E. 1984. Wound healing and wound care. In *Principles of Surgery*, edited by Schwartz, S.I., G.T. Shires, F.C. Spencer, and E.H. Storer. New York: McGraw-Hill.

Peacock Jr, E.E. and W. Van Winkle, Jr. 1976. *Wound Repair*. Philadelphia: W.B. Saunders.

Peehl, D.M. and R.G. Ham. 1980. Clonal growth of human keratinocytes with small amounts of dialyzed serum. *In Vitro* 16:526–540.

Peppas, N.A. and R. Langer. 1994. New challenges in biomaterials. *Science* 263: 1715–1720.

Petersen, M.J., D.T. Woodley, G.P. Stricklin, and E.J. O'Keefe. 1989. Constitutive production of procollagensae and collagenase inhibitor by human keratinocytes in culture. *J. Invest. Dermatol.* 92:156–159.

Petersen, M.J., D.T. Woodley, G.P. Stricklin, and E.J. O'Keefe. 1990. Enhanced synthesis of collagenase by human keratinocytes cultured on type I or type IV collagen. *J. Invest. Dermatol.* 94:341–346.

Pierce, G.F., J.V. Berg, R. Rudolph, J. Tarpley, and T.A. Mustoe. 1991. Platelet-derived growth factor-BB and transforming growth factor beta 1 selectively modulate glycosaminoglycans, collagen and myofibroblasts in excisional wounds. *Am. J. Pathol.* 138:629–646.

Pierce, G.F., J.E. Tarpley, D. Yanagihara, T.A. Mustoe, G.M. Fox, and A. Thomason. 1992. Platelet-derived growth factor (BB homodimer), transforming growth factor-b1, and basic fibroblast growth factor in dermal wound healing. *Am. J. Pathol.* 140:1375–1388.

Pierschbacher, M.D. and E. Ruoslahti. 1984a. The cell attachment activity of fibronectin can be duplicated by small synthetic fragments of the molecule. *Nature (London)* 309:30–33.

Pierschbacher, M.D. and E. Ruoslahti. 1984b. Variants of the cell recognition site of fibronectin that retain attachment-promoting activity. *Proc. Natl. Acad. Sci. USA* 81:5985–5988.

Piez, K.A., A.H. Reddi, and Eds. 1984. *Extracellular Matrix Biochemistry*. Elsevier: New York.

Pinkus, H. 1952. Examination of the epidermis by the strip method of removing horny layers II: Biometric data on regeneration of the human epidermis. *J. Invest. Dermatol.* 19:431–441.

Pittenger, M.F., A.M. Mackay, S.C. Beck, R.K. Jaiswal, R. Douglas, J.D. Mosca, M.A. Moorman, D.W. Simonetti, S. Craig, and D.R. Marshak. 1999. Multilineage potential of adult human mesenchymal stem cells. *Science* 284:143–147.

Podratz, J.L., E.H. Rodriguez, E.S. DiNonno, and A.J. Windebank. 1998. Myelination by Schwann cells in the absence of extraxellular matrix assembly. *Glia* 23:383–388.

Polezhaev, L.V. 1972. *Loss and Restoration of Regenerative Capacity in Tissues and Organs of Animals*. Jerusalem: Keter Press.

Politis, M.J., K. Ederle, and P.S. Spencer. 1982. Tropism in nerve regeneration in vivo. Attraction of regenerating axons by diffusible factors derived from cells in distal nerve stumps of transected peripheral nerves. *Brain Res.* 253:1–12.

Prockop, D.J. 1997. Marrow stromal cells as stem cells for nonhematopoietic tissues. *Science* 276:71–74.

Prunieras, M. 1975. Culture of the skin: How and why. *Int. J. Dermatol.* 14:12–22.

Prunieras, M., G. Moreno, Y. Dosso and F. Vinzens. 1976. Studies of guinea pig cell cultures V: Co-cultures of pigmented melanocytes and albino keratinocytes, a model for the study of pigmented transfer. *Acta Dermatovener (Stockholm)* 56:1–9.

Prunieras, M., M. Regnier, and M. Schlotterer. 1979. Nouveau procede de culture des cellules epidermiques humaines sur derme homologue ou heterologue: Preparation de greffons recombines. *Ann. Chir. Plast.* 24:357–362.

Pudenz, R.H. 1958. Experimental and clinical observations on the shunting of cerebrospinal fluid into the circulatory system. *Clin. Neurosurg.* 5:98–115.

Puolakkainen, P.A., D.R. Twardzik, J.E. Ranchalis, S.C. Pankey, M.J. Reed, and W.R. Gombotz. 1995. The enhancement in wound healing by transforming growth factor-β1(TGF-β1) depends on the topical delivery system. *J. Surg. Res.* 58:321–329.

Purdue, G.F., J.L. Hunt, J.M. Still Jr, E.J. Law, D.N. Herndon, I.W. Goldfarb, W.R. Schiller, J.F. Hansbrough, W.L. Hickerson, H.N. Himel, et al. 1997. A multicenter clinical trial of a biosynthetic skin replacement, Dermagraft-TC, compared with cryopreserved human cadaver skin for temporary coverage of excised burn wounds. *J. Burn Care Rehab.* 18:52–57.

Racine-Samson, L., D.C. Rockey, and D.M. Bissell. 1997. The role of alpha1beta1 integrin in wound contraction. A quantitative analysis of liver myofibroblasts in vivo and in primary culture. *J. Biol. Chem.* 272:30911–30917.

Ramirez, A.T., H.S. Soroff, M.S. Schwartz, J. Mooty, E. Pearson, and M.S. Raben. 1969. Experimental wound healing in man. *Surg. Gynecol. Obst.* 128(2):283–293.

Regan, M.C. and A. Barbul. 1991. Effect of wound fluid on local and systemic immune responses. In *Clinical and Experimental Approaches to Dermal and Epidermal Repair: Normal and Chronic Wounds*, edited by Barbul, A., M. Caldwell, W. Eaglstein, T. Hunt, D. Marshall, E. Pines, and G. Skover. New York: Alan R. Liss.

Regauer, S. and C. Compton. 1990. Cultured keratinocyte sheets enhance spontaneous re-epithelia-lization in a dermal explant model of partial-thickness wound healing. *J. Invest. Dermatol.* 95:341–346.

Regauer, S., G.R. Seiler, Y. Barrandon, K.W. Easley, and C.C. Compton. 1990. Epithelial origin of cutaneous anchoring fibrils. *J. Cell Biol.* 111:2109–2115.

Regnier, M. and M. Prunieras. 1974. Studies on guinea pig skin cell cultures III: Minimum cell numbers for establishment. *Acta dermatovener (Stockholm)* 54:339–342.

Regnier, M., P. Vaigot, S. Michel, and M. Prunieras. 1985. Localization of bullous pemphigoid antigen (BPA) in isolated human keratinocytes. *J. Invest. Dermatol.* 85:187–190.

Rheinwald, J.G. and H. Green. 1975a. Formation of a keratinizing epithelium in culture by a cloned cell line derived from a teratoma. *Cell* 6:317–330.

Rheinwald, J.G. and H. Green. 1975b. Serial cultivation of strains of human epidermal keratinocytes: The formation of keratinizing colonies from single cells. *Cell* 6:331–343.

Rich, K.M., T.D. Alexander, J.C. Pryor, and J.P. Hollowell. 1989. Nerve growth factor enhances regeneration through silicone chambers. *Exp. Neurol.* 105:162–170.

Rigal, C., M.-T. Pieraggi, C. Vincent, C. Prost, H. Bouissou, and G. Serre. 1991. Healing of full-thickness cutaneous wounds in the pig I: Immunohistochemical study of epidermodermal junction regeneration. *J. Invest. Dermatol.* 96:777–785.

Roberts, A.B. and M.B. Sporn. 1996. Transforming growth factor-β. In *The Molecular and Cellular Biology of Wound Repair*, edited by Clark, R.A.F. New York: Plenum Press.

Roberts, A.B., M.B. Sporn, R.K. Assoian, J.M. Smith, M.S. Roche, U.F. Heine, L. Liotta, V. Falanga, J.H. Kehrl, and A.S. Fauci. 1986. Transforming growth factor beta: Rapid induction of fibrosis and angiogenesis in vivo and stimulation of collagen formation. *Proc. Natl. Acad. Sci. USA* 83:41678–4171.

Robinson, P.H., B. van der Lei, H.J. Hoppen, J. Leenslag, A.J. Pennings, and P. Nieuwenhuis. 1991. Nerve regeneration through a two-ply biodegradable nerve guide in the rat and the influence of ACTH4-9 nerve growth factor. *Microsurg.* 12:412–419.

Rodriguez, F.J., E. Verdu, D. Ceballos, and X. Navarro. 2000. Nerve guides seeded with autologous Schwann cells improve nerve regeneration. *Exp. Neurol.* 161:571–584.

Rosdy, M., A. Pisani, and J.-P. Ortonne. 1993. Production of basement membrane components by a reconstructed epidermis cultured in the absence of serum and dermal factors. *Br. J. Dermatol.* 129:227–234.

Ross, M.H. and E.J. Reith. 1969. Perineurium: Evidence for contractile elements. *Science* 165:604–606.

Ross, R. and E.P. Benditt. 1961. Wound healing and collagen formation I: Sequential changes in componenets of guinea pig skin wounds observed in the electron microscope. *J. Biophys. Biochem. Cytol.* 11:677–700.

Ross, R. and G. Odland. 1968. Human wound repair II: Inflammatory cells, epithelial-mesenchymal interrelations, and fibrogenesis. *J. Cell Biol.* 39:152–168.

Ross, R. and A. Vogel. 1978. The platelet-derived growth factor. *Cell* 14:203–210.

Roy, P., W.M. Petroll, C.J. Chuong, H.D. Cavanaugh, and J.V. Jester. 1999. Effect of cell migration on the maintenance of tension on a collagen matrix. *Ann. Biomed. Engin.* 27:721–730.

Röyttä, M. and V. Salonen. 1988. Long-term endoneurial changes after nerve transection. *Acta Neuropathol. (Berlin)* 76:35–45.

Rubin, E. and J.L. Farber, eds. 1988. *Pathology.* Philadelphia: J.B. Lippincott.

Rudolph, R. 1975. Skin graft preparation and wound contraction. *Surg. For.* 26:560–562.

Rudoph, R. 1979. Location of the force of wound contraction. *Surg. Gynecol. Obst.* 148:547–551.

Rudolph, R. 1980. Contraction and the control of contraction. *World J. Surg.* 4:279–287.

Rudolph, R. and L. Klein. 1973. Healing processes in skin grafts. *Surgery Gynecol. Obst.* 136:641–654.

Rudolph, R., S. Gruber, M. Suzuki, and M. Woodward. 1977. The life cycle of the myofibroblast. *Surg. Gyn. Obst.* 145:389–394.

Rudolph, R., J. Abraham, T. Vecchione, S. Guber, and M. Woodward. 1978. Myofibroblasts and free silicon around breast implants. *Plast. Reconstr. Surg.* 62:185–196.

Rudolph, R., W.J. McClure, and M. Woodward. 1979a. Contracile fibroblasts in chronic alcoholic cirrhosis. *Gastroenterol.* 76:704–709.

Rudolph, R., J.C. Fisher, and J.L. Ninneman. 1979b. *Skin Grafting*. Boston: Little, Brown.

Rudolph, R., J. Van de Berg, and P. Ehrlich. 1992. Wound contraction and scar contracture. In *Wound Healing*, edited by Cohen, I.K., R.F. Diegelmann, and W.J. Lindblad. Philadelphia: W.B. Saunders.

Rutka, J.T., G. Apodaca, R. Stern, and M. Rosenblum. 1988. The extracellular matrix of the central and peripheral nervous systems structure and function. *J. Neurosurg.* 69:155–170.

Ryan, G.B., W.J. Cliff, G. Gabbiani, C. Irle, P.R. Statkov, and G. Majno. 1974. Myofibroblasts in human granulation tissue. *Hum. Pathol.* 5:55–67.

Sabolinski, M.L., O. Alvarez, M. Aulettea, G. Mulder, and N.L. Parenteau. 1996. Cultured skin as a "smart material" for healing wounds experience in venous ulcers. *Biomater.* 17:311–320.

Salonen, V., M. Lehto, A. Vaheri, H. Aro, and J. Peltonen. 1985. Endoneurial fibrosis following nerve transection. An immunohistological study of collagen types and fibronectin in the rat. *Acta Neuropathol. (Berl.)* 67:315–321.

Salonen, V., M. Röyttä, and J. Peltonen. 1987a. The effects of nerve transection on the endoneurial collagen fibril sheaths. *Acta Neuropathol. (Berl.)* 74:13–21.

Salonen, V., J. Peltonen, M. Röyttä, and I. Virtanen. 1987b. Laminin in traumatized peripheral nerve: Basement membrane changes during degeneration and regeneration. *J. Neurocytol.* 16:713–720.

Saltzman, W.M. 2000. Cell interactions with polymers. In *Principles of Tissue Engineering*, edited by Lanza, R.P., R. Langer, and J. Vacanti. San Diego: Academic Press.

Santos, P.M., J. Winterowd, G.G. Allen, M.A. Bothwell, and E.W. Rubel. 1991. Nerve growth factor: Increased angiogenesis without improved nerve regeneration. *Otolaryngol.-Head Neck Surg.* 105:12–25.

Sasagasako, N., M. Ohno, and R.H. Quarles. 1999. Evidence for regulation of myelin protein synthesis by contact between adjacent Schwann cell plasma membranes. *Dev. Neurosci.* 21:417–422.

Sawai, T., N. Usui, K. Sando, Y. Fukui, S. Kamata, A. Okada, N. Taniguchi, N. Itano, and K. Kimata. 1997. Hyaluronic acid of wound fluid in adult and fetal rabbits. *J. Pediatr. Surg.* 32:41–43.

Sawhney, C.P. and H.L. Monga. 1970. Wound contraction in rabbits and the effectiveness of skin grafts in preventing it. *Brit. J. Plast Surg.* 23:318–321.

Scaravilli, F. 1984. Regeneration of the perineurium across a surgically induced gap in a nerve encased in a plastic tube. *J. Anat.* 139:411–424.

Schaffer, C.J., L. Reinisch, S.L. Polis, G.P. Stricklin, and L.B. Nanney. 1997. Comparisons of wound healing among excisional, laser-created and standard thermal burns in porcine wounds of equal depth. *Wound Rep. Regen.* 5:52–61.

Scherman, P., G. Lundborg, M. Kanje, and L.B. Dahlin. 2000. Sutures alone are sufficient to support regeneration across a gap in the continuity of the sciatic nerve in rats. *Scand. J. Plast. Reconstr. Surg. Hand Surg.* 34:1–8.

Schiro, J.A., B.M.C. Chan, W.R. Roswit, P.D. Kassner, A.P. Pentland, M.E. Hemler, A.Z. Eisen, and T.S. Kupper. 1991. Integrin α2β1(VLA-2) mediates reorganization and contraction of collagen matrices by human cells. *Cell* 67:403–410.

Schmitz, J.P. and J.O. Hollinger. 1986. The critical size defect as an experimental model for craniomandibulofacial nonunions. *Clin. Orth.* 205:299–308.

Schmitz, J.P., Z. Schwartz, J.O. Hollinger, and B.D. Boyan. 1990. Characterization of rat calvarial nonunion defects. *Acta Anat.* 138:185–192.

Schürch, W., T.A. Seemayer, and G. Gabbiani. 1998. The myofibroblast. A quarter century after its discovery. *Am. J. Surg. Pathol.* 22:141–147.

Schwartz, S.M., M.B. Stemerman, and E.P. Benditt. 1975. The aortic intima II: Repair of the aortic lining after mechanical denudation. *Am. J. Pathol.* 81:15–42.

Seckel, B.R., T.H. Chiu, E. Nyilas, and R.L. Sidman. 1984. Nerve regeneration through synthetic biodegradable nerve guides: Regulation by the target organ. *Plast. Reconstr. Surg.* 74:173–181.

Seyer, J.M. and R. Raghow. 1992. Hepatic fibrosis. In *Wound Healing*, edited by Cohen, I.K., R.F. Diegelmann, and W.J. Lindblad. Philadelphia: W.B. Saunders.

Shafritz, T.A., L.C. Rosenberg, and I.V. Yannas. 1994. Specific effects of glycosaminoglycans in an analog of extracellular matrix that delays wound contraction and induces regeneration. *Wound Rep. Reg.* 2:270–276.

Shah, M., D.M. Foreman, and M.W.J. Ferguson. 1992. Control of scarring in adult wounds by neutralizing antibody to transforming growth factor b. *Lancet* 339:213–214.

Shah, M., D.M. Foreman, and M.W. Ferguson. 1994. Neutralising antibody to TGF-b1,2 reduces cutaneous scarring in adult rodents. *J. Cell Sci.* 107:1137–1157.

Shah, M., D.M. Foreman, and W.J. Ferguson. 1995. Neutralization of TGF-b1 and TGF-b2 or exogenous addition of TGF-b3 to cutaneous rat wounds reduces scarring. *J. Cell Sci.* 108:985–1002.

Shapiro, F. 1988. Cortical bone repair. *J. Bone Joint Surg.* 70-A:1067–1081.

Sheridan, R.L., M. Hegarty, R.G. Tompkins, and J.F. Burke. 1994. Artificial skin in massive burns: Results to ten years. *Eur. J. Plast. Surg.* 17:91–93.

Siironen, J., M. Sandberg, V. Vuorinen, and M. Röyttä. 1992a. Expression of type I and III collagens and fibronectin after transection of rat sciatic nerve. Reinnervation compared to denervation. *Lab Invest.* 67:80–87.

Siironen, J., M. Sandberg, V. Vuorinen, and M. Röyttä. 1992b. Laminin B1 and collagen type IV gene expression in transected peripheral nerve: Reinnervation compared to denervation. *J. Neurochem.* 59:2184–2192.

Sikorski, R. and R. Peters. 1997. Xenotransplanters turn xenovirologists. *Science* 276:1893.

Silver, F.H., I.V. Yannas, and E.W. Salzman. 1978. Glycosaminoglycan inhibition of collagen induced platelet aggregation. *Thromb. Res.* 13:267–277.

Silver, F.H., I.V. Yannas, and E.W. Salzman. 1979. In vitro blood compatibility of glycosaminoglycan-precipitated collagens. *J. Biomed. Mater. Res.* 13:701–716.

Singer, I.I. 1979. The fibronexus: A transmembrane association of fibronectin-containing fibers and bundles of 5 nm microfilaments in hamster and human fibroblasts. *Cell* 16:675–685.

Singer, I.I., D.W. Kawka, D.M. Kazazis, and R.A.F. Clark. 1984. In vivo co-distribution of fibronectin and actin fibers in granulation tissue: Immunofluorescence and electron microscope studies of the fibronexus at the myofibroblast surface. *J. Cell Biol.* 98:2091–2106.

Slack, J.M.W. 2000. Stem cells in epithelial tissues. *Science* 287:1431–1433.

Smola, H., H.J. Stark, G. Thiekotter, N. Mirancea, T. Drieg, and N.E. Fusenig. 1998. Dynamics of basement membrane formation by keratinocyte-fibroblast interactions in organotypic skin culture. *Exp. Cell Res.* 239:399–410.

Solter, D. and J. Gearhart. 1999. Putting stem cells to work. *Science* 283:1468–1470.

Somasundaram, K. and K. Prathrap. 1970. Intra-uterine healing of skin wounds in rabbit foetuses. *J. Pathol.* 100:81–86.

Son, Y.-J. and W.J. Thompson. 1995. Schwann cell processes guide regeneration of peripheral axons. *Neuron* 14:125–132.

Sopher, D. 1975. A study of wound healing in the foetal tissues of the cynomolgus monkey. *Lab. Anim. Handbooks* 6:327–335.

Spector, M., I. Heyligers, and J.R. Roberson. 1993. Porous polymers for biological fixation. *Clin. Orth.* 235:207–219.

Spence, R.J. 1998. The use of Integra for contracture release. *Burn Care Rehabil.* 19:S173.

Spilker, M.H. 2000. Peripheral nerve regeneration through tubular devices. Ph.D. thesis. Massachusettts Institute of Technology.

Staiano-Coico, L., J.G. Krueger, J.S. Rubin, S. D'limi, V.P. Vallat, L. Valentino, T.F. III, A. Hawes, G. Kingston, M.R. Madden, et al. 1993. Human keratinocyte growth factor effects in a porcine model of epidermal wound healing. *J. Exp. Med.* 178:865–878.

Stark, H.J., M. Bauer, D. Breitkreutz, N. Mirancea, and N. Fusenig. 1999. Organotypic keratinocyte cocultures in defined medium with regular epidermal morphogenesis and differentiation. *J. Invest. Dermatol.* 112:681–691.

Steer, C.J. 1995. Liver regeneration. *FASEB J.* 9:1396–1400.

Stelnicki, E.J., J. Arbeit, D.L. Cass, C. Saner, M. Harrison, and C. Largman. 1998. Modulation of the human homeobox genes PRX-2 and HOXB13 in scarless fetal wounds. *J. Invest. Dermatol.* 111:57–63.

Stelnicki, E.J., V. Doolabh, S. Lee, F.G. Baumann, M.T. Longaker, and S. Mackinnon. 2000. Nerve dependency in scarless fetal wound healing. *Plast. Reconstr. Surg.* 105:140–147.

Stemerman, M.B. 1973. Thrombogenesis of the rabbit arterial plaque: An electron microscopic study. *Am. J. Pathol.* 73:7–18.

Stemerman, M.B. and R. Ross. 1972. Experimental arteriosclerosis I: Fibrous plaque formation in primates, an electron microscopic study. *J. Exp. Med.* 136:769–793.

Stemerman, M.B., T.H. Spaet, F. Pitlick, J. Cintron, I. Lejnieks, and M.L. Tiell. 1977. Intimal healing. The pattern of reendothelialization and intimal thickening. *Am. J. Pathol.* 87:125–142.

Stenn, K.S. and R. Malhotra. 1992. Epithelialization. In *Wound Healing*, edited by Cohen, I.K., R.F. Diegelmann, and W.J. Lindblad. Philadelphia: W.B. Saunders.

Stern, R., M. McPherson, and M.T. Longaker. 1990. Histologic study of artificial skin used in the treatment of full-thickness thermal injury. *J. Burn Care & Rehab.* 11:7–13.

Stevens, M.P. 1990. *Polymer Chemistry.* New York: Oxford University Press.

Stocum, D.L. 1995. *Wound Repair, Regeneration and Artificial Tissues.* Austin: R.G. Landes.

Stone, P.A. and J.W. Madden. 1975. Biological factors affecting wound contraction. *Surg. Forum* 26:547–548.

Stopak, D. and A.K. Harris. 1982. Connective tissue morphogenesis by fibroblast traction I: Tissue culture observations. *Dev. Biol.* 90:383–398.

Stoschek, C.M., L.B. Nanney, and J.L.E. King. 1992. Quantitative determination of EGF-R during epidermal wound healing. *J. Invest. Dermatol.* 99:645–649.

Straile, W.E. 1959. The expansion and shrinkage of mammalian skin near contracting wounds. *J. Exp. Zool.* 141:119–131.

Strichartz, G.S. and B.G. Covino. 1990. Local anesthetics. In *Anesthesia*, edited by Miller, R.D. New York: Churchill Livingstone.

Sunderland, S. 1978. *Nerves and Nerve Injuries*. New York: Churchill Livingstone.

Sunderland, S. 1990. The anatomy and pathology of nerve injury. *Muscle & Nerve* 13:771–784.

Swann, D.A., H.G. Garg, C.J. Hendry, H. Hermann, E. Siebert, S. Sotman, and W. Stafford. 1988. Isolation and partial characterization of dermatan sulfate proteoglycans from post-burn scar tissues. *Collagen Rel. Res.* 8:295–313.

Swartzendruber, D.C., P.W. Wertz, D.J. Kitko, K.C. Madison, and D.T. Downing. 1989. Moleular models of the intercellular lipid lamellae in mammalian stratum corneum. *J. Invest. Dematol.* 92:251–257.

Sylvester, M.F., I.V. Yannas, E.W. Salzman, and M.J. Forbes. 1989. Collagen banded fibril structure and the collagen-platelet reaction. *Thromb. Res.* 55:135–148.

Takashima, A., R.E. Billingham, and F. Grinnell. 1986. Activation of rabbit keratinocyte fibronectin receptor function in vivo during wound healing. *J. Invest. Dermatol.* 86:585–590.

Taniguchi, S. and T. Hirone. 1983. Synthesis of basal lamina by epidermal cells in vitro. *Curr. Probl. Dermatol.* 11:127–133.

Taniuchi, M., H.B. Clark, and E.M. Johnson. 1986. Induction of nerve growth factor receptors by Schwann cells after axotomy. *Proc. Natl. Acad. Sci. USA* 83:4094–4098.

Taniuchi, M., H.B. Clark, H.B. Schweitzer, and E.M. Johnson. 1988. Expression of nerve growth factor receptors by Schwann cells of axotomized peripheral nerves: Ultrastructural location, suppression of axon contact, and bonding properties. *J. Neurosci.* 8:664–681.

Tanzer, M.L. 1973. Cross-linking of collagen. *Science* 180:561–566.

Tarpila, E., R. Ghassemifar, D. Fagrell, and A. Berggren. 1997. Capsular contracture with textured versus smooth saline-filled implants for breast augmentation: A prospective clinical study. *Plast. Reconstr. Surg.* 99:1934–1939.

Taskinen, H.S., J. Heino, and M. Röyttä. 1996. The dynamics of beta 1 integrin expression during peripheral nerve regeneration. *Acta Neuropathol. (Berlin)* 89:144–151.

Tassava, R.A. and C.L. Olsen. 1982. Higher vertebrates do not regenerate digits and legs because the wound epidermis is not functional: A hypothesis. *Differentiation* 22:151–155.

Taylor, A.C. and J.J. Kollros. 1946. Stages in the normal development of Rana pipiens larvae. *Anat. Rec.* 94:7–13.

Terzis, J.K. 1987. *Microreconstruction of Nerve Injuries*. Philadelphia: W.B. Saunders.

Terzis, J.K. and K.J. Smith. 1987. Repair of severed peripheral nerves: Comparison of the "de Medinacelli" and standard microsuture methods. *Exp. Neurol.* 96:672–680.

Thomas, P.K. 1963. The connective tissue of peripheral nerve: An electron microscope study. *J. Anat.* 97:35–44.

Thomas, P.K. 1988. Clinical aspects of PNS regeneration. In *Advances in Neurology*, edited by Waxman, S.G. New York: Raven Press.

Thomas, P.K. and D.G. Jones. 1967. The cellular response to nerve injury II: Regeneration of the perineurium after nerve section. *J. Anat.* 101:45–55.

Thomas, P.K. and Y. Olsson. 1975. Microscopic anatomy and function of the connective tissue components of peripheral nerve. In *Peripheral Neuropathy*, edited by Dyck, P.J., P.K. Thomas, and E.H. Lambert. Philadelphia: W.B. Saunders.

Thomson, R.C., A.K. Shung, M.J. Yaszemski, and A.G. Mikos. 2000. Polymer scaffold processing. In *Principles of Tissue Engineering*. 2nd ed, edited by Lanza, R.P., R. Langer, and J. Vacanti. San Diego: Academic Press, pp. 251–262.

Timpl, R. 1984. Immunology of the collagens. In *Extracellular Matrix Biochemistry*, edited by Piez, K.A. and A.H. Reddi. New York: Elsevier.

Tinois, E., J. Tiollier, M. Gaucherand, H. Dumas, M. Tardy, and J. Thivolet. 1991. In vitro and post-transplantation differentiation of human keratinocytes grown on the human type IV collagen film of a bilayered substitute. *Exp. Cell Res.* 193:310–319.

Tiscornia, O.M., J.H. Jacobson, and D.A. Dreiling. 1965. Microsurgery of the canine pancreatic duct: Experimental study and review of previous approaches to the management of pancreatic duct pathology. *Surgery* 58:58–72.

Tobolsky, A.V. 1960. *Properties and Structure of Polymers*. New York: Wiley.

Tompkins, R.G., J.F. Hilton, J.F. Burke, D.A. Scoenfeld, M.T. Hegarty, C.C. Bondoc, W.C.Q. Jr, G.E. Behringer, and F.W. Ackroyd. 1989. Increased survival after massive thermal injuries in adults: Preliminary report using artificial skin. *Child Care Med.* 17:734–740.

Tountas, C.P., R.A. Bergman, T.W. Lewis, H.E. Stone, J.D. Pyrek, and H.V. Mendenhall. 1993. A comparison of peripheral nerve repair using an absorbable tubulization device and conventional suture in primates. *J. App. Biomater.* 4:261–268.

Trinkaus, J.P. 1969. *Cells into Organs*. Englewood Cliffs, NJ: Prentice-Hall.

Troxel, K. 1994. Delay of skin wound contraction by porous collagen-GAG matrices. Ph.D. thesis, Massachusetts Institute of Technology, Cambridge, MA.

Tsao, M.C., B.J. Walthall, and R.G. Ham. 1982. Clonal growth of normal human epidermal keratinocytes in a defined medium. *J. Cell Physiol.* 110:219–229.

Tsonis, P.A. 1996. *Limb regeneration*. New York: Cambridge University Press.

Tsuboi, R. and D.R. Rifkin. 1990. Recombinant basic fibroblast growth factor stimulates wound healing in healing-impaired db/db mice. *J. Exp. Med.* 172:245–251.

Tsunenaga, M., Y. Kohno, I. Horii, S. Yasumoto, N.H. Huh, T. Tachikawa, S. Yoshiki, and T. Kuroki. 1994. Growth and differentiation properties of normal and transformed human keratinocytes in organotypic culture. *Jpn. Cancer Res.* 85:238–244.

Uitto, J., A. Mauviel, and J. McGrath. 1996. The dermal-epidermal basement membrane zone in cutaneous wound healing. In *The Molecular and Cellular Biology of Wound Repair*, edited by Clark, R.A.F. New York: Plenum Press.

Ushiki, T. and C. Ide. 1986. Three-dimensional architecture of the endoneurium with special reference to the collagen fibril arrangement in relation to nerve fibers. *Arch. Histol. Jpn.* 49:553–563.

Utley, D.S., S.L. Lewin, E.T. Cheng, A.N. Verity, D. Sierra, and D.J. Terris. 1996. Brain-derived neurotrophic factor and collagen tubulization enhance functional recovery after peripheral nerve transection and repair. *Arch. Otolaryngol. Head Neck Surg.* 122:407–413.

Uzman, B.G. and G.M. Villegas. 1983. Mouse sciatic nerve regeneration through semipermeable tubes: A quantitative model. *J. Neurosci. Res.* 9:325–338.

Valentini, R.F. 1995. Nerve guidance channels. In *The Biomedical Engineering Handbook*, edited by Bronzino, J.D. Boca Raton: CRC Press.

Valentini, R.F., P. Aebischer, S.R. Winn, and P.M. Galletti. 1987. Collagen- and laminin-containing gels impede peripheral nerve regeneration through semipermeable nerve guidance channels. *Exp. Neurol.* 98:350–356.

Van der Rest, M. and R. Garrone. 1991. Collagen family of proteins. *FASEB J.* 5:2814–2823.

Vaughan, M.B., E.W. Howard, and J.J. Tomasek. 2000. Transforming growth factor beta1 promotes the morphological and functional differentiation of the myofi-broblast. *Exp. Cell Res.* 25:180–189.

Vert, M. and S.M. Li. 1992. Bioresorbability and biocompatibility of aliphatic poly-esters. *J. Mater. Sci. Mater. Med.* 3:432–446.

Vert, M., P. Christel, F. Chabot, and J. Leray. 1984. Bioresorbable plastic materials for bone surgery. In *Macromolecular Biomaterials*, edited by Hastings, G.W. and P. Ducheyne. Boca Raton: CRC Press.

Vogel, G. 1999. Harnessing the power of stem cells. *Science* 283:1432–1434.

Volkman, R. 1893. Über die Regeneration des quergestreiften Muskelgewebes beim Menschen und Säugethier. *Beitr. Pathol. Anat. Allg. Pathol.* 12:233.

Vorontsova, M.A. and L.D. Liosner. 1960. *Asexual Propagation and Regeneration.* London: Pergamon Press.

Vracko, R. 1972. Significance of basal lamina for regeneration of injured lung. *Virchows Arch. (Pathol. Anat.)* 355:264–274.

Vracko, R. 1974. Basal lamina scaffold: Anatomy and significance for maintenance of orderly tissue structure. *Am. J. Pathol.* 77:313–346.

Vracko, R. and E.P. Benditt. 1972. Basal lamina: The scaffold for orderly cell replacement. *J. Cell Biol.* 55:406–419.

Wall, P.D. and M. Gutnick. 1974. Ongoing activity in peripheral nerves: The physiology and pharmacology of impulses originating from a neuroma. *Exp. Neurol.* 43:580–593.

Wallace, H. 1981. *Vertebrate Limb Regeneration.* New York: Wiley.

Walter, M.A., R. Kurouglu, J.B. Caulfield, L.O. Vasconez, and J.A. Thompson. 1993. Enhanced peripheral nerve regeneration by acidic fibroblast growth factor. *Lymphokine Cytokine Res.* 12:135–141.

Wang, G.H. 1975. Collagen-mucopolysaccharide interaction. M. S. thesis, Massachusetts Institute of Technology, Cambridge, MA.

Wasserman, D., M. Sclotterer, A. Toulon, C. Cazalet, M. Marien, B. Cherruau, and P. Jaffray. 1988. Preliminary clinical studies of a biological skin equivalent in burned patients. *Burns* 14:326–330.

Watts, G.T., G.C. Grillo, and J. Gross. 1958. Studies in wound healing II: The role of granulation tissue in contraction. *Ann. Surg.* 148:153–160.

Weiss, P. 1944. The techology of nerve regeneration: A review. Sutureless tubulation and related methods of nerve repair. *J. Neurosurg.* 1:400–450.

Weiss, P. and A.C. Taylor. 1944a. Impairment of growth and myelination in regenerating nerve fibers subject to constriction. *Proc. Soc. Exp. Biol. NY* 55:77–80.

Weiss, P. and A.C. Taylor. 1944b. Further experimental evidence against "neurotropism" in nerve regeneration. *J. Exp. Zool.* 95:233–257.

Welch, M.P., G.F. Odland, and R.A.F. Clark. 1990. Temporal relationships of F-actin bundle formation, collagen and fibronectin matrix assembly, and fibronectin receptor expression to wound contraction. *J. Cell Biol.* 110:133–145.

Wells, M.R., K. Kraus, D.K. Batter, D.G. Blunt, J. Weremowitz, S.E. Lynch, H.N. Antoniades, and H.-A. Hansson. 1997. Gel matrix vehicles for growth factor application in nerve gap injuries repaired with tubes: A comparison of Biomatrix, collagen and methylcellulose. *Exp. Neurol.* 146:395–402.

Whitby, D.J. and M.W. Ferguson. 1991. Immunohistochemical localization of growth factors in fetal wound healing. *Dev. Biol.* 147:207–215.

Whitworth, I.H., R.A. Brown, C. Dore, C.J. Green, and G. Terenghi. 1995. Orientated mats of fibronectin as a conduit material for use in peripheral nerve repair. *J. Hand Surg.* 20B:429–436.

Whitworth, I.H., R.A. Brown, C.J. Dore, P. Anand, C.J. Green, and G. Terenghi. 1996. Nerve growth factor enhances nerve regeneration through fibronectin grafts. *J. Hand Surg.* 21B:514–522.

Wickelgren, I. 1996. Muscling transplants into mice. *Science* 273:33.

Wille Jr, J.J., M.R. Pittelkow, G.D. Shipley, and R.E. Scott. 1984. Integrated control of growth and differentiation of normal human prokeratinocytes cultured in serum-free medium: Clonal analyses, growth kinetics, and cell cycle studies. *J. Cell Physiol.* 121:31–44.

Williams, A.K., M.B. Bunge, and P.M. Wood. 1982. The development of perineurium in culture. *J. Cell Biol.* 95:2a.

Williams, L.R. 1987. Exogenous fibrin matrix precursors stimulate the temporal progress of nerve regeneration within a silicone chamber. *Neurochem. Res.* 12:851–860.

Williams, L.R. and S. Varon. 1985. Modification of fibrin matrix formation in situ enhances nerve regeneration in silicone chambers. *J. Comp. Neurol.* 231:209–220.

Williams, L.R., F.M. Longo, H.C. Powell, G. Lundborg, and S. Varon. 1983. Spatial-temporal progress of peripheral nerve regeneration within a silicone chamber: Parameters for a bioassay. *J. Comp. Neurol.* 218:460–470.

Williams, L.R., H.C. Powell, G. Lundborg, and S. Varon. 1984. Competence of nerve tissue as distal insert promoting nerve regeneration in a silicone chamber. *Brain Res.* 293:201–211.

Williams, L.R., N. Danielsen, H. Muller, and S. Varon. 1987. Exogenous matrix precursors promote functional nerve regeneration across a 15-mm gap within a silicone chamber in the rat. *J. Comp. Neurol.* 264:284–290.

Wilson, C.J. and L.E. Dahners. 1988. An examination of the mechanism of ligament contracture. *Clin. Orthop.* 227:286–291.

Winter, G.D. 1972. Epidermal regeneration studied in the domestic pig. In *Epidermal Wound Healing*, edited by Maibach, H.L. and D.T. Rovee. Chicago: Year Book Medical Publishers.

Woodley, D.T. 1989. Covering wounds with cultured keratinocytes. *JAMA* 262:2140–2141.

Woodley, D.T. 1996. Repithelialization. In *The Molecular and Cellular Biology of Wound Repair*, edited by Clark, R.A.F. New York: Plenum Press.

Woodley, D.T. and R.A. Briggaman. 1988. Re-formation of the epidermal-dermal junction during wound healing. In *The Molecular and Cellular Biology of Wound Repair*, edited by Clark, R.A.F. and P.M. Henson. New York: Plenum Press.

Woodley, D.T., T. Kalebec, A.J. Banes, W. Link, M. Prunieras, and L. Liotta. 1986. Adult human keratinocytes migrating over nonviable dermal collagen produce collagenolytic enzymes that degrade type I and type IV collagen. *J. Invest. Dermatol.* 86:418–423.

Woodley, D.T., H.D. Peterson, S.R. Herzog, G.P. Stricklin, R.E. Burgeson, R.A. Briggaman, D.J. Cronce, and E.J. O'Keefe. 1988a. Burn wounds resurfaced by cultured epidermal autografts show abnormal reconstitution of anchoring fibtils. *JAMA* 259:2566–2571.

Woodley, D.T., P.M. Bachmann, and E.J. O'Keefe. 1988b. Laminin inhibits keratinocyte migration. *J. Cell Physiol.* 136:140–146.

Woodley, D.T., R.A. Briggaman, S.R. Herzog, A.A. Meyers, H.D. Peterson, and E.J. O'Keefe. 1990. Characterization of "neo-dermis" formation beneath cultured human epidermal autografts transplanted on muscle fascia. *J. Invest. Dermatol.* 95:20–26.

Woodley, D.T., P.M. Backmann, and E.J. O'Keefe. 1991. The role of matrix components in human keratinocyte re-epithelialization. In *Clinical and Experimental Approaches to Dermal and Epidermal Repair: Normal and Chronic Wounds*, edited by Barbul, A., M. Caldwell, W. Eaglstein, T. Hunt, D. Marshall, E. Pines, and G. Skover. New York: Alan R. Liss.

Woolley, A.L., J.P. Hollowell, and K.M. Rich. 1990. Fibronectin-laminin combination enhances peripheral nerve regeneration across long gaps. *Otolaryngol. Head Neck Surg.* 103:509–518.

Wornom, I.L. and S.R. Buchman. 1992. Bone and cartilaginous tissues. In *Wound Healing*, edited by Cohen, I.K., R.F. Diegelmann, and W.J. Lindblad. Philadelphia: W.B. Saunders.

Worst, P.K.M., E.A. Valentine, and N.E. Fusenig. 1974. Formation of epidermis after reimplantation of pure primary epidermal cell cultures from perinatal mouse skin. *J. Natl. Cancer Inst.* 53:1061–1064.

Wu, L., Y.L. Yu, R.D. Galiano, S.I. Roth, and T.A. Mustoe. 1997. Macrophage colony-stimulating factor accelerates wound healing and upregulates TGF-b1 mRNA levels through tissue macrophages. *J. Surg. Res.* 72:162–169.

Xu, A.S.L., T.L. Luntz, J.M. Macdonald, H. Kubota, E. Hsu, R.E. London, and L.M. Reid. 2000. Lineage biology and liver. In *Principles of Tissue Engineering*, edited by Lanza, R.P., R. Langer, and J. Vacanti. San Diego: Academic Press.

Xu, J. and R.A.F. Clark. 1996. Extracellular matrix alters PDGF regulation of fibroblast integrins. *J. Cell Biol.* 132:239–249.

Xu, J. and R.A.F. Clark. 2000. Integrin regulation in wound repair. In *Scarless Wound Healing*, edited by Garg, H.G. and M.T. Longaker. New York: Marcel Dekker.

Yamada, K.M., J. Gailit, and R.A.F. Clark. 1996. Integrins in wound repair. In *The Molecular and Cellular Biology of Wound Repair*, edited by Clark, R.A.F. New York: Plenum Press.

Yamaguchi, Y., D.M. Mann, and E. Ruoslahti. 1990. Negative regulation of transforming growth factor-b by the proteoglycan decorin. *Nature* 346:281–284.

Yamauchi, M. and G. Mechanic. 1988. Cross-linking of collagen. In *Collagen*, edited by Nimni, M.E. Boca Raton: CRC Press.

Yang, L., C.X. Qui, A. Ludlow, M.W. Ferguson, and G. Brunner. 1999. Active transforming growth factor-beta in wound repair: Determination using a new assay. *Am. J. Pathol.* 154:105–111.

Yannas, I.V. 1972a. Characterization techniques for the molecular design of polymeric implants. Paper read at *Proc. Biom. Mater. Conf.*, National Science Foundation, Brighton, UT, November 9, 1972.

Yannas, I.V. 1972b. Collagen and gelatin in the solid state. *Revs. Macromol. Chem.* C7:49–104B.

Yannas, I.V. 1981. Use of artificial skin in wound management. In *The Surgical Wound*, edited by Dineen, P. Philadelphia: Lea & Febiger.

Yannas, I.V. 1988. Regeneration of skin and nerves by use of collagen templates. In *Collagen: Biotechnology*, edited by Nimni, M. Boca Raton: CRC Press.

Yannas, I.V. 1990. Biologically active analogs of the extracellular matrix. *Angew. Chem. (Engl. Ed.)* 29:20–35.

Yannas, I.V. 1997. Models of organ regeneration processes induced by templates. *Ann. N. Y. Acad. Sci.* 831:280–293.

Yannas, I.V. 2000. Synthesis of organs: In vitro or in vivo? *Proc. Natl. Acad. Sci. USA* 97:9354–9356.

Yannas, I.V. and A.V. Tobolsky. 1967. Crosslinking of gelatine by dehydration. *Nature* 215:509–510.

Yannas, I.V. and C. Huang. 1972. Visoelastic distinction between helical and coiled macromolecules. *Macromol.* 5:99–100.

Yannas, I.V. and J.F. Silver. 1975. Thromboresistant analogs of vascular tissue. *Polym. Prepr. Am. Chem. Soc.* 16(2):529–534.

Yannas, I.V. and J.F. Burke. 1980. Design of an artificial skin I. Basic design principles. *J. Biomed. Mater. Res.* 14:65–81.

Yannas, I.V., N.-H. Sung, and C. Huang. 1972. Resolution of components of the optical rotation tensor of collagen. *J. Phys. Chem.* 76:2935–2937.

Yannas, I.V., J.F. Burke, C. Huang, and P.L. Gordon. 1975a. Suppression of in vivo degradability and of immunogenicity of collagen by reaction with glycosaminoglycans. *Polym. Prepr. Am. Chem. Soc.* 16(2):209–214.

Yannas, I.V., J.F. Burke, C. Huang, and P.L. Gordon. 1975b. Correlation of in vivo collagen degradation rate with in vitro measurements. *J. Biomed. Mater. Res.* 9:623–628.

Yannas, I.V., J.F. Burke, C. Huang, and P.L. Gordon. 1977. Multilayer membrane useful as synthetic skin. US Patent 4,060,081. Washington, DC: United States Patent Office.

Yannas, I.V., J.F. Burke, M. Umbreit, and P. Stasikelis. 1979. Progress in design of an artificial skin. *Fed. Proc. Am. Soc. Exp. Biol.* 38:988.

Yannas, I.V., J.F. Burke, P.L. Gordon, C. Huang, and R.H. Rubinstein. 1980. Design of an artificial skin II: Control of chemical composition. *J. Biomed. Mater. Res.* 14:107–131.

Yannas, I.V., J.F. Burke, M. Warpehoski, P. Stasikelis, E.M. Skrabut, D. Orgill, and D.J. Giard. 1981. Prompt, long-term functional replacement of skin. *Trans. Am. Soc. Artif. Intern. Organs* 27:19–22.

Yannas, I.V., J.F. Burke, D.P. Orgill, and E.M. Skrabut. 1982a. Wound tissue can utilize a polymeric template to synthesize a functional extension of skin. *Science* 215:174–176.

Yannas, I.V., J.F. Burke, D.P. Orgill, and E.M. Skrabut. 1982b. Regeneration of skin following closure of deep wounds with a biodegradable template. *Trans. Soc. Biomater.* 5:24–27.

Yannas, I.V., D.P. Orgill, E.M. Skrabut, and J.F. Burke. 1984. Skin regeneration with a bioreplaceable polymeric template. In *Polymeric Materials and Artificial Organs*, edited by Gebelein, C.G. Washington, DC: American Chemical Society.

Yannas, I.V., D.P. Orgill, J. Silver, T.V. Norregaard, N.T. Zervas, and W.C. Schoene. 1985. Polymeric template facilitates regeneration of sciatic nerve across 15 mm gap. *Trans. Soc. Biomater.* 8:146, 1985.

Yannas, I.V., D.P. Orgill, J. Silver, T. Norregaard, N.T. Zervas, and W.C. Schoene. 1987a. Regeneration of sciatic nerve across 15-mm gap by use of a polymeric template. In *Advances in Biomedical Materials*, edited by Gebelein, C.G. Washington, DC: American Chemical Society.

Yannas, I.V., E. Lee, D.P. Orgill, A. Ferdman, E.M. Skrabut, and G.F. Murphy. 1987b. De novo synthesis of skin. *Proc. Am. Chem. Soc. Div. Polym. Mat.* 57:28–32.

Yannas, I.V., T.V. Norregaard, J. Silver, N.T. Zervas, J.F. Kirk, and M.J. Colt. 1987c. Relations between properties of collagen-glycosaminoglycan graft and morphology of regenerating nerve. Part I. *Trans. Soc. Biomater.* 10:6.

Yannas, I.V., A.S. Chang, C. Krarup, R. Sethi, T.V. Norregaard, and N.T. Zervas. 1988. Conduction properties of peripheral nerves regenerated by use of copolymer matrices with different biodegradation rates. *Soc. Neurosci. Abs.* 14:165.

Yannas, I.V., E. Lee, D.P. Orgill, E.M. Skrabut, and G.F. Murphy. 1989. Synthesis and characterization of a model extracellular matrix which induces partial regeneration of adult mammalian skin. *Proc. Natl. Acad. Sci. USA* 86:933–937.

Yannas, I.V., A.S. Chang, S. Perutz, C. Krarup, T.V. Norregaard, and N.T. Zervas. 1991. Requirement for a 1-mm pore channel opening during peripheral nerve regeneration through a biodegradable chemical analog of ECM. In *Biotechnology and Polymers*, edited by Gebelein, C.G. New York: Plenum.

Yannas, I.V., J. Colt, and Y.C. Wai. 1996. Wound contraction and scar synthesis during development of the amphibian *Rana catesbeiana*. *Wound Rep. Reg.* 4:31–41.

Young, J.Z. 1948. Growth and differentiation of nerve fibers. *Symp. Soc. Exp. Biol. Growth* 2:57–74.

Yuspa, S.H., D.L. Morgan, R.J. Walker, and R.R. Bates. 1970. The growth of fetal mouse skin in cell culture and transplantation to F1 mice. *J. Invest. Dermatol.* 55:379–389.

Zahir, M. 1964. Contraction of wounds. *Brit. J. Surg.* 51:456–461.

Zeitz, M., A. Ruiz-Torres, and H.-J. Merker. 1978. Collagen metabolism in granulating wounds of rat skin. *Arch. Dermatol. Res.* 263:207–214.

Zhao, Q., L.B. Dahlin, M. Kanje, and G. Lundborg. 1992. The formation of a "pseudo-nerve" in silicone chambers in the absence of regenerating axons. *Brain Res.* 592:106–114.

Zochodne, D.W. and C. Nguyen. 1997. Angiogenesis at the site of neuroma formation in transected peripheral nerve. *J. Anat.* 191:23–30.

Index